Mechanism and
Management of Headache

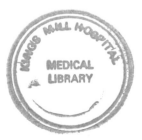

Mechanism and Management of Headache

Sixth edition

JAMES W LANCE, AO, CBE, MD, Hon DSc, FRCP(London), FRACP, FAA
*Consultant Neurologist, Institute of Neurological Sciences, The Prince Henry and
Prince of Wales Hospitals and Emeritus Professor of Neurology,
University of New South Wales, Sydney, Australia.*

PETER J. GOADSBY, BMedSc, MB, BS, MD, PhD, DSc, FRACP, FRCP
*Wellcome Senior Research Fellow and Professor of Clinical Neurology,
Institute of Neurology, University College London and Consultant Neurologist,
The National Hospital for Neurology and Neurosurgery, Queen Square, London, UK.*

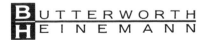

OXFORD   AUCKLAND   BOSTON   JOHANNESBURG   MELBOURNE   NEW DELHI

Butterworth-Heinemann
An imprint of Elsevier Science Limited
Robert Stevenson House,
1–3 Baxter's Place, Leith Walk,
Edinburgh EH1 3AF

First published 1969
Second edition 1973
Third edition 1978
Fourth edition 1982
Fifth edition 1993
Sixth edition 1998
Paperback edition 2000
Reprinted 2002

British Library Cataloguing in Publication Data
A catalogue record for this book is available from the British Library

Library of Congress Cataloging in Publication Data
A catalog record for this book is available from the British Library

ISBN 0 7506 4935 6

Typeset by David Gregson Associates, Beccles, Suffolk
Printed and bound in Great Britain by The University Press, Cambridge

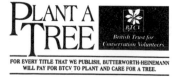

Contents

Preface to the sixth edition

While the principles of managing headache have altered little since the last edition of this book, advances in research and treatment have made a new edition mandatory. Current views on pathophysiology have been summarized and new medications evaluated. The aim is to provide a practical guide for clinicians dealing with one of humankind's most common and distressing ailments, backed up by references for those who want to pursue particular topics. Headache is a serious cause of disability and sufferers from headache deserve all the help that we can give them.

James W. Lance
Peter J. Goadsby

Preface to the first edition

About once a month, until the age of 70 years, George Bernard Shaw suffered a devastating headache which lasted for a day. One afternoon, after recovering from an attack, he was introduced to Nansen and asked the famous Arctic explorer whether he had ever discovered a headache cure.

'No,' said Nansen with a look of amazement.

'Have you ever tried to find a cure for headaches?'

'No.'

Well, that is a most astonishing thing!' exclaimed Shaw. 'You have spent your life in trying to discover the North Pole, which nobody on earth cares tuppence about, and you have never attempted to discover a cure for the headache, which every living person is crying aloud for.*

It is easy for a person who has never been troubled with headaches to lose patience with those who are plagued by them. The reaction of the virtuous observer may pass through a phase of sympathetic concern to one of frustrated tolerance and, finally, to a mood of irritation and resentment in which the recurrence of headaches is attributed to a defective personality or escape from unpleasant life situations. The sound sleeper is traditionally intolerant of the insomniac and the speedy of bowel is just a little contemptuous of the constipated. In short, we tend to consider ourselves as the norm and to look quizzically at those whose physiological or psychological processes are at variance with our own. Such an attitude often persists in spite of years of advanced education and scientific training. To make it clear that I am not numbering myself among the righteous, I must state that I am not subject to headache and that my spirits often sink when confronted with a succession of patients whose contorted expressions testify to a lifetime of headache misery. This is about the only circumstance which I find likely to provoke headache in myself – I suppose on the principle that if you can't beat them, join them!

It would be foolish to deny that the workings of the mind are of great importance in the production of headache, but they are only part of the story.

My interest in migraine was first aroused when working at the Northcott Neurological Centre in Sydney. Each patient with migraine gave a history that was a little different from the others but all were variations on a clearly recognizable theme. It seemed that all the clues were there to point the way to the understanding of the mechanism of migraine. These thoughts led to studies of the clinical features and natural history of migraine and, later, to laboratory work which now suggests that migraine is an hereditary recurrent metabolic disturbance. If this be the case, a patient cannot be held responsible for having migraine attacks any more than a

* Pearson, H. (1942). *Bernard Shaw*. pp. 242–243. London, Collins

woman for having menstrual periods. The treatment of migraine has improved with better understanding of the syndrome but knowledge of the migraine mechanism and its treatment still leave much to be desired.

Mysteries remain in the problem of tension headache although the place of psychological factors is much more obvious in this group than in migraine and an association with chronic over-contraction of muscle is almost universal. However, many tense, frowning people do not get headaches and the explanation for those that do must go beyond a catalogue of undesirable personality traits and bad luck in cards or love. Migraine and tension headache are given most space in this small book because they are common complaints, not always easy to diagnose and treat, and worry patients and their medical attendants. Other common forms of headache such as those arising from eye-strain or sinusitis are not emphasized as much, because their mechanism and management are more straightforward. Serious acute head-aches which betoken some hazardous intracranial condition are described sufficiently to assist in diagnosis, but not dealt with at length since their management usually becomes the prerogative of the specialist neurological unit.

This book is designed to be relatively easy armchair reading for the general practitioner, senior medical student or others who may be interested in the mech-anism of headache or concerned with the practical management of headache prob-lems. The neurologist may find something of interest in the chapters on tension headache and migraine. References are listed for those who wish to read in greater depth.

The present concept of headache mechanisms depends to a great extent on the work of the late Harold G. Wolff and his colleagues, which is described in Wolff's monograph *Headache and Other Head Pain*. The reader is referred to this work for aspects of headache which are passed over lightly here. The subject may not have all the excitement of a detective story but the talents of the great detectives of fiction would not be lost in trying to unravel some of the complexities of headache.

J.W.L.

Acknowledgements

Studies of clinical aspects, pathophysiology and treatment of headache have been conducted at The Prince Henry and Prince of Wales Hospitals, Sydney, and more recently at the National Hospital for Neurology and Neurosurgery, London, for over thirty years. Those who have been or are presently engaged in the research programme include:

R. D. Adams
H. Angus-Leppan
M. Anthony
A. Bahra
P. Boers
N. Bogduk
D. A. Curran
B. Daher
P. D. Drummond
J. W. Duckworth
V. Gordon
M. Hellier
H. Hinterberger
K. L. Hoskin
H. Kaube
Y. E. Knight
G. A. Lambert
G. D. A. Lord

A. Lowy
N. Marlowe
A. May
J. Michalicek
J. Misbach
E. Mylecharane
B. Olausson
J. Peralta
R. D. Piper
F. Ragaglia
R. J. Storer
T. Shimomura
B. W. Somerville
P. J. Spira
A. Srikiatkhachorn
K. M. A. Welch
A. S. Zagami

We are most grateful to this happy blend of neurologists, pharmacologists, anatomists, physiologists, biochemists and psychologists for many years of stimulating association, and to our neurosurgical colleagues for their friendly collaboration in managing headache and other problems.

The research programme has been supported by the National Health and Medical Research Council of Australia and has been generously assisted by grants from the J. A. Perini Family Trust, the Adolph Basser Trust, The Australian Brain Foundation, The Migraine Trust, Sandoz AG, Basel (now Novartis), Glaxo-Wellcome (Australia) and Warren and Cheryl Anderson. Peter J. Goadsby particularly wishes to acknowledge the generous support of the Wellcome Trust, and the privilege of contributing to this book.

The manuscript has been prepared by Patricia Miller, Carol Flecknoe and Sophie Ryan. The anatomical diagrams were drawn by Dr N. Bogduk and Mr Marcus

Cremonese. All photographs were prepared by the Department of Medical Illustration, University of New South Wales.

We are grateful to the editors of the following publications for permission to reproduce tables and figures from papers by our colleagues and ourselves: *Annals of Neurology*; *Archives of Neurology*; *Brain*; *Cephalagia*; *Clinical and Experimental Neurology* (Sydney, Adis Press); *Headache*; *Journal of Neurological Sciences*; *Journal of Neurology, Neurosurgery and Psychiatry*; *Neurology*; *Migraine and Other Headaches* (New York, Charles Scribner's Sons); *Migraine: a Spectrum of Ideas* (Oxford, Oxford University Press); *Medical Journal of Australia*; *Research and Clinical Studies in Headache* (Karger of Basel and New York); *Wolff's Headache and Other Head Pain* (5th Edn, New York, Oxford University Press).

Chapter 1

The history of headache

Among the brilliant frescoes in the Brancacci chapel in Florence painted by Masaccio in the fifteenth century is the Expulsion from the Garden of Eden. Adam and Eve are depicted with expressions of agony, Adam clasping his head with both hands, as the sad couple walk away. Was this the first headache since creation? A number of possible causes spring to mind.

To adopt an evolutionary approach one might speculate that the susceptibility to headache developed with the assumption of an upright posture. We have heard reports of a gorilla in Toronto Zoo who episodically curls up into a ball, shielding her eyes from the light and refusing to eat normally. The discovery of trepanned skulls with regrowth of bone shows that some Stone Age patients survived the trepanning procedure but does not tell us whether headache was the indication for operation.

Written accounts date from about 3000 BC: Alverez (1945) quotes a couplet from a Sumerian poem in which, in some sort of heaven or Abode of the Blessed,

The sick-eyed says not 'I am sick-eyed'
The sick-headed (says) not 'I am sick-headed'

Also poetic, and more specific, is a reference to headache from Babylonian literature of about the same period (Sigerist, 1955; McHenry, 1969).

Headache roameth over the desert, blowing like the wind,
Flashing like lightning, it is loosed above and below;
It cutteth off him who feareth not his god like a reed,
Like a stalk of henna it slitteth his thews.
It wasteth the flesh of him who hath no protecting goddess,
Flashing like a heavenly star, it cometh like the dew;
It standeth hostile against the wayfarer, scorching him like the day,
This man it hath struck and
Like one with heart disease he staggereth,
Like one bereft of reason he is broken,
Like that which has been cast into the fire he is shrivelled,
Like a wild ass .... his eyes are full of cloud,
On himself he feedeth, bound in death;
Headache whose course like the dread windstorm none knoweth,
None knoweth its full time or its bond.

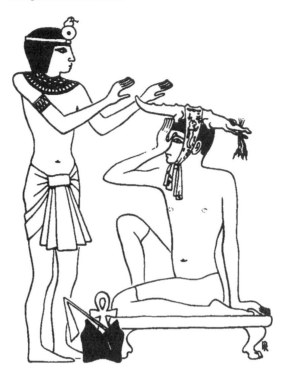

Figure 1.1 An interpretation of the treatment of migraine in 1200 BC. A clay crocodile with magic herbs in its mouth was bound to the patient's head. Drawing by P. Cunningham, reproduced by permission of J. Edmeads

The Atharvaveda, one of the four sacred Vedas of the Hindus, was written some time around the tenth century BC. One hymn reads:

> O physician, do thou release this man from headache, free him from cough which has entered into all his limbs and joints. One should resort to forests and hills for relief from diseases resulting from excessive rains, severe wind and intense heat.
>
> (Chand, 1982)

The main source of information about ancient Egyptian medicine is the Ebers Papyrus, said to have been found between the legs of a mummy in the necropolis of Thebes. The purchase and translation of this momentous and lengthy document (30 cm wide and 20.23 metres long) was arranged by George Ebers, Professor of Egyptology in Leipzig, after whom the papyrus was named (Von Klein, 1905). It has been estimated that the Ebers Papyrus, which mentions migraine, neuralgia and shooting head pains, was written or transcribed from earlier medical documents in approximately 1550 BC. The papyrus is obviously based on earlier writings since one prescription was written for King Usaphais who reigned in 2700 BC (Major, 1930). There are another six papyri on medical matters in existence. I am indebted to Dr John Edmeads for an artist's impression of the advice given to headache sufferers in those days (Figure 1.1). A clay crocodile was firmly bound to the head of the patient, with herbs being placed in the mouth of the crocodile. Since those archaic times we have dispensed with the clay crocodile and now give the herbs directly to the patient, but the principle of binding the temples remains sound.

Greek medicine may be said to have started with Aesculapius, who probably lived about 1250 BC and became so successful in his practice as a physician that the supply of souls to the underworld was imperilled. For this reason, at the request of Pluto, Zeus destroyed Aesculapius with a thunderbolt. After his death, he became revered as a god and temples dedicated to healing of the sick were known throughout Greece as Asklepia. Guthrie (1947) mentions that one of the cures recorded on stone tablets at Epidaurus was Case Number 29, a young man named Agestratos who suffered from insomnia on account of headaches. He fell asleep in the temple and dreamt that Aesculapius cured him of his headache, then taught him to wrestle. The next day he departed cured and, shortly afterwards, was victor in wrestling at the Nemean games.

Egyptian medicine was probably known to Hippocrates (460 BC) who first described visual symptoms associated with migraine (Critchley, 1967).

> Most of the time he seemed to see something shining before him like a light, usually in part of the right eye; at the end of a moment, a violent pain supervened in the right temple, then in all the head and neck, where the neck is attached to the spine . . . . Vomiting, when it became possible, was able to divert the pain and render it more moderate.

Other forms of headache, such as those caused by exercise and sexual intercourse, were noted by Hippocrates (Adams, 1939) and are inserted later in appropriate parts of this text.

The story of migraine was elaborated by Roman authors. Cornelius Celsus, a friend of the Emperor Tiberius, described how headache could be induced by drinking wine or by the heat of a fire or the sun (Critchley, 1967). Aretaeus, born in Cappodocia (now a region of Turkey) in about AD 80, enlarged on previous descriptions of migraine by commenting that pain is often restricted to one half of the head and that afflicted patients:

> . . . flee the light; the darkness soothes their disease; nor can they bear readily to look upon or hear anything agreeable; their sense of smell is vitiated, neither does anything agreeable to smell delight them, and they have also an aversion to fetid things; the patients, moreover, are weary of life and wish to die.
>
> (Adams, 1841)

Galen (AD 131–201) introduced the term 'hemicrania' for unilateral headache, attributing it to 'the ascent of vapours, either . . . . too hot or too cold'. 'Hemicrania' was later transformed to the Old English 'megrim' and French 'migraine'. The galenical view of four humours that govern health and disease persisted for many centuries but was expressed in terms that could be given a modern interpretation by Paul of Aegina, a Greek physician at the medical school of Alexandria who wrote in AD 600 : 'Headache, which is one of the most serious complaints, is sometimes occasioned by an intemperament solely; sometimes by redundance of humours, and sometimes by both.' (Adams, 1844).

The treatment of headache by the application of hot iron or by applying garlic to an incision in the temple was advocated by the Arabian physician Abu'l Oasim (Abulcasis), born in Spain in AD 936 (Critchley, 1967). Critchley also quotes the Persian Avicenna (AD 980–1037) as saying: 'Little does it concern the patient that there is an underlying cause to be treated if the practitioner proves unable to relieve his pain'.

An illuminated manuscript of the twelfth century by the Abbess Hildegard of Bingen describes recurrent visual phenomena which may well have been migraine equivalents: 'I saw a great star, most splendid and beautiful, and with it an exceeding multitude of falling sparks with which the star followed southward . . . . and suddenly they were all annihilated, being turned into black coals . . . . and cast into the abyss so that I could see them no more.' (Critchley, 1967). She explained that her headaches were unilateral because nobody could stand it if they were on both sides of the head (Isler, 1993).

Transient sensory loss and weakness on the left side of the body accompanying severe headache was described by Charles Le Pois in 1618 (Riley, 1932). In 1684 Dr Willis' *Practice of Physicke*, published in London nine years after the death of Thomas Willis (1621–1675), includes two chapters on headache (reproduced by Knapp, 1963, 1964). Headache is 'a disease which falls upon . . . . sober and intemperate, the empty and the full-bellied, the fat and the lean, the young and the old, yea upon men and women of every age, state or condition'. Willis pointed out that the source of pain is not the brain, cerebellum or medulla because 'they want sensible fibres' but rather distension of the vessels which 'pulls the nervous fibres one from another and so brings to them painful corrugations or wrinklings'. He described the provocation of headache by wine, overeating, lying in the sun, passion, sexual activity, long-sleeping, 'scirrhous tumours growing to the meninges' and 'other diseases of an evil conformation'. He comments on 'ravenous hunger' as a premonitory symptom of migraine and the nausea and vomiting which follows on the headache.

Willis' views on therapy do not live up to the expectation aroused by his clinical observations. He starts with sage but joyless advice about avoiding wine, spiced meats, baths, sexual intercourse ('Venus') and violent motions of the mind and body, before advocating enemas, the letting of blood and application of leeches, and then proceeding to a bizarre polypharmacy. While few would take umbrage at the use of vinegar, nutmeg and rosemary (a decoction of the dried leaves made with spring water), some would raise eyebrows at pills of amber, crab's eyes and coral, while most would draw the line at millipedes and woodlice. Perhaps they might still find a place in the management of the really difficult patients since 'we ought not to omit or postpone the use of millipedes or woodlice, for that the juice of them, wrung forth, with the distilled water, also a powder of them prepared, often bring notable help, for the curing of old and pertinacious headaches'. In fairness to Willis, he also administered anodynes and hypnotics to those in need.

The Swiss physician Wepfer (1620–1695) noted the alternation of migraine from one side of the head to the other in some cases, attributing migraine to relaxation of the vessels. In 1669 he observed the visual auras of migraine. Because this description was not published until 1727, long after his death, he was pre-empted by Vater who published a dissertation on hemianopic migraine scotomas in 1723 (Isler, 1993).

Descriptions of migraine multiplied in the eighteenth and nineteenth centuries, the most comprehensive being the work of Liveing (1873), from whose treatise 'On megrim, sick-headache and some allied disorders', many of the following statements and quotations are stolen, with some additions from Riley (1932), Critchley (1967) and Schiller (1975). Fordyce, in 'De Hemicrania' (published 1758) observed occasional premonitory depression, polyuria during the attack and the association with menstruation which had been reported by Johannis Van der Linden in 'De hemicrania menstrua' (published 1660). Fothergill in 1778 described the visual disturbances of classical migraine and was the first to use the term 'fortification spectra' to describe their zigzag appearance: 'after breakfast, if much toast and butter has been used, it begins with a singular kind of glimmering in the sight; objects swiftly changing their apparent position, surrounded with luminous angles like those of a fortification'. Fothergill considered that 'the headache proceeds from the stomach, not the reverse'. He blamed certain foods, particularly 'melted butter, fat meats, spices, meat pies, hot buttered toast and malt liquors when strong and hoppy'. In 1796 Erasmus Darwin, the grandfather of Charles Darwin, suggested a trial of centrifugal force for the relief of headache, which, as he quaintly added, 'cannot be done in private practice, and which I therefore recommend to some hospital physician'. 'What might be the consequence of whirling a person with his head next to the centre of motion, so as to force the blood from the brain into the other parts of the body?' This challenge was taken up 150 years later by Harold G. Wolff, using a man-carrying centrifuge, with success.

James Ware, in 1814, described bouts of fortification spectra without a headache ensuing, later called 'metastases of migraine' by Tissot (Critchley, 1967) but now known as migraine equivalents. Brief episodes of hemianopia without headache were described by Wollaston in 1824 and of scintillating scotomas by Parry in 1825. In 1865 Sir George Airy described his visual hallucinations as 'nearly resembling those of a Norman arch'. A similar form of migraine manifested itself in one of Sir George's sons, Hubert Airy, who introduced the term 'teichopsia' for fortification spectra and illustrated his own experience in coloured plates which were reproduced by Liveing (1873). Dysphasia with migraine was reported by Tissot, Parry, G. B. Airy and others (Schiller, 1975).

In 1837, Labarraque implicated noise as a cause of migraine in the following words:

> We all know that it is not everyone who can, with impunity, do himself the pleasure of assisting at certain theatrical representations where the glory of France is daily celebrated with noise and smoke. And how many good citizens are there not, tried patriots, whom the threatening of a migraine infallibly brought on by the unaccustomed din of drums and military music, forcibly hinders from taking part in our civic fêtes, and joining their companies on grand review days.

Marshall Hall wrote in 1849 that 'Nothing is so common – nothing is viewed as of such trifling import – as the seizure termed "sick-headache". Yet I have known "sick-headache" issue in paroxysmal attacks of a very severe nature, both apoplectic and epileptic'. (Schiller, 1975).

The fact that the pain of migraine 'mounts synchronously with the pulse of the temporal artery' was noted by Dubois-Reymond in 1859. His artery on the affected side was 'like a firm cord to the touch', his eye was 'small and reddened with a dilated pupil and his face became pale and warm, although his ear on the side of headache became red and hot toward the end of the attack'. His headaches were worse when he indulged 'in vast and uninterrupted mental exertions' but ceased completely on hiking trips. Parry in 1825 and later Mollendorf in 1867 observed that compression of the carotid artery made the headache disappear (Schiller, 1975). The concept of the pathophysiology of migraine was thus swinging to a vascular rather than a neural cause, although Liveing (1873) drew the analogy with epilepsy and regarded disorders of the local circulation as 'among the least constant and regular of the phenomena'. He was supported later by Hughlings Jackson (1890) who believed migraine to be a form of sensory epilepsy with the headache and vomiting as an epiphenomenon (Schiller, 1975). Liveing's classic monograph 'On megrim, sick headache and some allied disorders' was reprinted in 1997 (with an introduction by Oliver Sacks) by Arts and Boeve, Nijmegen, to commemorate the Eighth Congress of the International Headache Society, held in Amsterdam.

At about the same time as Liveing, P. W. Latham (1872) expressed the view that the disturbance of vision was due to defective supply of blood to one side of the brain from the contraction of the cerebral arteries after which 'the action of the sympathetic is exhausted . . . . the vessels become distended, the head throbs' (Schiller, 1975).

Sir Samuel Wilks (1872) gave an admirable dissertation on migraine which 'runs in families, and is due to a particular nervous temperament'. He states that 'whatever produces a strong impression on the nervous system of such a one predisposed will cause an attack, and it may thus be induced in a hundred different ways'. He lists as provocative factors a visit to the theatre, a dinner party, a loud noise, an hour's visit to a picture gallery, looking through a microscope, odours of various kinds (such as of spring flowers), exposure of the body to the sun or a strong wind, and various moral causes and worry – 'moving a single step out of the even tenor of their way'. The various influences 'alter the current of blood through the head: thus, while the face is pale, the larger vessels are throbbing, the head is hot, and the remedies which instinct suggests are cold and pressure to the part'. He recommends a wet bandage around the head, profound quiet, and, if possible, sleep. He discounts the use of drugs, in discussing a powder sent to him by a friend from Vancouver's Island: 'Alas! It must be catalogued with all the other remedies for sick-headache – it was useless.'

But help was at hand. An article appeared in the *British Medical Journal* of 1868 by Edward Woakers: 'On ergot of rye in the treatment of neuralgia', which term included hemicrania. A derivative of ergot (ergotin) was isolated in 1875 and was used by Eulenburg who regarded migraine as being of two types: 'pale' or sympatheticotonic and 'red' or sympatheticoparalytic (Schiller, 1975). Gowers (1893) considered that ergot was of use combined with bromide in patients whose face flushed or did not change colour during an attack but preferred the vasodilator nitroglycerine for those who became pale. He also advocated prophylactic therapy using a solution of nitroglycerine (1%) in alcohol combined with other agents, subsequently known as 'Gowers' mixture'. He recognized that 'a hypodermic injection of morphia often acts no better than other sedatives' and employed bromide and Indian hemp to relieve the acute attack of headache. Gowers disparaged the use of ergotin which did no more than 'lessen the throbbing intensification of the pain', commenting that 'drugs that cause contraction of the arteries are almost powerless'. He discussed the use of caffeine, local applications to the head and neck, hot baths of mustard and water to the feet and, finally, electrical stimulation of the sympathetic chain ('the value of the treatment is, to say the least, seldom perceptible').

In 1925, the Swiss chemist Rothlin isolated ergotamine which was introduced into clinical practice by 1928 when Tzanck wrote a paper on 'Le traitment des migraines par le tartrate d'ergotamine' (Schiller, 1975). Ergotamine tartrate became established as the preferred treatment for acute migraine headache after the report by Graham and Wolff (1938) and the subsequent studies of Wolff and his colleagues (Wolff, 1963).

From that time, the history of migraine, and of headache in general, blends with the present in forming the substance of this book. The International Headache Society was formed in 1983 to foster a systematic approach to the causes and treatment of headaches and has been responsible for a comprehensive classification of headaches, guide-lines for clinical trials and biennial scientific congresses. The history of headache is still in the process of being written for, in the words of Gowers, 'When all has been said that can be, mystery still envelops the mechanism of migraine'.

References

Adams, F. (1841). *The Extant Works of Aretaeus, the Cappodocian.* p. 294. London, Sydenham Society

Adams, F. (1844). *The Seven Books of Paulus Aegineta.* p. 350. London, Sydenham Society

Adams, F. (1939). *The Genuine Works of Hippocrates.* Baltimore, Williams and Wilkins

Alverez, W. C. (1945). Was there sick headache in 3000 B.C.? *Gastroenterology* 5, 524

Chand, D. (1982) *The Atharvaveda* (Sanskrit text with English translation). p. 10. New Delhi, Munshiram Manoharlal

Critchley, M. (1967). Migraine from Cappadocia to Queen Square. In *Background to Migraine*, Vol. 1. pp. 28–38. London, Heinemann

Gowers, W. (1893). *Diseases of the Nervous System*, Vol. 2. pp. 836–866. Philadelphia, P. Blakiston, Son & Co.

Graham, J. R. and Wolff, H. G. (1938). Mechanism of migraine headache and action of ergotamine tartrate. *Arch. Neurol. Psychiat., Chicago* 39, 737–763

Guthrie, D. (1947). *A History of Medicine.* p. 44. New York, Thomas Nelson and Sons

Isler, H. (1993) Historical background. In *The Headaches*, Eds J. Olesen, P. Tfelt-Hanson and K. M. A. Welch, pp. 1–8. New York, Raven Press

Knapp, R. D. Jr (1963). Reports from the past. 2. *Headache* 3, 112–122

Knapp, R. D. Jr (1964). Reports from the past. 3. *Headache* 3, 143–155

Liveing, E. (1873). *On Megrim, Sick-Headache and Some Allied Disorders: A Contribution to the Pathology of Nerve-Storms.* London, J. and A. Churchill

Major, R. H. (1930). The Papyrus Ebers. *Ann. Med. Hist.* (New Series) 2, 547–555

McHenry, L. C. Jr (1969). *Garrison's History of Neurology.* p. 451. Springfield, Illinois, Charles C. Thomas

Riley, H. A. (1932). Special article: Migraine. *Bull. Neurol. Inst. N.Y.* 2, 429–544

Schiller, F. (1975). The migraine tradition. *Bull. Hist. Med.* 49, 1–19

Sigerist, H. E. (1955). *A History of Medicine. Vol. 1. Primitive and Archaic Medicine.* p. 451. New York, Oxford University Press

Von Klein, C. H. (1905). The medical features of the Papyrus Ebers. *J. Am. Med. Ass.* **45**, 1928–1935

Wilks, S. (1872). On sick-headache. *Br. Med. J.* **1**, 8–9

Wolff, H. G. (1963). *Headache and Other Head Pain.* pp. 259–265. New York, Oxford University Press

Chapter 2

Recording the patient's case history

The most satisfying aspect of dealing with headache problems is that diagnosis can often be established solely by taking a systematic case history. When the pattern of illness is clearly recognizable, such as migraine, tension or cluster headache, this does not absolve the clinician from undertaking a physical examination but it may avoid unnecessary investigations and inappropriate treatment. On the other hand, the evolution of the disorder may sound a warning that some serious local or systemic disturbance is in progress and that action should be taken urgently. It must be admitted that there are some patients whose headaches blur traditional boundaries and defy rigid classification. In such instances, the history at least sets the clinician's thought processes in motion. If it does not provide the whole answer, it provides the clues from which the answer may finally be derived. This is part of the challenge to the knowledge, intellect and art of the clinician.

Some clinicians prefer to let patients tell their story without interruption and show commendable restraint by reserving their questions until the end. It may be preferable to guide the patient gently so that the history unfolds neatly and the plot is not obscured by irrelevant side-issues. This is theoretically less desirable but works well in practice and saves a lot of time. The history of headache, like any pain history, is most conveniently recorded under headings that bring out the characteristics to enable recognition of the major diagnostic categories. If there is more than one type of headache, such as the combination of migraine and tension headache, it is helpful to record the characteristics of each separately, perhaps in parallel down the page so that the diagnosis of each type becomes clear.

A systematic case history

Age of onset

The length of the patient's illness separates possible cases into acute, subacute and chronic groups, which reduces the number of diagnoses to be considered as described in Chapters 4 and 18.

Frequency and duration of headaches

These two factors define the temporal pattern of headache, which is important for establishing the diagnosis and setting a baseline for assessment of therapy. It is important to ensure that responses from patients are consistent. For example, patients may state that they have three headaches every week, possibly as three separate episodes each lasting for a day or as a single attack persisting for three days. Again, patients often say that they suffer several headaches each day when they really mean that they have a continuous tendency to headache, relieved by analgesics for some hours at a time.

Ask about relapses and remissions. Patients may have periods of freedom for weeks, months or years, characteristically in cluster headache, but also in some patients with migraine and trigeminal neuralgia. If headaches do recur in bouts, enquire whether there is more than one attack of pain in each 24 hours, how long each lasts and whether it tends to appear at any particular time of the day or night.

Time of onset

It is important to determine whether headaches habitually arouse patients from sleep or are present on awakening. If so, ask about any premonitory symptoms that may have been experienced the previous day. When headaches develop during the day-light hours, enquire about any neurological symptoms (aura) immediately preceding the onset of pain.

Mode of onset

Early warning symptoms

Most patients at first deny any premonitory sensations, but one-quarter recall them when prompted. This does require some leading questions. 'The day before you wake up with headache do you ever feel elated, "on top of the world" or as though you can fly through the day's work effortlessly?'. 'Do you ever feel unusually hungry or have a craving to eat sweet foods?'. Less commonly, patients may feel irritable, drowsy and yawn a lot. It is important to unearth such warning symptoms because they help to confirm the diagnosis of migraine and also to plan the timing of medication. Ergotamine tartrate or some prophylactic agent can be taken on retiring that night to anticipate and prevent the appearance of headache the next day.

Aura

Migraine headache is sometimes preceded by focal neurological symptoms, in which case it is called 'migraine with aura' or 'classical migraine'. The most common symptoms are visual disturbances such as flashes of light, rippling or zigzag sensations with impairment or even loss of vision. These may affect one half or both of the visual fields simultaneously or may spread slowly across the field of vision (fortification spectra, scintillating scotomas). The aura usually develops over 5–10 minutes, persists for 20–45 minutes, then subsides as the headache begins, although such symptoms sometimes continue, or even arise, during headache. Paraesthesiae, hemiparesis or aphasia may also be symptoms of the aura. Nausea may sometimes precede headaches.

Site and radiation of pain

Is the headache usually unilateral or bilateral? Is it localized to the orbital, frontal, temporal or occipital region? Does it radiate to other areas? Does the pain spread to involve the shoulder and arm on the affected side? Is it ever felt in the ipsilateral lower limb as well?

Quality

Does the headache seem to originate deep to the orbit or within the cranium or is it felt superficially in the skin or scalp? Is it stabbing, constant or throbbing? The term 'throbbing' has to be defined because many patients use it loosely to describe a severe pain that waxes and wanes without any relationship to the pulse. I usually enquire: 'does the pain get worse with each heart beat?' or, when really desperate, tap my own temple rhythmically with a pen and ask: 'does it go boom, boom, boom with your pulse?'. If the headache is consistent does it feel like pressure inside the head, a weight on top of the head or a band around the head?

A sudden explosive onset ('thunderclap headache') is typical of subarachnoid haemorrhage and acute pressor responses, but can occasionally occur in migraine.

Associated symptoms

Gastrointestinal disturbances, such as nausea, vomiting, diarrhoea and abdominal pain, are common in migraine but may sometimes accompany severe headaches from other causes.

Photophobia has two components. One is an expression of general hypersensitivity of the special senses – lights seem brighter, sounds seem louder and smells seem stronger. The second component is ocular pain on exposure to light, felt only on the side affected by headache (Drummond, 1986).

Neurological symptoms, associated with diminished cerebral blood flow, may originate in the cerebral cortex as described for the aura. Loss of concentration, confusion and impairment of memory are common events and may rarely develop into stupor or coma. Hindbrain symptoms such as vertigo, dysarthria, ataxia and incoordination are common. Circumoral paraesthesiae can be a symptom of migraine but can also be caused by hyperventilation, which is often associated with headache (see Appendix A). Faintness on standing or fainting, as the result of postural hypotension, is also quite common (Selby and Lance, 1960).

An ipsilateral ocular Horner's syndrome (ptosis, miosis and impaired thermoregulatory sweating in the supraorbital region) develops often in cluster headache, occasionally in migraine, and may persist between attacks. Ptosis is usually more prominent than miosis. On the side affected by cluster headache, the eye commonly reddens and lacrimates while the nostril blocks or runs. The ipsilateral forehead occasionally sweats excessively during attacks of cluster headache because the skin area vacated by sympathetic nerves has been reinervated by parasympathetic fibres originally destined for the lacrimal gland.

Migraine patients may comment on distended arteries or veins in the temple, pallor (rarely flushing), dark coloration under the eyes and swelling of the face with their headaches. The hands, feet or whole body may feel cold.

Scalp tenderness and hyperaesthesia may develop during headache and persist for some days afterwards.

Precipitating factors

Can the patient identify any trigger factor for headaches or do they recur regardless of circumstances? Common trigger factors include:

- Stress (migraine and tension-type headache)
- Relaxation after stress (migraine)
- Phases of the menstrual cycle (premenstrual and midcycle in migraine)
- Excessive afferent stimuli (glare, flickering light, noise, strong perfumes, and even having a haircut may bring on migraine and some tension-type headaches)
- The ingestion of alcohol, vasodilator drugs or specific foods (migraine)
- Excessive intake of tea or coffee (caffeine-withdrawal headache)
- Exercise (migraine and exertional vascular headaches)
- Sexual activity ('benign sex headaches')
- Coughing (intracranial vascular headaches and 'benign cough headaches')
- Posture, neck movements (upper cervical syndrome and tension-type headache)
- Talking, chewing, swallowing, touching the face (trigeminal neuralgia).

Aggravating factors

Is the headache made worse by jolting, jarring of the head, sudden movements, coughing or straining? A positive answer suggests an intracranial vascular origin which is typical of raised intracranial pressure or a space-occupying lesion but can also have a more banal cause such as hangover. Postural headache, present on standing and eased by lying down, suggests a low cerebrospinal fluid pressure.

Relieving factors

Most migraine patients prefer to lie down in a darkened room and try to sleep whereas cluster headache patients usually stand or pace about. Migraine and cluster headache may be eased temporarily by local pressure or the application of hot or cold packs. Tension-type headache may be relieved by alcohol or marijuana. Migraine ceases after the first trimester of pregnancy in about two-thirds of patients.

Previous treatment

Any form of treatment tried previously should be listed with a note about its success or failure. This list may include psychological counselling, relaxation training, biofeedback therapy, hypnosis, chiropractic, acupuncture and the use of transcutaneous nerve stimulation (TENS). In making a record of medications used in acute treatment or prophylaxis, it is important to ascertain the dosage whenever possible. Some patients may have been prescribed subtherapeutic doses whereas others may have been consuming vast amounts of ergotamine or analgesics without supervision. Therapy for co-existing conditions may also be relevant as bromocriptine, cyclosporin, vasodilators, cholesterol-lowering agents, antidepressants of the specific serotonin reuptake inhibitor type and various other medications can cause headache.

General health

It is important to determine at the outset whether headache is one facet of a systemic disease or whether it may be regarded as an isolated problem. Impairment of general health with loss of weight raises the possibility of chronic infections (tuberculous or cryptococcal meningitis, acquired immune deficiency syndrome – AIDS), malignancy, blood dyscrasias, vasculitis, connective tissue and endocrine disorders. The association of headache with general malaise, night sweats, joint and muscle pains (polymyalgia rheumatica) should make one think of temporal arteritis.

System review

It is always helpful to ask leading questions concerning each bodily system at the conclusion of the history of the present illness. In a patient with headache, the eyes, ears, nose and throat, teeth and neck should be included in this review. The chronic obstruction of one or other nostril by vasomotor rhinitis or chronic respiratory tract infection may suggest the possibility of sinusitis. The eye may become proptosed with retro-orbital tumours or a mucocele projecting into the orbit from the frontal sinus. Dimness of vision and 'haloes' seen around lights may mark the onset of glaucoma. Complaints of impaired eyesight may draw attention to compression of the visual pathways. Papilloedema may be symptomless or the patient may notice blurring of vision on bending the head forwards. In contrast, visual loss is severe in retrobulbar neuritis associated with a central scotoma.

A space-occupying lesion or other intracranial disturbance, such as progressive hydrocephalus, becomes much more likely if the recent onset of headache is associated with any of the following symptoms:

- Drowsiness at inappropriate times
- Vomiting without apparent cause
- Fits
- Sudden falling attacks, in which consciousness may be retained
- Progressive neurological deficit of any kind, for example, mental deterioration, impairment of senses of smell, vision or hearing. It is remarkable how a unilateral nerve deafness may be present for years without being complained of, or even noticed, by the patient
- Double vision

- Weakness or sensory impairment of the face or limbs on one or other side
- Disturbed coordination or loss of balance, with or without vertigo
- Polyuria and polydipsia
- Progressive change in pituitary function. Symptoms suggesting hypopituitarism are asthenia, diminished libido, reduction of body hair, lessened shaving frequency in men, premature cessation of menstruation in women, the skin becoming soft and finely wrinkled in both sexes, and the delay of pubescence in the child. On the other hand, hyperpituitarism may be responsible for excessive growth and early pubescence in the young, and deepening of the voice and enlargement of the jaw and hands in adults.

Past health

Head and neck injuries at any time in the past may be of relevance. Subdural haematoma may follow a blow on the head which the patient considered trivial.

A number of episodes of 'encephalitis' or any severe headache with neck stiffness should arouse suspicion of bleeding from a cerebral angioma or leakage of fluid from a craniopharyngioma or other cystic lesion. A useful additional point in the diagnosis of subarachnoid haemorrhage is the development of spinal root pains in the back, buttocks and thighs some hours or days after the onset of headache, which is caused by blood tracking down the subarachnoid space to the cauda equina.

Past infections, particularly tuberculosis, should be recorded. Old tuberculous lesions may be reactivated by immunosuppressant therapy or AIDS, and an impaired immune response makes the patient vulnerable to toxoplasmosis, cryptococcal meningitis, progressive multifocal leucoencephalopathy and primary lymphoma of the brain. Sinusitis and recurrent ear infections are also of potential relevance, particularly in children.

Vomiting attacks and motion sickness in childhood are often precursors of migraine in later life. A past history of asthma in a migraine patient cautions against the use of beta-blockers in management.

Episodes of depression or other psychiatric disturbance may be related to the patient's present illness.

Family history

Both migraine and tension headache run in families but there is less tendency for cluster headache to do so. Information may be gained about a familial tendency to malignancy, tuberculosis, hypertension and other disorders, which may relate to the problem of headache.

Personal background

Occupation
Exposure at work to toxic or vasodilator substances, such as dry cleaning fluids, may have direct relevance to the problem of headache. Some infections, such as brucellosis, leptospirosis and Q fever are liable to occur in abattoir workers. and crypto-

coccosis (torulosis) in those handling birds, particularly pigeons. Noise, flickering light, small video screens, unpleasant smells and harsh air-conditioning may contribute to an unfavourable work environment, quite apart from the tedium of a boring job. The workplace may have lost its appeal for a number of other reasons. The pressure of uninspired or heavy-handed management, the inability to see the end-result of one's labour, falling behind in the race for promotion, difficulty in adapting to changing techniques, financial insecurity and the fear of retrenchment are all potential causes of occupational stress. The waning of old skills may cause anxiety in the years before retirement and when the retirement finally comes it may remove an important source of motivation and take much of the zest from life. The outlook is not entirely gloomy. Many people enjoy their work and many even enjoy their years of retirement.

Personal or family problems
Every stage of development abounds in potential sources of anxiety but it must be borne in mind that stress by itself is usually not enough to cause headache. The fault lies more often in failure to adapt to a situation that would not trouble most people. It is therefore important to determine any source of worry and then assess whether the patient's reaction to it is realistic.

Problems in childhood range from physical, mental or sexual abuse to natural concerns about relationships with parents, siblings and peers, success or failure in school work and sporting activities, and the making and breaking of friendships. Unrealistic goals set by parents for their children may lead to feelings of inadequacy and frustration on both sides. The self-confidence and rate of progress of a child depends largely on the attitude of parents and teachers. Some childhood headaches can be cured by changing schools. Parental separation or divorce, or a strained marriage continuing for the sake of the children, are common causes of insecurity, tension and behaviour disturbances among children. It requires patient and devoted teamwork between husband and wife to bring up a family successfully at the best of times.

The miraculous transformation of the body at puberty may give rise to feelings other than joy and wonder to the transformee. Puberty may arrive too early or too late. Children may grow too much or too little. The outward and visible signs of their sexuality may seem too large or too small. They may be inadequately prepared for the onset of menstruation or may be unnecessarily laden with guilt about masturbation. As though acne were not enough! Their increasing desire for independence often conflicts with parental guide-lines and the perceived need to conform to their ethnic customs as well as the rigours of a school curriculum.

Sexual problems may be important at any age. The containment within accepted social bounds of the sexual vigour of youth, and the maintenance of satisfactory sexual life in marriage during the mature middle years plus the tensions of work and child-raising may each bring difficulties. The unmarried of any age may be troubled by the instability of their sexual and social relationships, and with the spectre of loneliness at the end of the line. A tactful enquiry about sexual preference should be made when appropriate because of possible conflicts arising from the homosexual lifestyle and the threat of AIDS.

Habits

The personal history also covers intake of alcohol, tea and coffee, medications, 'recreational drugs' and smoking. The daily consumption of analgesics or ergotamine tartrate can transform intermittent headaches into chronic daily headache. Drinking more than six cups of tea or coffee each day may cause rebound headache from caffeine withdrawal. Alcohol, monosodium glutamate and vasodilator drugs induce headache in susceptible people. Certain foods, missed meals or 'sleeping-in' at weekends may be identified as trigger factors for headache.

Emotional state

As the personal history is taken, some insight is usually gained into whether the patient's symptoms are exaggerated by loneliness and introspection, or whether they are being played down by one who has an active and interesting life. The history is a second-hand experience, which is coloured by the emotional expression of the person telling the story. While the story is being recorded it may be possible to discern whether the patient reacts to problems with physical manifestations of tension by frowning, clenching the jaws or holding the head and neck rigidly. It is important to look for symptoms of depression, such as loss of interest in work, home life or personal affairs; or staying at home and not wanting to see friends or continue with previous activities. Depressive symptoms are important to recognize because their treatment may play a big part in restoring pleasure to life, quite apart from relieving the headache, which is often a reflection of the depressive state.

References

Drummond, P D. (1986). Quantitative assessment of photophobia in migraine and tension headache. *Headache* **26**, 465–469

Selby, G. and Lance, J. W. (1960). Observations on 500 cases of migraine and allied vascular headache. *J. Neurol. Neurosurg. Psychiat.* **23**, 23–32

Chapter 3

Types of headache

It often comes as a surprise to the general public and even some medical students that there are many varieties of headache. To many, a headache is a headache and that is that. When headaches are caused by some recognizable structural change or pathological process they can be sorted readily into appropriate categories; the task becomes more difficult when we are dealing with symptoms but no physical signs and our understanding of headache mechanisms is incomplete. In such cases, no help is usually forthcoming from specialized investigations and scanning techniques. The classification of each headache must then be undertaken in the same way that we make our clinical diagnosis, by recording and analysing the case history, including the site, nature, pattern of recurrence and accompanying symptoms.

The system first used was based on the recommendations of the Ad Hoc Committee on Classification of Headache (Friedman *et al.*, 1962). This was a useful start but many of the definitions employed by the Committee were qualified by adjectives such as 'commonly' or 'sometimes'. This is difficult to avoid when headache patterns are variable, when the characteristics of one may merge into another or when two or more types of headache may coexist. Drummond and Lance (1984) compared a computer classification of headache symptoms with the clinical diagnosis in 600 patients attending their neurology clinic. They found that migraine with aura and cluster headache emerged as clearly defined syndromes but that those designated clinically as 'migraine without aura' and 'tension headache' differed in the number rather than the nature of supposedly migrainous symptoms; this suggests that there was a spectrum of 'idiopathic headache' with episodic 'migraine' at one end and frequently occurring 'tension headache' at the other. For example, the headache was unilateral in almost 60 per cent of those attacks recurring from once a month to several times each week but was still unilateral in approximately 20 per cent of patients with daily headache. The latter group included patients who had previously suffered from migraine ('transformed migraine'). Other observers (Rasmussen et al., 1991) have found a clear distinction between the symptoms of migraine and tension headache.

The International Headache Society (IHS) has made a brave attempt to define and provide diagnostic criteria for headache disorders, cranial neuralgias and facial pain (Headache Classification Committee of the International Headache Society, 1988). This classification is tentative and is subject to revision if some of its premises are found wanting. The following summary is based on the IHS classification but the original publication should be consulted for details.

1. Migraine (see Chapters 6–9)

1.1 Migraine without aura
This episodic headache used to be called common migraine and is typically unilateral, associated with nausea, photophobia and sensitivity to sound.

1.2 Migraine with aura
Migrainous headaches preceded by neurological symptoms were termed 'classic' or 'classical' migraine in the past but the IHS Committee considered that, to avoid any possibility of confusion, 'migraine with aura' was preferable. The aura is commonly a visual disturbance that may affect both visual fields simultaneously, such as blurring, rippling, spots or flashes, but in some cases moves slowly over one or both fields of vision as a zigzag pattern, leaving areas of impaired vision. These auras are known as fortification spectra or scintillating scotomas and are discussed in detail in Chapter 6.
   Varieties of 'migraine with aura' included familial hemiplegic migraine, basilar migraine (when aura symptoms arise from the brain stem and occipital lobes) and episodes consisting solely of the aura without any headache ('migraine equivalents').

1.3 Ophthalmoplegic migraine
A rare condition in which paresis of one or more of the ocular motor nerves (third, fourth or sixth cranial nerves) accompanies migrainous headache. This diagnosis can only be made after other causes of compression of these nerves has been excluded.

1.4 Retinal migraine
In retinal migraine, the visual disturbance is confined to one eye and the headache then develops behind that eye. This variety is very uncommon and a structural ocular lesion must be ruled out.

1.5 Childhood periodic syndromes
The IHS Committee recognized that certain recurrent symptoms in childhood could be associated with migraine or be precursors of migraine in later life. Those nominated were 'benign paroxysmal vertigo' and 'alternating hemiplegia of childhood'. The authors would delete the latter which is a progressive disorder leading to a dystonic state and would add abdominal pain or vomiting recurring without an organic explanation (abdominal migraine, 'bilious attacks').

1.6 Complications of migraine
Prolonged migrainous headache, continuing for days or weeks (status migrainosus) and permanent ischaemic damage to the nervous system (migrainous infarction) are listed as complications.

2. Tension-type headache (see Chapter 10)

2.1 Episodic
Recurrent attacks of a tight, pressing sensation in the head, usually bilateral. The

episodes are usually precipitated by physical or mental stress and a subvariety is associated with excessive muscle contraction and muscle tenderness.

2.2 Chronic
Chronic tension-type headache recurs 15 or more days in a month, commonly every day. It has the same heavy or tight quality as the episodic variety and may or may not be associated with overactivity of the jaw and facial muscles. Other forms of chronic daily headache may develop from episodic migraine attacks ('transformed migraine') or start suddenly for no apparent reason ('new daily persistent headache').

3. Cluster headache and paroxysmal hemicrania (see Chapter 11)

3.1 Cluster headache
Attacks of unilateral pain, centred on the orbital or periorbital region, usually lasting 15–180 minutes and recurring up to eight times a day. The pain is usually severe and is accompanied by redness and lacrimation of the eye and nasal congestion on the affected side. The disorder characteristically recurs in bouts lasting weeks or months, separated by a period of freedom for months or years (episodic cluster headache). If attacks continue for a year or more without remission, the condition is known as chronic cluster headache. Previous names for this disorder include ciliary neuralgia, migrainous neuralgia and Horton's histaminic cephalalgia.

3.2 Chronic paroxysmal hemicrania (CPH)
CPH has the same characteristics as cluster headache but recurs as brief episodes, usually lasting 5–20 minutes, from five to 30 times in each 24-hour period. It is said to respond specifically to indomethacin. An episodic form has also been described. Short-lasting unilateral neuralgiform headache attacks with conjunctival injection, tearing, sweating and rhinorrhoea (SUNCT syndrome) may also be a variation of cluster headache.

4. Miscellaneous headaches unassociated with a structural lesion (see Chapter 12)

4.1 Idiopathic stabbing headache
Transient stabs of pain in the head ('icepick pains') that occur spontaneously in the absence of organic disease of underlying structures.

4.2 External compression headache
Headache resulting from continued stimulation of peripheral nerves by pressure from a hat or tight band such as the goggles worn during swimming training ('swim goggle headache').

4.3 Cold stimulus headache
Headache caused by exposure of the unprotected head to a low environmental temperature, for example, subzero weather or diving into cold water. Headache caused by the ingestion of cold substances ('ice-cream headache').

4.4 Benign cough headache
Headache precipitated by coughing in the absence of any intracranial disorder.

4.5 Benign exertional headache
Headache brought on by exercise. Some varieties have been given specific names such as 'weightlifter's headache'.

4.6 Headache associated with sexual activity
Headache arising during sexual intercourse or masturbation, often as a dull ache increasing with sexual excitement, becoming intense with orgasm, but sometimes as an explosive headache at the time of orgasm without warning. Care must be taken to exclude an underlying organic cause such as aneurysm. A rare form of postural headache after intercourse has also been described.

5. Headache associated with head trauma (see Chapter 13)

5.1 Acute post-traumatic headache
Headache occurring less than 14 days after head injury and ceasing within 8 weeks of trauma.

5.2 Chronic post-traumatic headache
Headaches persisting for more than 8 weeks after head injury.

6. Headache associated with vascular disorders (see Chapter 14)

6.1 Acute ischaemic cerebrovascular disease
Headaches accompanying transient ischaemic attacks or thromboembolic stroke.

6.2 Intracranial haematoma
Headaches with intracranial, subdural or extradural haematomas.

6.3 Subarachnoid haemorrhage
A severe headache of sudden onset, usually associated with neck stiffness, caused by rupture of an intracranial aneurysm or arteriovenous malformation.

6.4 Unruptured vascular malformation
Headache caused by enlargement of an intracranial aneurysm. Whether an unruptured arteriovenous malformation ever causes headache is uncertain.

6.5 Arteritis
Giant cell arteritis (temporal arteritis, Horton's disease) causes headache by inflammation of the scalp arteries. It is often associated with polymyalgia rheumatica.

6.6 Carotid or vertebral artery pain
Dissection of carotid or vertebral arteries gives rise to ipsilateral pain in the neck and head, often associated with neurological signs of ischaemia in the affected arterial

territory. Carotidynia is the term given to pain and tenderness over the carotid artery without evidence of a structural lesion. Ipsilateral postendarterectomy headache has been described.

6.7 Venous thrombosis
Headache associated with thrombosis of one of the major intracranial veins or venous sinuses, often accompanied by raised intracranial pressure, focal neurological deficits or seizures.

6.8 Arterial hypertension
Acute pressor responses may be caused by phaeochromocytoma, acute nephritis, malignant hypertension, eclampsia or medications (for example, a patient taking sympathomimetic drugs while being treated with monoamine oxidase inhibitors). Moderate chronic hypertension does not cause headache.

7. Headache associated with non-vascular intracranial disorders (see Chapter 15)

7.1 High cerebrospinal fluid pressure
Headache is a feature of communicating and non-communicating hydrocephalus with high cerebrospinal fluid (CSF) pressure. In the absence of any obstruction to the CSF pathways, the condition is called 'benign intracranial hypertension'.

7.2 Low cerebrospinal fluid pressure
A postural headache, worse on standing and relieved by lying, may develop after lumbar puncture or result from other causes of a CSF leak.

7.3 Intracranial infection
Meningitis and encephalitis are associated with headache from meningeal irritation.

7.4 Intracranial sarcoidosis and other non-infectious inflammatory diseases

7.5 Headache associated with intrathecal injections
An example is the headache following the insertion of air into the CSF in the now out-moded technique of pneumo-encephalography.

7.6 Intracranial neoplasms
Cerebral tumours may cause headache by displacing blood vessels or obstructing the flow of CSF.

8. Headache associated with substances or their withdrawal (see Chapter 12)

8.1 Headache induced by acute substance use or exposure
Examples are the headaches induced by vasodilator agents, such as nitrates, nitrites or calcium channel blockers, and the inhalation of volatile hydrocarbons used in dry cleaning and similar processes.

8.2 Headache induced by chronic substance use or exposure
The daily ingestion of ergotamine tartrate or analgesics may induce headache.

8.3 Headache from substance withdrawal (acute use)
'Hangover' headache following the excessive consumption of alcohol is cited as an example but this may depend upon the action of toxic metabolites rather than the withdrawal of alcohol.

8.4 Headache from substance withdrawal (chronic use)
'Rebound' headache following the withdrawal of ergotamine tartrate, caffeine or narcotics.

8.5 Headache associated with substances but with uncertain mechanism
Oral contraceptives, for example, may increase the tendency to vascular headaches.

9. Headache associated with non-cephalic infection (see Chapter 12)

9.1 Viral infections

9.2 Bacterial infections
Localized or systemic (septicaemia).

10. Headache associated with metabolic disorder (see Chapter 12)

10.1 Hypoxia
Headaches associated with a Pa_{O_2} less than 70 mmHg. This section includes headaches developing at high altitudes and those following sleep apnoea.

10.2 Hypercapnia
Headaches associated with a Pc_{O_2} above 50 mmHg in the absence of hypoxia.

10.3 Mixed hypoxia and hypercapnia

10.4 Hypoglycaemia
Headache precipitated by a blood glucose of less than 2.2 mmol/litre (40 mg%).

10.5 Dialysis
Headache during or after haemodialysis.

11. Headache or facial pain associated with disorder of neck, cranial or extracranial structures (see Chapter 16)

11.1 Cranial bones
Diseases of the skull such as osteomyelitis, multiple myeloma and Paget's disease may cause headache.

11.2 Neck
Occipital headache can be referred from the upper cervical spine. A constant pain in the back of the neck and head, aggravated by bending the neck backwards, has been described as 'retropharyngeal tendinitis'.

Some patients with lax atlanto-axial joints experience a sharp pain in the upper neck on sudden neck turning, associated with numbness in the occiput and the ipsilateral half of the tongue ('neck–tongue syndrome'). The reason for this is that proprioceptive fibres from the tongue enter the central nervous system through the second cervical root, which is compromised by extreme neck rotation.

11.3 Eyes
Acute glaucoma may cause pain in the eye and forehead. Refractive errors and disorders of ocular balance may be factors promoting headache.

11.4 Ears
Disorders of the middle ear may cause neuralgic pain, classified under heading 12.

11.5 Nose and sinuses
Headache and facial pain may be caused by obstruction of the nasal sinuses.

11.6 Teeth, jaws and related structures
Disorders of the teeth usually cause facial pain but are rarely responsible for headache.

11.7 Temporomandibular joint disease
Dysfunction of the temporomandibular joint may refer pain to the temple and adjacent areas of the face (Costen's syndrome).

12. Cranial neuralgias, nerve trunk pain and deafferentation pain (see Chapter 17)

12.1 Constant pain of cranial nerve origin
Compression or distortion of sensory cranial nerves (trigeminal, nervus intermedius, glossopharyngeal, vagus) or the upper three cervical roots may refer pain to the appropriate area. Optic neuritis, diabetic oculomotor nerve palsy and Tolosa–Hunt syndrome (orbital fissure granuloma) may be associated with pain in the orbit or frontal region. Herpes zoster infection affecting the first division of the trigeminal nerve or the geniculate ganglion refers pain to the forehead or ear respectively and may be followed by postherpetic neuralgia.

12.2 Trigeminal neuralgia
Shock-like pains limited to one or more divisions of the trigeminal nerve. Trigger points and trigger factors can usually be identified. The condition may be symptomatic of trigeminal nerve compression by blood vessels or tumours, or of a central lesion, such as multiple sclerosis.

12.3 Glossopharyngeal neuralgia

Stabbing pains felt in the ear and base of the tongue, often provoked by swallowing, talking or coughing. Like trigeminal neuralgia, it may also be symptomatic of a structural lesion.

12.4 Nervus intermedius neuralgia

A rare disorder characterized by brief paroxysms of pain felt deeply in the external auditory canal.

12.5 Superior laryngeal neuralgia

A rare condition in which paroxysms of severe pain are felt in the lateral aspect of the throat and under the ear, precipitated by swallowing, shouting or turning the head.

12.6 Occipital neuralgia

Jabbing or constant pain, with or without altered sensation, associated with the distribution of one greater occipital nerve. The affected nerve is tender to palpation.

12.7 Central causes of head and facial pain

Persistent pain may follow lesions of the trigeminal nerve (analgesia dolorosa) or disorder of the central pain pathways in the quintothalamic tract or thalamus (thalamic pain).

12.8 Facial pain not fulfilling the criteria for groups 11 and 12

Persistent facial pain not associated with physical signs or a demonstrable organic cause (atypical facial pain).

The list of possible causes of headache appears formidable but, by following the principles put forward in the following chapters, a satisfactory clinical diagnosis can usually be made to the gratification of both doctor and patient.

References

Drummond, P. D. and Lance, J W. (1984). Clinical diagnosis and computer analysis of headache symptoms. *J. Neurol. Neurosurg. Psychiat.* **47**, 128–133

Friedman, A. P., Finley, K. M., Graham, J. R, Kunkle, E. C., Ostfeld, A. M. and Wolff, H. G. (1962). Classification of headache. The Ad Hoc Committee on the Classification of Headache. *Arch. Neurol.* **6**, 173–176

Headache Classification Committee of the International Headache Society (1988). Classification and diagnostic criteria for headache disorders, cranial neuralgias and facial pain. *Cephalalgia* **8** (Suppl. 7), 9–96

Rasmussen, B. K., Jensen, R. and Olesen, J. (1991). A population-based analysis of the diagnostic criteria of the International Headache Society. *Cephalalgia* **11**, 129–134

Chapter 4

Diagnosis based on the history

The case history and its interpretation are the most important factors in headache diagnosis. Information about the nature of the headache obtained under each descriptive subheading makes a contribution to the differential diagnosis. Each feature will now be considered in turn to evaluate its significance.

Age of onset

The length of time a patient has been troubled by headache is the first guide as to whether the symptom portends some malignant or progressive neurological disorder that requires further investigation. At one end of the scale, the sudden onset of severe headache, possibly followed by impairment of consciousness or focal neurological signs, suggests some serious illness, such as subarachnoid haemorrhage or meningitis. At the other end of the scale, a patient who has had headaches regularly for many years is likely to have some form of vascular headache (migraine or one of its variants) or chronic tension-type headache. The first attack of migraine that a patient experiences may be confusing unless it is preceded by characteristic symptoms, and may suggest systemic infection, encephalitis or meningitis.

Between the very acute and very chronic headaches lie the most difficult to interpret, those that have developed over some days, weeks or months. The subacute headache may have a relatively simple explanation, such as sinusitis, but one must be on guard against less common but more life-threatening conditions, such as subdural haematoma, cerebral tumour or other causes of increased intracranial pressure, and, in those over 55 years of age, the insidious onset of temporal (giant cell) arteritis.

Frequency and duration of headaches

These two variables establish the temporal pattern, which is important in the diagnosis of recurrent headache. In this group the main conditions to be considered are migraine, cluster headache, trigeminal neuralgia (tic douloureux) and tension-type headache (see Figure 4.1).

Migraine may recur irregularly at intervals of months or years but commonly a pattern has become established by the time a patient seeks medical advice. The headache may be linked to the menstrual cycle or recur one or more times each

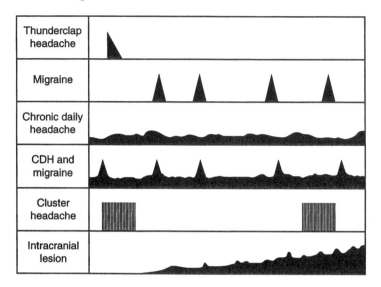

Figure 4.1 Temporal patterns of headache; chronic daily headache (CDH)

week without any obvious cause, sometimes disappearing during pregnancy, holidays, admission to hospital or other periods of prolonged rest. The headache may last from a few hours to several days, but is usually followed by a period of freedom from headache before the next attack starts.

Cluster headache, on the other hand, has an intriguing periodicity. It commonly recurs in bouts lasting from 2 weeks to 3 months and then vanishes completely for 3 months to as long as 4 years. During a bout, the headache returns one, two or more times in 24 hours, and lasts from 10 minutes to several hours on each occasion. The fact that the pain persists for this length of time clearly distinguishes it from trigeminal neuralgia, which recurs as transient jabs of pain, each lasting a fraction of a second, although the jabs may be repetitive. The two disorders are mentioned together because they are commonly confused in general practice. Many patients with cluster headache are referred with the provisional diagnosis of trigeminal neuralgia, probably because the pattern of cluster headache is not widely known. One point that the conditions have in common is the tendency to spontaneous remission for months or years. The distinction between the two is important because the mechanism and treatment of each are entirely different.

Some 20 per cent of cluster headache patients suffer from a chronic form, recurring regularly without periods of remission. In this case, the distinction from migraine depends on the rapidity of onset, relative brevity of each attack and the autonomic disturbances described in Chapters 2 and 11. Rare variations of cluster headache, with many brief episodes developing each day, are known as episodic or chronic paroxysmal hemicrania (CPH) and, with still shorter duration, as the SUNCT (Short-lasting Unilateral Neuralgiform headache attacks with Conjunctival injection, Tearing, sweating and rhinorrhoea) syndrome.

Tension-type headache is set apart from those just considered by the absence of any paroxysmal quality or periodicity about its course. While acute forms of tension headache may appear at the end of a stressful day in a busy office or a household of screaming children, the usual story is that there is always a headache lurking in the background. Such patients have some sort of headache all day and every day. There is a form of headache intermediate between this undulating pattern and the paroxysms of migraine in which surges of more severe throbbing headache become superimposed every few days or weeks on an otherwise monotonous background of constant discomfort. Most of these patients have previously experienced episodic migraine and are considered to have 'transformed migraine'.

Time of onset

Migraine headache commonly awakens the patient in the early hours of the morning but may come on at any time of the day. Cluster headache tends to recur punctually at certain times of the day or night, often one or two hours after the patient goes to sleep. Hypnic headaches are an unusual variety awakening the patient, usually elderly, from sleep and are often preventable by a nocturnal dose of lithium. Tension-type headache may be present on waking but more often starts on getting up and about.

The time of onset is important from the therapeutic as well as the diagnostic point of view. If headaches awaken the patient from sleep consistently, preventive medication is best taken the night before.

Mode of onset

Early warning symptoms
A change of mood, such as an unwarranted elation or irritability, excessive yawning or a craving to eat sweet foods, are harbingers of migraine and should be recognized by the patient as a signal to take medication that night to ward off the headache threatening the next day.

Aura
An aura before migraine headache is the exception rather than the rule but, when it does occur, it places the diagnosis beyond reasonable doubt. The symptoms comprising the aura usually develop gradually over some minutes, persist for 10 to 45 minutes and then subside slowly. The most common aura is a visual disturbance with positive features (flashes, zigzags, circles of light or rippling vision) and negative features (patchy scotomas, hemianopia, bilateral blurring or tunnel vision). One may follow the other as in the classical fortification spectra (scintillating scotomas), in which shimmering or jittering zigzag figures pass slowly over one or both visual fields leaving behind areas of impaired vision. Other focal neurological symptoms, such as paraesthesiae, hemiparesis and dysphasia, may develop during the aura.

Acute onset
Headaches usually develop and increase in severity slowly, whether or not they are

preceded by an aura. If headache strikes suddenly 'like a blow to the head' ('thunderclap headache'), one must think of subarachnoid haemorrhage, fulminant meningitis or encephalitis, obstruction of the cerebral ventricles or a rapid rise in blood pressure such as that which occurs in phaeochromocytoma, although migraine and orgasmic headaches may present in this manner.

Site

Headache is commonly unilateral in migraine (about two-thirds), cluster headache and trigeminal neuralgia (which are almost always unilateral), local changes in the eye, sinuses, skull or scalp, and expanding lesions of one cerebral hemisphere. An aneurysm of the internal carotid artery may cause pain behind one eye by enlarging without rupturing. Subarachnoid haemorrhage from an aneurysm or angioma may start with local pain but headache usually becomes generalized and spreads to the back of the neck. Space-occupying lesions may cause unilateral pain by displacement of vessels, but headache becomes bilateral if cerebrospinal fluid (CSF) pathways are obstructed. The site of headache is not reliable as a means of localizing a cerebral tumour. The headache of internal carotid dissection or thrombosis is unilateral, whereas vertebrobasilar disorders may refer pain to the occipital area bilaterally. Scalp vessels may be involved separately in temporal arteritis so that pain is limited to the distribution of a specific artery.

Migraine headache often starts in one temple or occipital region (Figure 4.2), then coalesces between these areas as a bar of pain before radiating over that half of the head or becoming generalized. It may spread to involve the neck and shoulder or, rarely, the entire half of the body on the affected side. Sometimes pain may be felt more below the eye, in which case it is termed 'lower-half headache' or facial migraine.

The pain of cluster headache characteristically involves the eye and frontal region on one side and may radiate to the occiput and the nostril, cheek and teeth on the same side (Figure 4.2), overlapping the distribution of 'lower-half headache'. The stabbing pains of trigeminal neuralgia are usually felt in the cheek or chin (second and third divisions) but start in the eye or forehead (first division) in about 5 per cent of cases. Tension-type headache is commonly bilateral but is unilateral in some 20 per cent of patients, particularly in those who are also subject to migraine. The pain arising from a temporomandibular joint may radiate up to the temple and down over the face on that side.

'Ice-cream headache' is usually felt in the midline but may be referred to one temple, particularly when the subject is prone to experience migraine in that site (see Chapter 13). The pain of sinusitis commonly overlies the affected areas.

Quality

Headache may be constant, pulsatile or stabbing. Migraine usually starts as a dull ache but may become pulsatile ('throbbing') as the intensity increases. The pain of cluster headache is described as deep, boring and intense. Trigeminal neuralgia is a shocklike stab or series of stabs. Tension-type headache is dull, constant, tight and

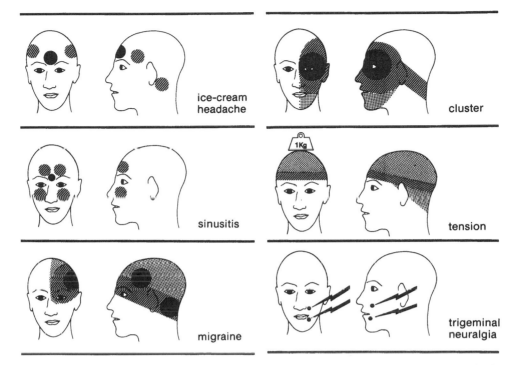

Figure 4.2 Sites of head and facial pain. (From Lance, 1986, by permission of the publishers, Charles Scribner's Sons, New York)

Regions commonly affected by six varieties of head pain are illustrated, with the usual intensity indicated as severe (black), moderate (diagonal lines) or a milder pressure sensation (stippled). Tension headache is often described as a feeling of weight on the head or a bandlike sensation around the head. The stabbing nature of trigeminal neuralgia is depicted by zigzag lines.

pressing like a band around the head or a weight on the head (Figure 4.2). Patients with tension-type headache and migraine may also be subject to sudden jabs of pain in the head ('ice-pick pains'), often felt in the site of their habitual headache.

Associated phenomena

The usual accompaniments of migraine and cluster headache are mentioned in Chapter 2 and described in more detail in Chapters 7 and 11, respectively. Tension-type headache is notable for the absence of these distinctive features, although most patients do complain of a constant mild photophobia.

The meningeal irritation of subarachnoid haemorrhage, meningitis and encephalitis causes a protective reflex muscle spasm of the extensor muscles of the neck, which is manifest clinically as neck rigidity.

The sudden headache caused by a colloid cyst blocking the flow of CSF in the third ventricle may be accompanied by a 'drop attack', a sudden loss of power in the legs, caused by compression of the midline reticular formation. Consciousness is not necessarily lost during drop attacks. With any space-occupying lesion, or progressive hydrocephalus, the patient may become drowsy, yawn frequently or vomit without preliminary nausea. Fits or other symptoms of focal cortical irritation may precede headache or appear as the headache intensifies. Diplopia may herald the onset of compression of the third cranial nerve, caused by an expanding intracranial mass forcing part of the temporal lobe downwards through the tentorial opening. Dilatation of the ipsilateral pupil can be a sinister sign of tentorial herniation requiring immediate action, but may also be seen, occasionally, in vertebrobasilar migraine.

Rigors and sweats in any acute infectious process, nasal obstruction and bony tenderness in sinusitis, and conjunctival and circumcorneal injection in ocular conditions, are all indications of the source of headache.

Precipitating or aggravating factors

Any intracranial vascular headache, whether it be caused by 'hangover', hypoglycaemia or intracranial tumour, will be made worse by jarring, sudden movements of the head, coughing, sneezing or straining. 'Cough headache' is not always associated with intracranial tumour but can be a benign, if unexplained, vascular syndrome in its own right. Bending the head forwards may bring on a severe paroxysmal headache in patients with a colloid cyst of the third ventricle, or other forms of obstructive hydrocephalus.

Sensitivity to light is a common feature of diffuse intracranial disturbance such as meningitis or encephalitis as well as migraine. Glare, loud noises and even strong odours are liable to initiate or worsen tension-type headache as well as migraine.

Exercise aggravates vascular headache of any type and the occasional individual may suffer disability as a result of exercise alone. Sexual intercourse may bring on tension-type or vascular headaches and has been known to precipitate subarachnoid haemorrhage.

Some people are liable to a dull headache on missing a meal and hypoglycaemia or dehydration may provoke a migraine attack in susceptible patients. Certain foods are said to induce migraine, but doubt has been cast on whether fatty foods, chocolate, oranges and other traditional migraine precipitants act specifically or by a psychological conditioning process. Vascular reactivity appears to be altered by hormonal changes, thus accounting for the association between migraine and menstruation, and its relief in some women during pregnancy.

Alcohol usually triggers cluster headache during a bout, but not at other times. It may also bring on migraine when the patient is in a susceptible phase (not in the refractory period after an attack has recently ended). Red wines in particular have been incriminated, but white wines are thought to be culpable in France.

The lightning jabs of trigeminal neuralgia may be brought on by talking, chewing, swallowing, shaving or even a puff of wind blowing on the face. Pain arising from the teeth is usually exacerbated by hot or cold fluids in the mouth; temporomandibular joint dysfunction is made worse by chewing or clenching the jaw. Chewing may cause pain in the temporal and masseter muscles ('claudication of the jaw muscles') when their blood supply is impaired by temporal arteritis.

Changes in barometric pressure may make the pain of sinusitis worse. Anyone who has ever had a cold when travelling by air and experienced pain from the sinuses during the aircraft's descent will be sufficiently impressed to carry a nasal decongestant in future.

The occipital headache of cervical spondylosis is understandably aggravated by neck movement. Tension-type headache may correlate with periods of turbulence caused by worry, anger or excitement, but in the chronic form it may persist inexorably, no matter how calm the waters. Migraine may occur at a time of stress but it more commonly follows some hours after relaxation from stress or even the following day, as in 'weekend migraine'.

Headache caused by low cerebrospinal fluid pressure develops when the patient stands and is relieved by lying down.

Relieving factors

Pressure on distended scalp arteries, and the use of hot or cold compresses, are often soothing in migraine and cluster headache. The migraine patient usually wishes to sit or lie in a darkened room whereas the cluster headache patient prefers to stand or pace the floor, holding one hand over the affected eye. Rebreathing into a paper bag or the inhalation of carbon dioxide at 10 per cent in air or oxygen is said to shorten the vasoconstrictive phase of migraine, and the inhalation of 100 per cent oxygen relieves most patients with cluster headache.

The pain of sinusitis is abolished when the sinuses are cleared by the relief of nasal obstruction. The avoidance of chewing on one side and excessive jaw clenching eases the pain of temporomandibular strain or arthritis.

Voluntary relaxation of forehead and jaw muscles will reduce the severity of tension-type headache and the use of alcohol may temporarily abolish it.

Paracetamol (acetaminophen) will sometimes stop the pain of migraine in childhood but usually not in adult life. Aspirin is useful in mild forms of head pain, alone or in combination with paracetamol or caffeine, and may prevent migraine if taken in effervescent or soluble form early in the attack after a drug to promote gastric absorption such as metoclopramide.

More specific methods of relieving headache will be discussed later in the appropriate chapters.

Conclusion

It is to be hoped that sufficient of the factors mentioned in this chapter will emerge during the taking of a case history to form a clear clinical impression of the headache pattern and an opinion about the group to which the headache belongs and its probable cause. Well-directed enquiries may bring out important points that the patient has neglected to mention. If the diagnosis is not evident after taking the case history, at least the clinician should know what to look for on physical examination and should also have formed an opinion as to whether the headache warrants further investigation.

Chapter 5

Physical examination

The case history may direct the clinician's attention to certain aspects of the physical examination, to look for signs of meningeal irritation, raised intracranial pressure or other signs of organic disease. Even if the story is typical of migraine, cluster headache or tension-type headache, a general examination should be performed. This will often be completely normal but it is important for both clinician and patient to know that it is normal. The emphasis of examination will naturally be on the head, neck and nervous system, but there are so many ways in which headache can be produced that other systems should not be neglected.

General appearance

The patient's demeanour while the history is being taken may give some indication of anxiety, depression or hypochondriacal exaggeration of symptoms. Sighing or yawning may betray a tendency to overbreathe. Other manifestations of nervous tension include frowning, thrusting forward or clenching of the jaw, restless movements and the transfer of a handkerchief from one moist palm to another. Occasionally the clinician may observe signs of an organic disorder – the large jaw and hands of acromegaly, a goitre obstructing the jugular venous outflow (see Figure 14.4), the large head of Paget's disease or the short neck that accompanies an anomaly of the craniospinal junction, such as platybasia and Arnold–Chiari malformation.

If a patient is suffering an attack of migraine at the time, the clinician may see undue pulsation of the temporal artery and its branches while the skin is pale with the area under the eyes becoming dark and puffy. The pupil on the affected side may constrict, although it dilates in rare instances of 'basilar artery migraine'. The changes are more striking during episodes of cluster headache, when an ocular Horner's syndrome (Figure 5.1) becomes apparent in about one-third of patients, often persisting between attacks. Thickened or thrombosed scalp arteries may be visible in patients with temporal arteritis.

Mental state

The mental state of the patient will have been assessed superficially during history-taking. Drowsiness, confusion or disorientation may indicate a space-occupying

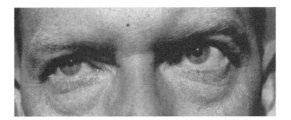

Figure 5.1 Ocular Horner's syndrome in cluster headache. Right ptosis and miosis is accompanied by conjunctional injection and lacrimation

lesion or diffuse cerebral disorder, such as meningitis or encephalitis. Focal cortical lesions can prevent normal appreciation of the body image or affect understanding of the written or spoken word, which might, therefore, give a false impression of general intellectual deterioration. Patients may be unable to express themselves in words, mime, or writing; to calculate or perform routine tasks; or distinguish between right and left because of a lesion of the dominant hemisphere. If cortical function is intact, the emotional tone of the patient must be assessed because it is often altered in patients with chronic headache.

Speech

If the patient is dysphasic, a note must always be made as to whether the patient is right- or left-handed. The left hemisphere is responsible for speech mechanisms in some 96 per cent of right-handed patients, and about 50 per cent of left-handers.

Skull

The skull should be examined if indicated by the case history. A search of the scalp may disclose local infection, a bone tumour, Paget's disease, or the hardened tender arteries of temporal arteritis. The bones overlying inflamed sinuses or mastoid processes become sensitive to percussion. Bulging of the fontanelles is a direct indication of increased intracranial pressure in infants. In children, the head circumference should be measured, because repeated recordings are of value in detecting progressive hydrocephalus. In adult life, a large head suggests hydrocephalus from aqueduct stenosis or another cause of obstruction of the CSF pathways.

Auscultation of the skull (listening over the orbits, temples and mastoid processes) may disclose a systolic bruit in the case of angioma, vascular tumours or stenosis of the cranial vessels. When the clinician is listening over the closed eyelids, patients should be requested to open the other eye and hold their breath to prevent eyelid flutter and breath sounds from obscuring a bruit. Skull bruits are often normal in children under 10 years of age and may be discounted unless loud and unilateral. An unexpected dividend from auscultation of the skull is that the sound of muscle contraction may be heard over the temporal and frontal muscles in patients who are unable to relax. The greater occipital nerve (see Figure 16.2) is tender to pressure in many patients with migraine or cluster headache as well as in those with occipital neuralgia and upper cervical syndromes.

The temporomandibular joints should be palpated while the jaw is opened and closed. Inserting a finger in each ear and pressing forwards on the joint will often elicit tenderness or crepitus.

Spine

The cervical spine is tested for mobility and localized tenderness. Resistance of the neck to passive flexion and Kernig's sign are usually present in meningeal irritation.

Gait and stance

An unsteady, wide-based gait may be observed as a result of a cerebellar disturbance. It may be the only indication of a midline cerebellar lesion in the early stages and may also be the presenting symptom of hydrocephalus because corticopontocere-bellar pathways become splayed over the enlarged lateral ventricles. In some cases of posterior fossa tumour, the head may be held to one side with the occiput tilted to the side of the lesion (Figure 5.2).

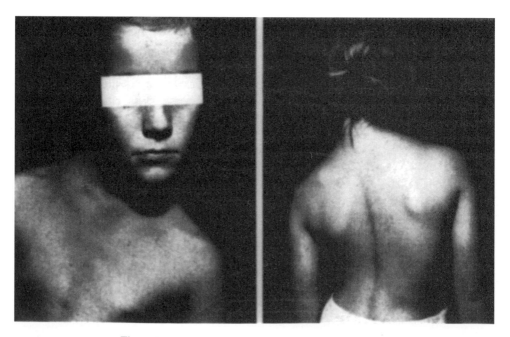

Figure 5.2 Head tilting to the side of a cerebellar tumour

Special senses

Smell

The nostrils are often blocked in rhinitis and sinusitis so that sense of smell cannot be adequately assessed. The sense of smell may be lost when the olfactory nerve is damaged by head injury or by a tumour in the vicinity of the olfactory groove. The sense of smell should always be tested when a patient's intellectual ability has deteriorated, because a frontotemporal tumour may cause both anosmia and mental confusion.

Vision

Circumcorneal injection may be observed in acute angle-closure glaucoma and increased intraocular pressure may give rise to a palpable firmness of the eye. The visual fields of those patients in whom the suspicion of an intracranial lesion has arisen should be tested to confrontation; and inattention to one half-field sought if the parietal lobe is thought to be involved.

The optic discs should be examined when appropriate for signs of optic atrophy or papilloedema. Swelling of the disc occurs in about 15 per cent of cases of retrobulbar (optic) neuritis but, unlike patients with papilloedema from raised intracranial pressure, central vision is severely impaired.

Optic atrophy may result from interference with the blood supply to the optic nerve, long-standing papilloedema, retrobulbar neuritis or compression of the optic nerve or the optic chiasma. Occasionally a sphenoid wing meningioma compresses one optic nerve and its surrounding subarachnoid space, and then expands sufficiently to increase intracranial pressure or to impair venous return from the other eye, so that papilloedema develops on the side opposite to the origin of the lesion. This combination of optic atrophy in one eye and papilloedema in the other (Foster–Kennedy syndrome) is rarely seen now because most tumours are detected early by computerized tomography (CT) or magnetic resonance imaging (MRI).

Subhyaloid haemorrhages may be observed after subarachnoid bleeding, and perivascular nodules may rarely be seen in tuberculous meningitis or disseminated lupus erythematosus. Circumscribed areas of choroidal atrophy may be a sign of toxoplasmosis.

Hearing

The eardrums should be inspected, particularly in children, when otitis media is suspected, because infection can spread centrally to cause thrombosis of the lateral sinus (otitic hydrocephalus) or to form an abscess of the temporal lobe or cerebellum. Conduction deafness is demonstrated by tuning fork tests in the case of otitis media or Eustachian catarrh. Unilateral nerve deafness should be investigated by audiometry, loudness-balance tests, brain stem auditory evoked responses, electronystagmography and CT scanning or MRI to ensure that an acoustic neuroma is not missed.

Other cranial nerves

A latent ocular imbalance may be unmasked by any infectious or debilitating illness and give rise to diplopia, which may be misinterpreted as indicating a paresis of one or other of the extraocular muscles. A sixth nerve palsy may be found on the side of a retro-orbital lesion, and bilateral sixth nerve palsies may develop with any case of acute hydrocephalus or cerebral oedema because the sixth nerves are compressed in their long intracranial course by the expanded brain.

Progressive enlargement of the pupil on one side, with or without other signs of a third nerve palsy, is an indication for immediate action because the third nerve may be compressed by any expanding lesion forcing the uncus and medial aspect of the temporal lobe downwards through the tentorial opening into the posterior fossa (tentorial herniation). It can be taken as a rule that the dilated pupil is always on the side of the expanding lesion (such as a subdural haematoma) and exceptions to this rule are rare. Inability to elevate and converge the eyes (Parinaud's syndrome) indicates compression of the midbrain from above by a tumour such as pinealoma, but it should be remembered that many elderly patients have difficulty in looking upwards.

The sudden onset of a third nerve palsy with pain behind the eye is most frequently caused by the sudden enlargement of an aneurysm, although this may also occur in the rare Tolosa–Hunt syndrome (Figure 5.3) (see Chapter 15) and ophthalmoplegic migraine (see Chapter 6).

If the patient's consciousness becomes impaired so that voluntary eye movements are no longer possible, the integrity of the third, fourth and sixth nerves may be tested by the 'doll's-eye manoeuvre'. When the head is rotated to one side, the eyes roll to the opposite side, thus producing the movements of lateral conjugate devia-

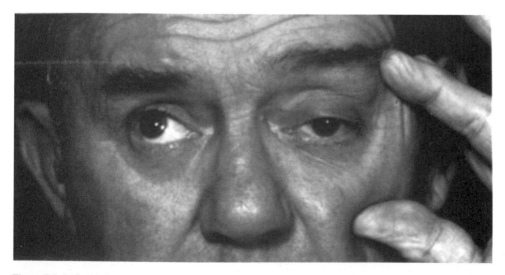

Figure 5.3 Left third cranial nerve palsy in a patient with Tolosa–Hunt syndrome. He is elevating his ptosed left eyelid with his fingers and looking to his right. The left eye fails to adduct

tion. Similarly, if the chin is pushed down on the chest the eyes elevate and if the head is extended the eyes roll downwards.

The presence of Horner's syndrome in cluster headache has already been mentioned, and it may also be seen occasionally in migraine. The pupil of one side may remain small between paroxysms of cluster headache or after a severe attack of migraine. Both pupils may be small in a pontine lesion and one pupil may dilate in 'basilar artery migraine'.

Any cranial nerve may be involved by direct compression. It is particularly important to test facial sensation carefully, including two-point discrimination on the lip, and to check the corneal responses in patients with trigeminal neuralgia. If there is any sensory deficit, the patient must be suspected of having a lesion compressing the trigeminal nerve, or a pontine plaque of multiple sclerosis.

If corticobulbar pathways are involved, weakness of the lower face will be detected and the jaw jerk and facial reflexes may increase. A bifrontal lesion will result in a pouting response to gentle tapping on the closed lips.

Motor system

Signs of an upper motor neurone or cerebellar disturbance may be detected with an expanding intracranial lesion. When the patient's arms are extended and the eyes are closed, the arm may slowly fall away on the affected side.

A hemiparesis is most commonly found on the side opposite to a cerebral lesion but in a minority of patients with a rapidly expanding mass, such as subdural haematoma, the hemiparesis is found on the same side as the lesion. The reason for this is that the growing mass pushes the midbrain over on to the tentorial edge so that the opposite cerebral peduncle is compressed. Since the pyramidal tracts cross below this level, the hemiparesis is on the same side as the causative lesion. Bilateral upper motor neurone signs may result from midbrain compression. A grasp reflex and palmomental response indicates a lesion of the opposite frontal lobe.

With a cerebellar lesion, the affected side is hypotonic. When the elbows are resting on a table with forearms vertical and wrist muscles relaxed, the hand hangs lower on the affected side. If the eyes are closed and the arms are lifted suddenly to a point at right angles to the body, the arm on the affected side overshoots and oscillates. The knee jerk is pendular on the affected side. Rapid and alternating movements are impaired and finger–nose and heel–shin coordination is defective. The gait is wide-based and halting, and the patient turns jerkily 'by numbers' and tends to stumble to the side of the lesion.

Sensory system

A parietal lobe disturbance may cause subtle sensory deficit with difficulty in discriminating two points or recognizing objects placed in the hand. Sensory inattention should be sought by touching both arms or legs simultaneously with the patient's eyes closed. Long sensory tracts may be involved with deeply placed cerebral lesions or brain stem disorders, resulting in a more clearcut sensory disturbance.

Sphincters and sexual functions

Urgency of micturition may appear with upper motor neurone lesions, and a casual approach towards the time and place of relaxing the sphincters may be a feature of frontal lobe disturbance. Impotence can result from a temporal lobe lesion or from testicular atrophy secondary to hypopituitarism. In patients with impaired penile erection it is helpful to ensure the integrity of the second and third sacral segments by testing the bulbocavernosus reflex.

General examination

Café au lait patches and cutaneous nodules, seen in Von Recklinghausen's disease (neurofibromatosis Type 1), indicate that there is an increased risk of phaeochromocytoma (about 1 per cent) and intracranial tumour (about 2 per cent). Cutaneous manifestations are less obvious, and may be absent in neurofibromatosis Type 2, which is characterized by bilateral acoustic neuromas. The observation of cutaneous angiomas raises the possibility of an intracerebral angioma. Peutz–Jeghers syndrome is an unusual familial condition characterized by dark pigmentation on the lips and buccal mucosa, which is associated with polyposis of the small intestine. There may be an increased tendency to intracranial tumour in this condition, as there is in polyposis coli, because we have seen such a patient with multiple intracranial meningiomas.

Smoothness of the skin, paucity of body hair and testicular atrophy or delayed development of secondary sexual characteristics in adolescents should be looked for as signs of pituitary deficiency. The breasts should be examined if the patient has noticed any lump.

Any scar in the skin warrants an enquiry about the nature of the removed lesion, as melanoma is notorious for presenting with metastases in the nervous system years after the primary tumour has been removed. Skin rashes are of importance in many infectious processes, such as meningococcaemia, glandular fever, secondary syphilis and the exanthemata associated with headache.

The association of a thin build with long fingers and toes and a high arched palate (Marfan's syndrome) carries an increased liability to intracranial aneurysms. Other inconsistent features include hypertension from coarctation of the aorta, congenital heart defects and congenital dislocation of the lenses of the eye, which transmits a noticeable quivering movement to the iris on sudden eye movements.

Enlargement of lymph glands or spleen is relevant to the problem of headache in patients with blood dyscrasias, infectious mononucleosis, AIDS and other infections. Ecchymoses and purpura may be observed in thrombocytopenic purpura with neurological complications.

Urine testing does not contribute to the solution of most headache problems but the presence of albuminuria or glycosuria may be relevant to some causes of headache. The finding of a cardiac valvular defect should suggest the possibility of cerebral emboli (from an atrial clot or subacute bacterial endocarditis) when transient cerebral episodes and headache are of recent onset.

Since most systemic disorders may have a neurological component, and most cerebral disorders may have headache as a symptom, there is no need to catalogue all the possible signs that could be unearthed by careful examination which may bear direct relevance to the problem of headache. Having said this, it must be added that the majority of patients complaining of chronic headache do not have physical signs that pertain to their main symptoms, unless we include constant muscular over-activity and the inability to relax, which is dealt with elsewhere. A number of other minor problems, which require attention, may be disclosed by a careful ex-amination; many of them may have been a source of worry to the patient although not mentioned in the original history. There is no better start to the reassurance of a patient than the knowledge that a proper physical examination has been carried out as part of a careful clinical assessment.

Chapter 6

Migraine: varieties

The word migraine is of French origin and derives from the Greek 'hemicrania' like the old English term 'megrim'. Although hemicrania literally means only half the head, migraine involves both sides of the head from its onset in about 40 per cent of patients. Another 40 per cent experience strictly unilateral headaches, and approximately 20 per cent have headaches that start on one side and later become generalized (Selby and Lance, 1960).

Definition

Migraine is essentially an episodic headache, usually accompanied by nausea and photophobia, which may be preceded by focal neurological symptoms (aura). The aura may be experienced without any ensuing headache; such attacks have in the past been called migraine equivalents. Skyhøj Olsen (1990) put forward the view that migraine with and without aura may share the same pathophysiology with the intensity of cerebral ischaemia determining the presence or absence of an aura (see Chapter 8). Russell et al. (1996) consider migraine with aura and migraine without aura as distinct clinical entities, finding the coexistence of the two varieties in only 3.5 per cent of males and 5.4 per cent of females. This figure is surprisingly low as it is common in clinical practice to find patients who have an aura at some stage of their lives and not at others, although the headache component retains the same characteristics (Centonze et al., 1997).

Because of the variability in the symptoms of migraine from one patient to another, and even between recurrent attacks in the same patient, the definition of migraine has always presented difficulties. These problems have been tackled systematically by the Headache Classification Committee of the International Headache Society (1988), which presented the following diagnostic criteria for migraine headache: the patient must have had five or more attacks of headache lasting 4–72 hours if untreated, with at least two of four features (unilaterality, pulsating quality, moderate or severe intensity, and aggravation by exertion), as well as nausea, with or without vomiting, or photophobia and phonophobia. Structural abnormalities or other causative lesions should have been excluded by the history, physical examination or, when indicated, by appropriate investigations.

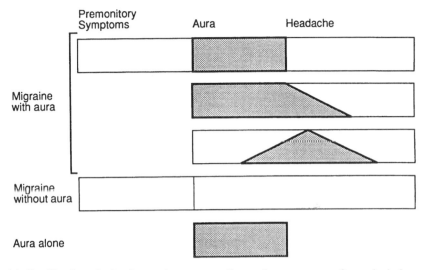

Figure 6.1 Classification of migraine syndromes according to the appearance of neurological symptoms (shaded areas) in relation to headache. Premonitory symptoms include changes in mood, alertness and appetite that may precede migraine by a day or so

These criteria have necessarily been made precise. It may be possible to make a presumptive diagnosis of migraine after one or two typical headaches but it would be unwise to include such a patient in a clinical trial. Some headaches with migrainous characteristics last less then 4 hours, particularly in children (Maytel *et al.*, 1995). If headaches persist for longer than 72 hours, the condition has been termed 'status migrainosus'. Variations in the symptomatology of migraine led to the allocation of attacks to subtypes of migraine under heading 1 in the classification of headache (see Chapter 3).

1.1 Migraine without aura ('common migraine')
Headache as described above without any focal neurological symptoms (Figure 6.1). The old term 'common migraine' will be used at times in this text for the sake of brevity.

1.2 Migraine with aura ('classical migraine')
Typical headaches preceded by neurological symptoms arising from the cerebral cortex or brain stem, usually developing gradually over 5–20 minutes and lasting less than 60 minutes (Figure 6.1).

1.2.1 Migraine with typical aura

1.2.2 Migraine with prolonged aura
Neurological symptoms persisting for more than 60 minutes with no abnormality being demonstrated by neuroimaging.

1.2.3 Familial hemiplegic migraine
Hemiparesis occurring during the attack. This condition is usually inherited as an autosomal dominant characteristic.

1.2.4 Basilar migraine
Aura symptoms arising from the territory supplied by the vertebrobasilar arterial system and its continuation as the posterior cerebral arteries (brain stem, cerebellum and occipital lobes).

1.2.5 Migraine aura without headache ('migraine equivalent')

1.2.6 Migraine with acute onset aura
The aura developing in less than 5 minutes.

1.3 Ophthalmoplegic migraine
Paresis of the third, fourth or sixth cranial nerves during migrainous headache.

1.4 Retinal migraine
Visual symptoms restricted to one eye.

1.5 Childhood periodic syndromes
May be precursors of, or associated with, migraine.

1.6 Complications of migraine

1.6.1 Status migrainosus
Attacks in which the headache phase exceeds 72 hours without headache-free intervals of more than 4 hours while the patient is awake.

1.6.2 Migrainous infarction
Aura exceeding 7 days or confirmation of infarction by neuroimaging.

1.7 Migrainous disorder not fulfilling the above criteria
An example is 'transformed migraine', i.e. headache meeting all of the requirements for the diagnosis of migraine except for frequency and duration, because such headaches may recur daily for months or years, often developing from typical episodic migraine headaches (Matthew, Reuveni and Perez, 1987).

Phases of migraine

Premonitory symptoms

The first indication of an impending migraine attack may be noticed 24 hours or more before headache begins (Figure 6.1). Of 50 patients questioned by Blau (1980), 17 said that changes in mood, alertness and appetite preceded headache by 1–24 hours. Drummond and Lance (1984) interviewed 530 patients with recurrent headache, ranging from typical migraine to tension-type headache, of whom 160 reported such premonitory symptoms. These patients suffered from headaches with migrainous characteristics and about half had associated focal neurological symptoms. Mood swings such as irritability or depression were noted by 86 patients and a feeling of elation by 54. Of 47 who mentioned hunger, 34 craved for sweet foods such as cake, biscuits and chocolate (which was specifically mentioned by 12 patients). Drowsiness and yawning were symptoms in 38 patients and thirst in 15. Premonitory symptoms probably arise in the hypothalamus, possibly as a result of changes in monoaminergic transmission, and culminate in migraine headache, with or without aura. It could be relevant that the $5HT_2$ antagonist, pizotifen, may cause euphoria, drowsiness and a craving to eat sweet foods.

Aura

The aura of migraine most often arises in the visual cortex of the occipital lobe. Visual hallucinations or scotomas form part of the attack in about one-third of all migraine patients. Fortification spectra are experienced by about 10 per cent of patients (Lance and Anthony, 1966) and were given this name because the zigzag appearance of the hallucination resembles a medieval fortified town viewed from above. The equivalent term teichopsia is derived from the Greek 'teichos', meaning a wall. The fortification figures are white more often than coloured and commonly shimmer or jitter as they expand across the visual field, leaving an area of impaired vision behind them, so-called 'scintillating scotomas'. Another 25 per cent of patients describe unformed flashes of light ('photopsia'), which usually remain in the same part of the visual field or are scattered across both visual fields. That the origin of such symptoms is from the visual cortex and not from the retina is clear from their distribution in the visual field and is confirmed by the fact that they occurred in a patient whose eyes had been removed (Peatfield and Rose, 1981).

Symptoms that arise in areas of cortex other than the occipital lobe are much less common. Unilateral paraesthesiae associated with hemiparesis or dysphasia is encountered in about 4 per cent of all migraine patients (Lance and Anthony, 1966). Russell and Olesen (1996) analysed the symptoms of 163 patients experiencing migraine with aura. Almost all had visual disturbances, 31 per cent had sensory symptoms spreading from hand and arm to the face, 18 per cent became aphasic and 6 per cent developed weakness on one side. Transient temporal or parietal lobe symptoms may form part of the migraine attack. Peatfield (1991) reported a patient who experienced *déjà vu* and a dreamlike state. Olfactory hallucinations of burning, cooking or unpleasant smells may also occur during the aura. Morrison (1990) reported that five of 46 patients studied had olfactory hallucinations, three had gustatory hallucinations and two experienced distortion of the body, head and neck with their migraine attacks. One of our patients described her fingers feeling 'as long as telegraph poles' and her mouth and teeth like 'a cave full of tombstones'. Charles Dodgson (Lewis Carroll) suffered from migraine and it has been suggested that the inspiration for illusions of vision and body image in *Alice in Wonderland* may have had a migrainous origin. The appeal of the story is little diminished by the knowledge that *Alice in Wonderland* was written before the author started to suffer from migraine. The auras of migraine are beautifully described and illustrated by Oliver Sacks (1992).

Headache

Migraine headache is primarily unilateral in two-thirds of patients and is bilateral in the remainder (Selby and Lance, 1960; Lance and Anthony, 1966). It may change from one side to the other in a single attack. The pain may be felt deeply behind the eye or in the inner angle of the eye, but more commonly involves the frontotemporal region. It may radiate backwards to the occiput and upper neck or even to the lower neck and shoulder. In other patients it starts as a dull ache in the upper neck and radiates forwards. In some patients it may remain limited to the vascular territory of frontal, temporal or occipital arteries. In others the pain affects mainly the face (lower-half headache, facial migraine). Facial migraine is usually unilateral and pain involves the nostril, cheek, gums and teeth. It may spread to the neck, ear or eye, in which case it may be confused with cluster headache. It differs from cluster headache in its pattern of recurrence, being without the remissions which usually occur between bouts of cluster headache, and with each episode lasting for 4 hours to several days. Guiloff and Fruns (1988) reported 22 patients with migraine or cluster headache who experienced pain in the upper or lower limbs on the same side as their headache, suggesting thalamic involvement in the genesis of such attacks.

It might be assumed that the headache of classical migraine would affect the side of the head overlying the hemisphere from which the focal neurological symptoms originated, but this is not always the case. Of 75 patients with unilateral paraesthesiae and unilateral headache, the headache developed on the same side as the paraesthesiae in 55 and on the opposite side in only 20 (Peatfield, Gawel and Rose, 1981). When these figures are pooled with other published reports, the numbers of patients with headache ipsi- and contralateral to the side of neurological symptoms are equal. A prospective study by Jensen et al. (1986) confirmed this important fact: aura symptoms were ipsilateral to the headache in 19 patients and contralateral in 19.

Migraine commonly starts as a dull headache, which may become throbbing in quality (increasing with each pulse) as the headache intensifies, and reverts to a constant pain later. Many migraine patients experience a constant headache that is never truly pulsatile. In addition, 42 per cent of patients are subject to sudden jabbing pains ('ice-pick pains') in the head, whether or not they have their characteristic headache at the time, compared with only 3 per cent of normal controls (Raskin and Schwartz, 1980).

Resolution

A feeling of exhaustion and lethargy may remain for several days after the cessation of headache. Blau (1987) described 'postdromes' of impaired concentration, irritability, sluggishness and diminished appetite for a day or more after the headache had gone. Less commonly, patients may experience euphoria and a craving for sweet foods, resembling the symptoms of the premonitory phase. Headache may recur briefly during the 'hangover phase' if patients bend forwards or shake their heads.

Variations on the theme of migraine

Hemiplegic migraine

Weakness or paralysis is an uncommon accompaniment of migraine and, when it occurs, is usually transient, resolving without evidence of infarction. Oedema of one cerebral hemisphere has been demonstrated on CT scanning during hemiplegia and an emission CT scan using Tc^{99m} revealed a striking accumulation of isotope over the affected hemisphere, indicating a breakdown of the blood–brain barrier (Harrison, 1981). Friberg et al. (1987) studied regional cerebral blood flow (rCBF) in three patients in whom hemiplegic migraine was induced by cerebral angiography. Focal hypoperfusion, preceded by hyperperfusion in two cases, developed in the frontal lobes and spread posteriorly. Rapid fluctuations in rCBF were observed, attributed to instability of cerebral vascular tone, which reached ischaemic levels on occasions.

CSF pleocytosis has been found at the height of hemiplegic migraine (Schraeder and Burns, 1980). This form of migraine may be inherited, usually as a dominant characteristic, when it is known as familial hemiplegic migraine. Either side of the body may be affected, sometimes alternately in successive episodes. Since the hemiplegia is often associated with dysphasia or other cortical symptoms it is probably of hemispheric origin in most instances and the finding that cerebral blood flow is reduced on the affected side supports this view (Staehelin Jensen et al., 1981b). Angiography demonstrated a local constriction of one internal carotid artery at the level of the skull base in one patient at the height of the attack (Staehelin Jensen et al., 1981b). On the other hand, some families are subject to attacks of hemiplegia without aphasia, and vertebral angiography in a patient from such a family showed a marked constriction of the basilar artery during an attack (Staehelin Jensen et al., 1981a). Other members of this family had dysarthria, dysphagia and drop attacks.

Fitzsimons and Wolfenden (1985) reported a family in which hemiplegic migraine was associated with coma and life-threatening cerebral oedema. Cerebellar ataxia followed each episode and eventually persisted. There have been a number of other reports in the literature of familial hemiplegic migraine associated with a cerebellar disturbance, which appears to be an hereditary cerebellar degenerative disorder rather than the result of ischaemia from repeated migraine attacks. This is explicable by the discovery that many families owe their susceptibility to hemiplegic migraine to a gene on chromosome 19, overlapping the locus for periodic cerebellar ataxia and another rare condition CADASIL. CADASIL (Cerebral Autosomal Dominant Arteriopathy with Subcortical Infarcts and Leukoencephalopathy) may present as familial hemiplegic migraine but usually progresses to pseudobulbar palsy associated with gross white matter changes demonstrated by MRI (Hutchinson et al., 1995).

Hemiplegia usually clears up over a period of 24 hours but death during an attack was reported by Guest and Woolf (1964), who found ischaemic changes in the cerebrum and brain stem, and also by Neligan, Harriman and Pearce (1977). In the case described by Neligan and colleagues, autopsy was performed 4 months after the initial episode as life had been maintained by mechanical ventilation;

microinfarcts were found in the cortex and basal ganglia, although the brain stem was apparently spared.

Hemiplegic migraine may thus be sporadic or familial, and arise from either cerebral hemisphere or brain stem disturbance. The association between migraine and stroke is discussed later in this chapter under the heading 'Migrainous infarction'.

Vertebrobasilar migraine

Symptoms arising from the brain stem, such as diplopia, vertigo, incoordination, ataxia and dysarthria, are neurological components of the migraine attack in about 25 per cent of patients (Lance and Anthony, 1966). Bickerstaff (1961a,b) pointed out that severe brain stem symptoms in migraine were often associated with faintness, fainting or sudden loss of consciousness, which he attributed to constriction of the basilar artery causing ischaemia of the midbrain reticular formation. This is supported by our own observations, since 7 per cent of patients with symptoms referable to the distribution of the vertebrobasilar arterial system had fainted on occasions during their attacks whereas none of those with symptoms arising from areas supplied by the carotid artery had done so (Lance and Anthony, 1966).

Photopsia and fortification spectra were found to occur as often in association with symptoms arising from either carotid or basilar territories. The frequency of hindbrain symptoms in migraine led Klee (1968) to conclude that 'the symptoms of migraine are primarily due to a dysfunction of the vertebrobasilar arterial system'. Symptoms indistinguishable from those of migraine, including fortification spectra and other visual disturbances, can be precipitated by vertebral angiography (Hauge, 1954).

A confusional state lasting up to several hours is not uncommon in juvenile migraine and probably results from general depression of cortical function. More specifically related to the vertebrobasilar circulation is a stuporose or comatose state lasting for up to 7 days, termed migraine stupor. We have encountered this condition in patients from 10 to 52 years of age (Lee and Lance, 1977). Most were associated with homonymous hemianopia, ataxia, incoordination and dysarthria, while one pupil dilated in some patients, all indicating a disturbance in the distribution of the vertebrobasilar arterial system and its posterior cerebral continuation. Confused, aggressive and hysterical behaviour was encountered at some stage of the illness in most patients.

Some children and adolescents subject to both basilar migraine and epilepsy have had interictal EEGs showing slow spike-wave complexes in the occipital region, blocking on visual attention (Camfield, Metrakos and Andermann, 1978; Panayiotopoulos, 1980). This presumably means that the occipital cortex is in a constant state of hyperexcitability, although the relationship of this to migrainous symptoms is uncertain. The grossly abnormal EEG distinguishes this syndrome, which appears to have a good prognosis, from other forms of basilar migraine in which the EEG is usually normal between attacks.

Migraine aura without headache

The waxing and waning of fortification spectra, scotomas, paraesthesiae, dysphasia and other symptoms of cortical or brain stem origin over a period of 10–60 minutes may occur without any headache following. This has been recognized in the past as a migraine equivalent or acephalgic migraine (Kunkel, 1986). Focal neurological symptoms in middle-aged and elderly patients may evolve and resolve slowly in a manner that suggests a migrainous rather than thromboembolic phenomenon. Fisher (1980) has called these episodes transient migrainous accompaniments (TMAs) to distinguish them from transient ischaemic attacks (TIAs). Although there is no significant difference in the vascular risk factors for migraine equivalents and TIAs, the former have less risk of subsequent vascular disease (Dennis and Warlow, 1992). A familial form of acephalgic migraine has been described (Shevell, 1997).

Ophthalmoplegic migraine

The recurrence of double vision with migraine, associated with signs of paresis of the extra-ocular muscles, has been termed ophthalmoplegic migraine. The third nerve is most commonly affected; paresis usually outlasts the migraine headache by days or weeks and may become permanent after repeated attacks. Walsh and O'Doherty (1960) pointed out that the literature had been confused by reports of patients in whom a clear cause of compression of the third, fourth or sixth nerves had eventually been established, and which could not therefore be considered as ophthalmoplegic migraine. They cited angiographic findings in four patients including two of their own, showing narrowing of the distal portion of the internal carotid artery consistent with swelling of the vessel wall. They suggested that paresis of the third, fourth and sixth cranial nerves could be caused either by direct vascular compression or by interference with flow in the vasa nervorum. The latter contention was supported by Vijayan (1980) who found that the pupillary reaction to light was partly or completely spared in two-thirds of the patients experiencing a third nerve palsy with migraine. He pointed out that angiography was usually normal and that direct compression would involve the peripherally situated pupillary fibres first whereas ischaemic neuropathy, as in diabetes, often spared pupillary reactions. Ophthalmoplegic migraine may therefore be regarded as a delayed ischaemic neuropathy. Dilatation of one pupil without paresis of extra ocular muscles (internal ophthalmoplegia) may be a feature of basilar migraine.

The condition must be distinguished from compression of the third, fourth or sixth cranial nerves by aneurysm or other space-occupying lesions so that the diagnosis can only be made after prolonged observation of the patient and exclusion of other conditions by carotid and vertebral angiography.

Retinal migraine and monocular blindness

This is a subdivision of classical migraine in which constriction of retinal arterioles impairs vision in one eye, with or without photopsia, usually preceding headache or a dull ache behind the affected eye. The condition is uncommon. Compression of the optic nerve and transient ischaemic attacks arising from the ipsilateral carotid artery must be excluded, particularly when monocular visual loss is not followed by headache.

Carroll (1970) presented case histories of ten women and five men with retinal migraine, seven of whom had experienced typical attacks of migraine at other times. One developed a permanent visual deficit. Ischaemic papillopathy has been described as a complication of migraine (McDonald and Sanders, 1971; Lee, Brazis and Miller, 1996). Coppeto et al. (1986) summarized 12 reported cases with permanent visual impairment and added two of their own. Occlusion of the central retinal artery and its branches with infarction and transient retinal oedema have been described most commonly but venous obstruction has also been reported in migraine patients.

In many cases, it is difficult to determine whether transient blindness in one eye is a migrainous variant or is thromboembolic in origin. Tomsak and Jergens (1987) reported 24 patients ranging from 19 to 61 years of age in whom cerebral angiography and cardiac investigation disclosed no source of emboli. Visual loss lasted from 30 seconds to 30 minutes, recurred from twice a year to twice a week, and was precipitated by bending over in eight patients and strenuous exercise in four. Seven patients had suffered from migraine previously. The differential diagnosis from other forms of amaurosis remains one of exclusion. Retinal migraine was included in a recent review of visual phenomena by Chronicle and Mulleners (1996).

Childhood periodic syndromes in IHS classification

The Headache Classification Committee of the International Headache Society (IHS) has recognized two conditions that may be precursors of, or associated with, migraine.

Benign paroxysmal vertigo of childhood
Basser (1964) reported episodic vertigo and nystagmus in ten girls and four boys, starting in the first 8 years of life and recurring on average every 6–8 weeks. Caloric tests demonstrated unilateral or bilateral vestibular abnormalities. The attacks ceased spontaneously after some months or years. A history of migraine was not recorded in any case, and the reason for considering this condition as a migrainous variant is obscure.

Alternating hemiplegia of childhood
Alternating hemiplegia has been described as a possible expression of migraine in childhood, but may terminate in a dystonic state and is clearly a separate entity.

Other periodic syndromes of childhood and adult life related to migraine

Recurrent neck pain
Episodic unilateral neck pain with tenderness of the carotid artery, responsive to ergotamine and sumatriptan, is probably a variant of migraine (De Marinis and Accornero, 1997). See also 'Carotidynia' in Chapter 14.

Abdominal migraine and vomiting attacks
Bille (1962) found that 20 per cent of migrainous children were subject to paroxysmal abdominal pains compared with 4 per cent of a control group and regarded these symptoms as a migraine equivalent. In a follow-up study only 1.5 per cent of migraine patients still had attacks of abdominal pain in later life at 30 years of age or more (Bille, 1981). A past history of vomiting attacks in childhood was found in 23 per cent of migraine patients compared with 12 per cent of patients subject to tension headache by Lance and Anthony (1966). Lundberg (1975) reported that 12 of 100 migraine patients suffered from recurrent abdominal pain and that some responded to antimigrainous therapy.

Cardiac migraine
The term 'cardiac migraine' was introduced by Leon-Sotomayor (1974) to demarcate a syndrome of classical migraine, chest pain and functional hypoglycaemia. During the prodrome of an attack, patients experienced palpitations, anxiety symptoms and chest pain that radiated on occasions to the inner aspect of the arm. This pain was reproduced in four of the patients during coronary angiography while segmental coronary spasm was demonstrated. The relationship of migraine headache to the episodes of coronary spasm is not clear from this report.

A group of 62 patients with 'variant angina' (episodic angina at rest associated with transient ST segment elevation and rapidly relieved by nitroglycerin) was studied by Miller *et al.* (1981). Migraine was diagnosed in 26 per cent of the patients with variant angina compared with 6 per cent of a 'coronary' control group and 10 per cent of a 'non-coronary' control group. Raynaud's phenomenon occurred in 26 per cent of the patients with variant angina in contrast to 5 per cent and 3 per cent of the two control groups. There may therefore be a tendency for spasm to occur in different vascular beds at different times in some patients. Atrial fibrillation has been reported to accompany attacks of migraine (Petersen, Scruton and Downie. 1977) and we have observed this association in one patient who proved to have a phaeochromocytoma. Hyperventilation is a common accompaniment of migraine headache (Blau and Dexter, 1980) and may give rise to symptoms such as tightness and pain in the chest, which might be misinterpreted as 'cardiac migraine'.

Anginal pain may be referred to the head. Headache on exertion relieved by rest may be a presenting symptom of cardiac ischaemia (Lance and Lambros, 1998; Lipton *et al.* 1997).

Benign recurrent vertigo
Vertigo is a common symptom of basilar migraine. Abnormalities of the vestibular system were found in 60 per cent of patients by Kayan and Hood (1984). Attacks of spontaneous vertigo not precipitated by movement and not accompanied by cochlear or neurological symptoms in young or middle-aged adults were called 'benign recurrent vertigo' by Slater (1979). This disorder shows some features in common with migraine including female preponderance, positive family history and precipitation by alcohol, lack of sleep and emotional stress.

Behan and Carlin (1982) reported 32 patients, seven males and 25 females, between 8 and 65 years of age, who experienced episodes of giddiness, sometimes associated with tinnitus, deafness, ataxia, nausea and headache, which responded to treatment with pizotifen and propranolol. The paroxysmal nature of these symptoms suggests that 'benign recurrent vertigo' may be caused by a disturbance of the internal auditory artery circulation allied to migraine. Viirre and Baloh (1996) reported the sudden onset of deafness in 13 patients whose migraine was associated with vertigo – a less benign manifestation.

Migraine stupor

Clouding of consciousness, faintness and syncope are not uncommon in migraine, but are often associated with postural hypotension. Less often, migraine may be accompanied by stupor or coma. Lee and Lance (1977) noted cases previously reported and described seven patients from 10 to 52 years of age who had become stuporose for periods varying from 12 hours to 5 days during attacks of migraine. The diagnosis of basilar migraine was suggested by the symptoms and signs that preceded or arose during the headache: dysarthria, ataxia, incoordination, paraesthesiae, dilatation of one pupil and homonymous hemianopia. However, ischaemia is not limited to the vertebrobasilar circulation. One of our patients developed unilateral motor seizures, which persisted for some days, and was left with a parietal lobe syndrome that took some months to recover from. Measurement of cerebral blood flow in an episode of migraine stupor demonstrated a severe, global reduction in cerebral blood flow (Hachinski *et al.*, 1977).

Acute confusional migraine

Selby and Lance (1960) reported that 3.5 per cent of their 500 patients had experienced a confusional state as part of their migraine attacks. One woman walked out of her house, forgetting all about her children. The condition was described in children by Gascon and Barlow (1970) and is probably not uncommon because Ehyai and Fenichel (1978) encountered five such instances in 100 successive migrainous children. Confusion lasts from 10 minutes to 20 hours, usually terminating in deep sleep. Disorientation and agitation may be thought at first to be hysterical phenomena if the headache is not a prominent feature. Attacks may be triggered by relatively minor blows to the head, particularly in children (Haas, Pineda and Lourie, 1975), in a manner comparable with footballer's migraine (Matthews, 1972; Bennett *et al.*, 1980). Confusion is probably the result of diffuse cerebral ischaemia, like a milder form of migraine stupor.

Transient global amnesia

The sudden loss of short-term memory and the inability to register memory for a period of hours, known as transient global amnesia (TGA), was described by Fisher and Adams (1964) and may occur in epilepsy, vertebrobasilar insufficiency and migraine. In the two latter cases, the probable cause is ischaemia of the entry portals for memory, comprising the hippocampus and temporal stem situated in the medial aspect of each temporal lobe, in territory supplied by the posterior cerebral artery. For memory loss to be complete, ischaemia would have to involve both sides together, suggesting that flow is reduced in the basilar artery and hence its posterior cerebral branches. Migraine was almost nine times as common as in a control situation in the study presented by Melo, Ferro and Ferro (1992) and significantly more common than a comparative group of patients with transient ischaemic attacks (Hodges and Warlow, 1990). The proposition that migrainous vasospasm may be responsible for TGA in some cases is strengthened by reports of both migraine and transient global amnesia occurring in siblings (Stracciari and Rebucci, 1986; Dupuis, Pierre and Gonsette, 1987) and by the finding of abnormalities in cerebral blood flow 1–5 days after an episode (Crowell et al., 1984). TGA is a frightening symptom but rarely recurs often and does not appear to be a risk factor for stroke (Hodges and Warlow, 1990).

Migrainous infarction

Ischaemic papillopathy and retinal infarction were referred to in connection with retinal migraine. The risk of cerebral infarction in migraine patients and the complex relationship between migraine and stroke have now been studied intensively. Welch and Levine (1990) have considered the problem under the following headings:

1. Coexisting stroke and migraine. The stroke occurs remote in time from a migraine attack.
2. Stroke with clinical features of migraine. An underlying structural lesion causes both neurological deficit and migrainous symptoms (symptomatic migraine).
3. Migraine-induced stroke. The stroke occurs during the course of a migraine attack with the neurological deficit being in the area corresponding to the origin of aura symptoms in previous migrainous episodes. Subdivisions of this category are those with and without risk factors, such as oral contraceptive use and cigarette smoking.

There have been many reports over the years of strokes in the third category. It is curious that vascular occlusion demonstrated by angiography involves large arteries or their branches, the posterior cerebral more often than the middle cerebral circulation, whereas the vascular changes associated with the migrainous aura presumably affect the cortical microcirculation because arteriography during an attack does not usually show any constriction of major vessels. Among almost 5000 patients diagnosed as having migraine or vascular headache at the Mayo Clinic over a 4-year period, there were 20 with migraine-associated strokes (Broderick and Swanson, 1987). Two patients had a second episode over a 7-year follow-up. The outlook for recovery was good, as 14 patients were left with only a mild deficit and four had completely recovered.

Henrich and Horwitz (1989) reported that migraine with aura carried an increased risk of ischaemic stroke (odds ratio 2.6). Merikangas et al. (1997) found that a history of migraine and 'severe non-specific headache' was a risk factor for stroke in general (odds ratio 1.5) whereas Carolei et al. (1996) concluded that, in the absence of other risk factors, migraine was of significance only in women below the age of 35. Tzourio et al. (1995) studied 72 women under the age of 45 years with ischaemic stroke, discerning an increased risk for patients suffering from migraine without aura (odds ratio 3) as well as those with aura (odds ratio 6.2).

The risk of stroke was greatly increased for migrainous patients who smoked more than 20 cigarettes a day (odds ratio 10.2) and for those using oral contraceptives (odds ratio 13.9). They calculated that the absolute risk of young women with migraine suffering a stroke was 19 per 100,000 per year.

An association between migraine and the presence of lupus anticoagulants (anti-phospholipid antibodies) has been reported (Levine et al., 1987) and could be relevant to the genesis of stroke, although Hering et al. (1991) found no association between anticardiolipin antibodies and migraine. Since various antiphospholipid antibodies cross-react, it is unlikely that their presence reported in other series can be attributed to migraine alone. They may be a manifestation of some associated disorder. Montagna et al. (1988a) found an elevated blood lactate on exertion in nine migraine patients, five of whom had suffered a migrainous stroke, and muscle biopsy disclosed ragged red fibres in one case, thus bringing up the possibility of mitochondrial disease underlying migrainous stroke. The syndrome of mitochondrial myopathy, encephalopathy, lactic acidosis and stroke-like episodes (MELAS syndrome) is a maternally inherited disorder associated with severe migraine (Montagna et al., 1988b; Goto et al., 1992), but there is no evidence for abnormalities of mitochondrial DNA in migraine with aura (Klopstock et al., 1996).

It may be concluded that prolonged cerebral oligaemia in migraine predisposes to a stroke in the ischaemic territory responsible for the aura (Bogousslavsky et al., 1988).

Persistent positive visual phenomena in migraine

Some patients with migraine may be left with visual disturbances seen as dots or flashes in both visual fields that continue indefinitely without evidence of infarction (Liu et al., 1995). One young patient of ours also had patchy scotomas and difficulty in maintaining concentration on a line of print that interfered seriously with his performance in school examinations. These migrainous sequelae have proved resistant to medication.

References

Basser, L. S. (1964). Benign paroxysmal vertigo of childhood. A variety of vestibular neuronitis. *Brain* **87**, 141–152

Behan, P. O. and Carlin, J. (1982). Benign recurrent vertigo. In *Advances in Migraine*, Ed. F. Clifford Rose. pp. 19–55. New York, Raven Press

Bennett, D. R., Fuenning, S. I., Sullivan, G. and Weber, J. (1980). Migraine precipitated by head trauma in athletes. *Am. J. Sports Med.* **8**, 202–205

Bickerstaff, E. R. (1961a). Basilar artery migraine. *Lancet* **1**, 15–17

Bickerstaff, E. R. (1961b). Impairment of consciousness in migraine. *Lancet* **2**, 1057–1059

Bille, B. (1962). Migraine in school children. *Acta Paediat. Scand.* **51** (Suppl. 136), 1–151

Bille, B. (1981). Migraine in childhood and its prognosis. *Cephalalgia* **1**, 71–75

Blau, J. N. (1980). Migraine prodromes separated from the aura: complete migraine. *Br. Med. J.* **281**, 658–660

Blau, J. N. (1987). Adult migraine: the patient observed. In *Migraine: Clinical and Research Aspects*, Ed. J. N. Blau. pp. 3–30. Baltimore, Johns Hopkins University Press

Blau, J. N. and Dexter, S. L. (1980). Hyperventilation during migraine attacks. *Br. Med. J.* **280**, 1254

Bogousslavsky, J., Regli, F., Van Melle, G., Payot, M. and Uske, A. (1988). Migraine stroke. *Neurology* **28**, 223–227

Broderick, J. P. and Swanson, J. W. (1987). Migraine-related strokes. Clinical profile and prognosis in 20 patients. *Arch. Neurol.* **44**, 868–871

Camfield, P. R., Metrakos, K. and Andermann, F. (1978). Basilar migraine, seizures and severe epileptiform EEG abnormalities. A relatively benign syndrome in adolescents. *Neurology* **28**, 584–588

Carolei, A., Marini, C., De Matteis, G. and the Italian National Research Council Study Group on Stroke in the Young (1996). History of migraine and risk of cerebral ischaemia in young adults. *Lancet* **347**, 1503–1506

Carroll, D. (1970). Retinal migraine. *Headache* **10**, 9–13

Centonze, V., Polito, B. M., Valerio, A., Cassiano, M. A., Amato, R., Ricchetti, G., Bassi, A., Valente, A. and Albano, O. (1997). Migraine with and without aura in the same patient: expression of a single clinical entity. *Cephalalgia* **17**, 585–587

Chronicle, E. P. and Mulleners, W. M. (1996). Visual system dysfunction in migraine : a review of clinical and psychophysical findings. *Cephalalgia* **16**, 525–535

Coppeto, J. R.. Lessell, S., Sciarra, R. and Bear, L. (1986). Vascular retinopathy in migraine. *Neurology* **36**, 267–270

Crowell, G. F., Stump, D. A., Biller, J., McHenry, C. J. Jr and Toole, J. F. (1984). The transient global amnesia–migraine syndrome. *Arch. Neurol.* **41**, 75–79

De Marinis, M. and Accornero, N. (1997). Recurrent neck pain as a variant of migraine. *J. Neurol. Neurosurg. Psychiat.* **62**, 669–670

Dennis, M. and Warlow, C. (1992). Migraine aura without headache: transient ischaemic attack or not? *J. Neurol. Neurosurg. Psychiat.* **55**, 437–440

Drummond, P. D. and Lance, J. W. (1984). Neurovascular disturbances in headache patients. *Clin. Exp. Neurol.* **20**, 93–99

Dupuis, M. J. M., Pierre, P. H. and Gonsette, R. E. (1987). Transient global amnesia and migraine in twin sisters. *J. Neurol. Neurosurg. Psychiat.* **50**, 816–824

Ehyai, A. and Fenichel, G. M. (1978). The natural history of acute confusional migraine. *Arch. Neurol.* **35**, 368–369

Fisher, C. M. (1980). Late-life migraine accompaniments as a cause of unexplained transient ischaemic attacks. *Can. J. Neurol. Sci.* **7**, 9–17

Fisher, C. M., and Adams, R. D. (1964). Transient global amnesia. *Acta Neurol. Scand.* **40** (Suppl. 9), 1–83

Fitzsimons, R. B. and Wolfenden, W. H. (1985). Migraine coma. Meningitic migraine with cerebral oedema associated with a new form of autosomal dominant cerebellar ataxia. *Brain* **108**, 555–577

Friberg, L., Olsen, T. S., Roland, P. E. and Lassen, N. A. (1987). Focal ischaemia caused by instability of cerebro-vascular tone during attacks of hemiplegic migraine. A regional cerebral blood flow study. *Brain* **110**, 917–931

Gascon, G. and Barlow, C. (1970). Juvenile migraine presenting as acute confusional state. *Pediatrics* **45**, 628–635

Goto, Y., Horai, S., Matsuoka, T., Koga, Y., Nihei, K., Kobayashi, M. and Nonaka, I. (1992). Mitochondrial myopathy, encephalopathy, lactic acidosis, and stroke-like episodes (MELAS). A correlative study of the clinical features and mitochondrial DNA mutation. *Neurology* **42**, 545–550

Guest, I. A. and Woolf, A. L. (1964). Fatal infarction of brain in migraine. *Br. Med. J.* **1**, 225–226

Guiloff, R. J. and Fruns, M. (1988). Limb pain in migraine and cluster headache. *J. Neurol. Neurosurg. Psychiat.* **51**, 1022–1031

Haas, D. C., Pineda. G. S. and Lourie, H. (1975). Juvenile head trauma symptoms and their relationship to migraine. *Arch. Neurol.* **32**, 727–730

Hachinski, V. C., Olesen, J., Norris, J. W., Larsen. B., Enevoldsen, E. and Lassen, N. A. (1977). Cerebral haemodynamics in migraine. *Can. J. Neurol. Sci.* **4**, 245–249

Harrison, M. J. G. (1981). Hemiplegic migraine. *J. Neurol. Neurosurg. Psychiat.* **44**, 652–653

Hauge, T. (1954). Catheter vertebral angiography. *Acta Radiol. Suppl.* **109**, 1–219

Headache Classification Committee, the International Headache Society (1988). Classification and diagnostic criteria for headache disorders, cranial neuralgias and facial pain. *Cephalalgia* **8** (Suppl. 7), 19–28

Henrich, J. B. and Horwitz, R. I. (1989). A controlled study of ischemic stroke risk in migraine patients. *J. Clin. Epidemiol.* **42**, 773–780

Hering, R., Couturier, G. M., Steiner, T. J., Asherson, R. A. and Clifford Rose, F. (1991). Anticardiolipin antibodies in migraine. *Cephalalgia* **11**, 19–21

Hodges, J. R. and Warlow, C. P. (1990). The aetiology of transient global amnesia. *Brain* **113**, 639–657

Hutchinson, M., O'Riordan, J., Javed, M. *et al.* (1995). Familial hemiplegic migraine and autosomal dominant arteriopathy with leukoencephalopathy (CADASIL). *Ann. Neurol.* **38**. 817–824.

Jensen, K., Tfelt-Hansen, P., Lauritzen, M. and Olesen, J. (1986). Classic migraine. A prospective reporting of symptoms. *Acta Neurol. Scand.* **73**, 359–362

Kayan, A. and Hood, J. D. (1984). Neuro-otological manifestations of migraine. *Brain* **107**, 1123–1142

Klee, A. (1968). *A Clinical Study of Migraine with Particular Reference to the Most Severe Cases.* p. 190. Copenhagen, Munksgaard

Klopstock, T., May, A., Seibel, P., Papagiannuli, E., Diener, H.C. and Reichmann H. (1996).Mitochondrial DNA in migraine with aura. *Neurology* **46**, 1735–1738

Kunkel, R. S. (1986). Acephalgic migraine. *Headache* **26**, 198–201

Lance, J. W. and Anthony, M. (1966). Some clinical aspects of migraine. *Arch. Neurol.* **15**, 356–361

Lance, J. W. and Lambros, J. (1998). Headache associated with cardiac ischaemia. *Headache* **38**, 315–316.

Lee, A. G., Brazis, P. W. and Miller, N. R. (1996). Posterior ischemic optic neuropathy associated with migraine. *Headache* **36**, 506–509.

Lee, C. H. and Lance, J. W. (1977). Migraine stupor. *Headache* **17**, 32–38

Leon-Sotomayor, L. A. (1974). Cardiac migraine – report of twelve cases. *Angiology* **25**, 161–171

Levine, S. R., Joseph, R., D'Andrea, G. and Welch, K. M. A. (1987). Migraine and the lupus anticoagulant. Case reports and review of the literature. *Cephalalgia* **7**, 93–99

Lipton, R. B., Lowenkopt, T., Bajwa, Z. H., Leekie, R. S., Ribeiro, S., Newman, L. C. and Greenberg, M. A. (1997). Cardiac cephalgia: a treatable form of exertional headache. *Neurology* **49**, 813–816

Liu, G. T., Schatz, N. J., Galetta, S. L., Volpe, N. J., Skobieranda, F. and Kosmorsky, G. S. (1995). Persistent positive visual phenomena in migraine. *Neurology* **45**, 664–668

Lundberg, P. O. (1975). Abdominal migraine – diagnosis and therapy. *Headache* **15**, 122–125

Mathew, N. T., Reuveni, U. and Perez, F. (1987). Transformed or evolutive migraine. *Headache* **27**, 102–106

Matthews, W. B. (1972). Footballer's migraine. *Br. Med. J.* **3**, 326–327

Maytal, J., Lipton, R., Young, M. and Schechter, A. (1995). International Headache Society criteria and childhood migraines. *Ann. Neurol.* **38**, 529–530

McDonald, W. I. and Sanders, M. D. (1971). Migraine complicated by ischaemic papillopathy. *Lancet* **ii**, 521–523

Melo, T. P., Ferro, J. M. and Ferro, H. (1992) Transient global amnesia, a case control study. *Brain* **115**, 261–270

Merikangas, K. R., Fenton , B. T., Cheng, S. H., Stolar, M. J. and Risch, N. (1997). Association between migraine and stroke in a large-scale epidemiological study in the United States. *Arch. Neurol.* **54**, 362–368

Miller, D., Waters, D. D., Warnica, W., Szlachcic, J., Kreeft, J. and Theroux, P. (1981). Is variant angina the coronary manifestation of a generalized vasospastic disorder? *New Engl. J. Med.* **304**, 763–766

Montagna, P., Gallassi, R., Medori, R., Govoni, E., Zeviani, M., Di Mauro, S., Lugaresi, E. and Andermann, F. (1988a). MELAS syndrome: characteristic migrainous and epileptic features and maternal transmission. *Neurology* **38**, 751–754

Montagna, P., Sacquegna, T., Martinelli, P., Cortelli. P., Bresolin, N., Maggio, M., Baldrati, A., Riva, R. and Lugaresi, E. (1988b). Mitochondrial abnormalities in migraine. Preliminary findings. *Headache* **28**, 477–480

Morrison, D. P. (1990). Abnormal perceptual experiences in migraine. *Cephalalgia* **10**, 273–277

Neligan, P., Harriman, D. G. F. and Pearce, J. (1977). Respiratory arrest in familial hemiplegic migraine: a clinical and neuropathological study. *Br. Med. J.* **2**, 732–734

Panayiotopoulos, C. P. (1980). Basilar migraine? Seizures and severe epileptic EEG abnormalities. *Neurology* **30**, 1122–1125

Peatfield, R. C. (1991). Temporal lobe phenomena during the aura phase of migraine. *J. Neurol. Neurosurg. Psychiat.* **54**, 371–372

Peatfield, R. C., Gawel, M. J. and Rose, F. C. (1981). Asymmetry of the aura and pain in migraine. *J. Neurol. Neurosurg. Psychiat.* **44**, 846–848

Peatfield R. C. and Rose, F. C. (1981). Migrainous visual symptoms in a woman without eyes. *Arch. Neurol.* **38**, 466

Petersen. J., Scruton, D. and Downie, A. W. (1977). Basilar artery migraine with transient atrial fibrillation. *Br. Med. J.* **4**, 1125–1126

Raskin, N. H. and Schwartz, R. K. (1980). Icepick-like pain. *Neurology* **30**, 203–205

Russell, M. B., and Olesen, J. (1996). A nosographic analysis of the migraine aura in a general population. *Brain* **119**, 355–361

Russell, M. B., Rasmussen, B. K., Fenger, K. and Olesen, J. (1996). Migraine without aura and migraine with aura are distinct clinical entities: a study of four hundred and eighty four male and female migraineurs from the general population. *Cephalalgia* **16**, 239–245

Sacks, O. (1992). *Migraine*. Berkeley, University of California Press

Schraeder, P. L. and Burns, R. A. (1980). Hemiplegic migraine associated with an aseptic meningeal reaction. *Arch. Neurol.* **37**, 377–379

Selby, G. and Lance, J. W. (1960). Observations on 500 cases of migraine and allied vascular headache. *J. Neurol. Neurosurg. Psychiat.* **23**, 23–32

Shevell, M. I. (1997). Familial acephalgic migraines. *Neurology* **48**, 776–777

Skyhøj Olsen, T. (1990). Migraine with and without aura: the same disease due to cerebral vasospasm of different intensity. A hypothesis based on CBF studies during migraine. *Headache* **30**, 269–272

Slater, R. (1979). Benign recurrent vertigo. *J. Neurol. Neurosurg. Psychiat.* **42**, 363–367

Staehelin Jensen. T., de Fine Olivarius, B., Kraft, M. and Hansen, H. J. (1981a). Familial hemiplegic migraine – a reappraisal and a long-term follow-up study. *Cephalalgia* **1**, 33–39

Stahelin Jensen, T., Voldby, B., de Fine Olivarius. B. and Tågehøj Jensen, F. (1981b). Cerebral haemodynamics in familial hemiplegic migraine. *Cephalalgia* **1**, 121–125

Stracciari, A. and Rebucci, G. G. (1986). Transient global amnesia and migraine: familial incidence. *J. Neurol. Neurosurg. Psychiat.* **49**, 716–719

Swanson, J. W. and Vick, N. A. (1978). Basilar artery migraine. Twelve patients, with an attack recorded electroencephalographically. *Neurology* **28**, 782–786

Tomsak, R. L. and Jergens, P. B. (1987). Benign recurrent transient monocular blindness: a possible variant of acephalgic migraine. *Headache* **27**, 66–69

Tzourio, C., Tehindrazanarivelo, A., Iglesias, S., Alperovitch, A., Chedru, F., d'Anglejan-Chatillon, J. and Bousser, M.-G. (1995). Case-control study of migraine and risk of ischaemic stroke in young women. *Brit. Med. J.* **310**, 830–833

Viire, E. S. and Baloh, R. W. (1996). Migraine as a cause of sudden hearing loss. *Headache* **36**, 24–28

Vijayan, N. (1980). Ophthalmoplegic migraine: ischaemic or compressive neuropathy? *Headache* **20**, 300–304

Walsh, J. P. and O'Doherty, D. S. (1960). A possible explanation of the mechanism of ophthalmoplegic migraine. *Neurology* **10**, 1079–1084

Welch, K. M. A. and Levine, S. R. (1990). Migraine-related stroke in the context of the International Headache Society classification of head pain. *Arch. Neurol.* **47**, 458–462

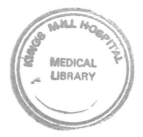

Chapter 7

Migraine: clinical aspects

The extent of the problem

Prevalence

The difficulty in defining and classifying migraine obviously extends to any survey of its prevalence, whether conducted by questionnaire or personal interview, because of the wide variation in the nature, frequency and severity of attacks. It is not uncommon to find patients who have had only one, two or three migrainous attacks in their lives. The frequency of attacks may therefore range from one in a lifetime to one almost every day.

Bille (1962) studied a group of almost 9000 Swedish children and found that the prevalence of migraine increased during childhood from 1 per cent at 6 years of age to 5 per cent at 11 years of age. Dalsgaard-Neilsen (1970) reported a higher prevalence than Bille for each age group in Danish children, increasing from 3 per cent at 7 years of age to 9 per cent at 15 years of age. He found that the prevalence for males remained at 11 per cent during adult life, and that for women reached 19 per cent by 40 years of age.

A survey of almost 15,000 people conducted in 1975 by the British Migraine Trust (Green, 1977) disclosed that 10 per cent of males and 16 per cent of females suffered from unilateral headache with migrainous characteristics. If bilateral headaches were included, the figures increased to 20 per cent and 26 per cent, respectively. In a telephone interview of some 10,000 people between 12 and 29 years of age in the USA, Linet et al. (1989) found that 3 per cent of males and 7.4 per cent of females had suffered from a migraine headache in the month before interview. A national migraine study of over 20,000 people in the USA showed that 17.6 per cent of women and 5.7 per cent of men experience severe migraine headaches (Stewart et al., 1992) with the prevalence in lower income groups being more than 60 per cent higher than those with an annual income of more than 30,000 dollars.

Using the diagnostic criteria for migraine of the International Headache Society, Rasmussen et al. (1991) reported that the lifetime prevalence of migraine in the Danish population was 8 per cent for men and 25 per cent for women. Comparable figures for France were 4 per cent and 11.9 per cent, respectively, when strict IHS criteria were used, but increased to 6.1 per cent and 17.6 per cent when 'borderline migraine' patients were included (Henry et al., 1992).

In specific groups of subjects, the prevalence is high. For example, a study of 97 narcotic addicts in a methadone treatment programme found that 21 per cent of males and 45 per cent of females had suffered from migraine, compared with 8 per cent and 18 per cent, respectively, of 617 university students used as a control population (Webster *et al.*, 1977). Of considerable interest is a survey of a rural community in Nigeria (Osuntokun, Bademosi and Osuntokun, 1982) which found a prevalence of 5 per cent in males and 9 per cent in females, increasing in females to 17 per cent during the reproductive years of life. In Nigeria, there is an association of migraine with the sickle-cell trait, that is patients with haemoglobin As (Osuntokun and Osuntokun, 1972).

A survey of citizens in the USA demonstrated striking differences in the prevalence of migraine in patients from various ethnic backgrounds. The prevalence in those of Caucasian, African and Asian origin was, respectively, 20.4, 16.2 and 9.2 per cent for women and 8.6, 7.2 and 4.2 per cent for men (Stewart, Lipton and Liberman, 1996).

Arregui *et al.* (1991) used the International Headache Society criteria in assessing the prevalence of migraine in Peru, which varied from 3.6 per cent at sea level to 12.4 per cent in the Andes, 14,200 feet above sea level, whereas tension headache was equally common at 9.5 per cent in both sites. Further studies are required to determine if the prevalence or severity of migraine alters when a simple village or farming existence is exchanged for life in a large city or when a subordinate job, in which the subject acts in a repetitive fashion under direction, is exchanged for one that involves frequent and difficult decision-making.

Morbidity and economic impact

Bille (1962) found that 42 per cent of migrainous children were subject to one or more attacks each month that were sufficiently severe to prevent the child from working. There was no significant difference in the hours lost from school by boys with migraine when compared with a control group, but migrainous girls lost a mean of 50 hours from school each term compared with 27 hours per term for girls who were not subject to headache.

A British Migraine Trust survey (Green, 1977) showed that migrainous patients were absent from work an average of 4 days each year because of headache. A study of 2000 headache sufferers in Finland found that 13 per cent had been absent from work in the previous year for this reason, 17 per cent of these for more than 7 days (Nikiforow and Hokkanen, 1979). In a random sample of 514 working people in the Republic of San Marino, 255 suffered from headache, 164 reported decreased efficiency as a result and 38 (7.4 per cent of the population and about 15 per cent of the headache group) were absent from work because of headache for a total of 338 working days (Benassi *et al.*, 1986). Of all working days lost because of illness, 8.4 per cent were due to headache.

Linet *et al.* (1989) reported that 6.1 per cent of males and 14 per cent of females from 12 to 29 years of age had missed part of a day or more from school or work because of their most recent headache. Department of Social Security data from the United Kingdom for the year ending April 1989 showed 43,800 days of sickness and 276,900 days of invalidity (Blau and Drummond, 1991). The authors comment that the social and economic impact of migraine is underestimated by certified days of illness, because many patients remain at work during an attack and others, such as housewives, would not be included. A Danish study of 119 migrainous subjects found that 43 per cent had missed 1–7 days from work in the preceding year. A general practitioner had been consulted by 56 per cent and a specialist by 16 per cent (Rasmussen, Jensen and Olesen, 1992). Stewart, Lipton and Simon (1996) examined work-related disability in 1663 migraine patients in the USA. The average number of working days missed each year was 3.8 for men and 8.3 for women. When reduced efficiency caused by headache was considered, 51 per cent of females and 38 per cent of males experienced 6 or more 'lost workday equivalents'.

The migraine patient

Sex and age distribution

It is apparent from the surveys of prevalence and morbidity that migraine affects women more than men. In the British Migraine Trust survey of almost 15,000 people (Green, 1977), unilateral headaches with migrainous features were experienced by women more than men in the ratio 3:2 and the mean age of onset was at 19 years of age. The age of onset of migraine was recorded in two series, each of 500 patients attending a neurological clinic in Sydney. Women comprised 60 per cent of the first series (Selby and Lance, 1960) and 75 per cent of the second (Lance and Anthony, 1966). The initial attack of migraine was experienced in the first decade of life by 25 per cent of patients (Figure 7.1) and was uncommon after 50 years of age. It may have its onset, often unrecognized, in infancy and also in advancing years when migrainous episodes may be confused with transient ischaemic attacks. Fisher (1980) has analysed migraine equivalents of late onset, which may appear even in

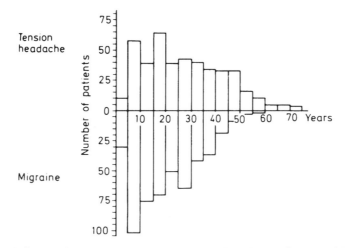

Figure 7.1 The age of onset of tension headache and migraine. (From Lance, Curran and Anthony, 1965, by permission of the editor of *The Medical Journal of Australia*)

a person's seventies, and has termed them transient migrainous accompaniments (TMAs).

Genetic background: the family history

When only parents and siblings were considered, 46 per cent of patients were found to have a family history of migraine, compared with 18 per cent of patients with tension headache used as a control group (Lance and Anthony, 1966). If grandparents were included, 55 per cent of patients had a positive family history (Selby and Lance, 1960). Green (1977) reported a positive family history in some 60 per cent of migraine patients and 16 per cent of normal controls. The relative most commonly affected was the mother (53 per cent), while the father was affected in 17 per cent, a sister in 17 per cent and a brother in 12 per cent of cases. Laurence (1987), in discussing the genetics of migraine, cites a risk of children developing the disorder as 70 per cent when both parents suffer from migraine, 45 per cent when one parent is affected, and 30 per cent when close relatives other than the parents have migraine. D'Amico et al. (1991) found at least one affected relative in 85 per cent of cases and postulated a 'sex-limited' transmission mode of inheritance to explain the female preponderance.

Comparisons of the prevalence of migraine in monozygotic and dizygotic twins in Australia (Merikangas, 1996) and in Sweden (Larson, Bille and Pederson, 1995) have shown that approximately half of the susceptibility to migraine is of genetic origin and that the other half is determined by environmental influences. Russell and Olesen (1995) found that the first-degree relatives of patients suffering migraine without aura (MO) had 1.9 times the risk of MO and 1.4 times the risk of migraine with aura (MA). The first-degree relatives of patients with MA had nearly four times the risk of MA but no increased risk of MO. Familial hemiplegic migraine is inherited as a dominant gene and is discussed further in Chapter 8.

Is there a 'migraine personality'?

Bille (1962) compared personality characteristics of migrainous school children with those of their peer groups. There was no demonstrable difference in social class, intelligence or ambition, or in such symptoms as nervous tics, nail-biting or nocturnal enuresis. There was a higher incidence of sleep disturbances and 'night terrors', temper tantrums, recurrent abdominal pains and motion sickness among the migrainous children. The migraine group performed more slowly in sensorimotor tests but with less errors than the control groups. They were more fearful, tense, sensitive and vulnerable to frustration. They were tidier and less physically enduring than their non-migrainous fellows. Guidetti et al. (1987) used a personality inventory to compare 40 migrainous children between 8 and 14 years of age with a control group, finding a significantly higher score for somatic concern, anxiety and depression, but no difference in the remaining 30 scores as indices of behaviour, achievement and adjustment. Many of the traits thought to be characteristic of childhood migraine can be found in children with other chronic pain disorders (Cunningham et *al.*, 1987). The migraine patient is not subject to more stress than a control group but reacts more to such stress (Henryk-Gutt and Rees, 1973).

The Minnesota Multiphasic Personality Inventory (MMPI), or variations on it, has been used repeatedly to assess migraine patients without being able to confirm the traditional view of the sufferer being a rigid perfectionist or indeed demonstrating any unequivocal departure from normality (Silberstein, Lipton and Breslau, 1995). A recent study by Breslau and Andreski (1995) found an association with neurotic traits once comorbidity of frank psychiatric disorders had been excluded. There is a significant association between migraine, anxiety and depression (Merikangas and Angst, 1996). Young adults with migraine were followed up by Breslau and Davis (1992) and found to develop panic attacks 12 times as often as non-migrainous control subjects and were four times more likely to develop major depression.

Is there any relationship between migraine and allergy?

Many anecdotal reports in the past have linked migraine with allergic disorders such as asthma, hay fever, hives and eczema. This possibility was examined prospectively in a comparative study of 500 migrainous patients and 100 patients with typical daily tension headache (Lance and Anthony, 1966). No significant difference in the family or personal history was found between the groups (Table 7.1). There is also no evidence that children with migraine are more prone to allergies than other children (Bille, 1962). Medina and Diamond (1976) were unable to demonstrate any difference in the prevalence of allergy or the plasma levels of immunoglobulin E (IgE) between migrainous and control groups. Merrett *et al.* (1983) studied the serum IgE and IgG_4 levels in groups of patients with so-called 'dietary migraine', non-dietary migraine and headache-free controls but found no significant difference between the groups.

Migraine and epilepsy

Speculation that migraine and epilepsy might share a common pathophysiology has continued for the past 100 years. Lance and Anthony (1966) undertook a prospective survey of patients referred to a headache clinic and could find no significant differ-

Table 7.1 Personal and family history of migraine, epilepsy, allergy and vomiting attacks in migraine and tension headache

	Personal history			*Family history*		
	Migraine (%)	*Tension (%)*	*Significance of difference*	*Migraine (%)*	*Tension (%)*	*Significance of difference*
Migraine	100.0	0	Not applicable	46.0	18	$P < 0.001$
Epilepsy	1.6	2	Not significant	2.4	3	Not significant
Allergy	17.4	13	Not significant	8.2	6	Not significant
Childhood vomiting	23.2	12	$P < 0.02$			

ence in the personal or family history of epilepsy between patients with migraine and those with tension headache (Table 7.1). Ottman and Lipton (1996) did not find an increased risk of epilepsy in the relatives of migrainous patients, with the exception of male children of female patients who carried a 1.8 times increased risk of epilepsy. Conversely there was no greater risk of migraine in the relatives of epileptic patients. Since this study was carried out in adults, it does not exclude an increased risk of migraine in childhood epilepsies. There is a significant association between migraine and epilepsy, particularly post-traumatic epilepsy (Ottman and Lipton, 1994), but this does not appear to have any genetic basis.

Andermann (1987), in his overview of a symposium on migraine and epilepsy, concluded that there was no genetic link between the two disorders in general but that some forms, such as benign Rolandic epilepsy, benign occipital epilepsy and, possibly, absence attacks, were associated with a higher than expected prevalence of migraine. Some patients who initially have epileptic attacks only during migraine may subsequently have seizures independent of migraine. In epileptic patients, the characteristic post-ictal headache may assume migrainous characteristics.

Panayiotopoulos (1987) has suggested the term 'childhood epilepsy with migrainous phenomena and occipital paroxysms' for those adolescent patients reported by him and by Campbell, Metrakos and Andermann (1978) with migraine, seizures and almost continuous occipital spike-wave paroxysms which were inhibited by opening the eyes and fixating on a target. The condition usually responds well to anticonvulsants although exceptions are recorded. Panayiotopoulos (1996) has drawn attention to differences in the visual auras of migraine, which are usually linear, zigzag, arcuate and relatively colourless, with those of occipital lobe epilepsy, which tend to be circular or of geometric shapes and multicoloured. He has never observed a migrainous aura triggering an epileptic fit in his experience of 600 patients.

Benign Rolandic epilepsy is a syndrome of nocturnal epilepsy in children associated with centrotemporal spike discharges in the EEG. It was found to be associated with migraine in 21 out of 30 cases reported by Bladin (1987), increasing to 24 out of 30 on follow-up. The seizures responded well to anticonvulsants but the headaches continued, even after the tendency to seizures subsided and anticonvulsants were withdrawn. Septien et al. (1991) reported that the prevalence of migraine was 63 per cent in Rolandic epilepsy, 33 per cent in absence epilepsy, 7 per cent in partial epilepsy and 9 per cent for those whose seizures followed cranial trauma.

Features of the migraine attack

The varieties of migraine and the phases of migraine attacks have been considered in Chapter 6. As well as the focal neurological symptoms and headache, which form the mainstay of migraine, there are intriguing accompaniments that require explanation.

Gastrointestinal disturbance

About 90 per cent of patients feel nauseated with their migraine headache and 75 per cent vomit with some attacks. The passage of one or more loose stools at this phase of the migraine attack is noted by about 20 per cent of patients (Lance and Anthony, 1966). These gastrointestinal symptoms are not a reaction to the pain of migraine because they may occur with comparatively mild headaches, particularly in children, and nausea may sometimes precede headache by an hour or so. A history of migraine is common in adults as well as children with recurrent vomiting attacks (Scobie, 1983) and migrainous adults often recall periodic vomiting attacks in child-hood (see Table 7.1). The mechanism of vomiting was discussed by Baker and Bernat (1985) who reported the case of a patient presenting with nausea and projectile vomiting who was later found to have a solitary metastasis involving the lateral tegmentum of the pons. This is near the 'vomiting centre' in the dorsolateral reticular formation of the medulla, which receives afferents from the chemoreceptor trigger zone in the area postrema in the floor of the caudal part of the fourth ventricle as well as directly from the gastrointestinal tract. The fact that the dopamine antago-nists metoclopramide, prochlorperazine and domperidone are effective in reducing nausea and vomiting in migraine and that the intravenous infusion of the 5-HT$_3$ antagonist granisetron at 40 µg/kg, reduced nausea more than a placebo during migraine headache (Rowat et al., 1991) implicates dopamine and 5HT receptors, although the mechanism remains uncertain.

Hyperacuity of the special senses

During migraine headache most patients are aware of an exaggeration of brightness of light (dazzle) and some feel pain on exposure to light (photophobia). Some 80 per cent of patients find light unpleasant and prefer to lie down in a darkened room (Selby and Lance, 1960).

> And screened in shades from days detested glare,
>   She sighs for ever on her pensive bed,
> Pain at her side, and megrim at her head.
>   (Rape of the Lock, Canto 4, Alexander Pope)

Moreover, about 80 per cent of patients are subject to phonophobia. They complain that their hearing becomes more acute during migraine headache so that the faintest sound seems to be louder and more disturbing (Kayan and Hood, 1984). A heigh-tened sense of smell is also common at this time.

Drummond (1986) determined that there were two components to photophobia. The first, a general sensitivity to glare, affected both eyes and persisted to some extent between attacks in comparison with headache-free controls. The second was light-induced pain that was greater on the side of unilateral headache in 19 out of 25 migrainous patients. He postulated that trigeminal and visual inputs interacted, probably in the thalamus, to produce the unilateral component whereas the background of bilateral photophobia shared a mechanism with phonophobia and osmophobia.

Kayan and Hood (1984) suggested that a transient disturbance of cochlear func-tion during migraine could cause phonophobia by loudness recruitment, a phenom-enon common in Ménière's disease. In this condition, auditory acuity is diminished at low noise levels but improves as sound intensity increases, whereas in migraine the slightest sound appears to be louder than normal as one aspect of a general hyper-acuity of the special senses. Auditory and visual discomfort thresholds decrease substantially during attacks of migraine, suggesting a disturbance of central sensory processing mechanisms (Woodhouse and Drummond, 1993).

Sensitivity to light has been reported as a symptom developing 3 months after infarction in the territory of one posterior cerebral artery, causing thalamic damage (Cummings and Gittinger, 1981), and the authors quote older reports in the litera-ture that thalamic lesions cause not only hyperpathia to common sensation but also dislike of light, noise, smells and tastes.

Hyperaesthesia and hyperalgesia

Hyperaesthesia of the face and scalp may have a mechanism akin to the increased acuity of the special senses mentioned above. Tenderness of the scalp is noticed by about two-thirds of patients, who may find it uncomfortable to lie on the affected side or to comb their hair (Selby and Lance, 1960).

Bakal and Kaganov (1977) found increased EMG activity in the frontal and neck muscles of migraine patients, during and between headaches, compared with tension headache patients and normal controls. During migraine headache, muscles in the areas afflicted by pain become tender to palpation (Tfelt-Hansen, Lous and Olesen, 1981) and headache is relieved by injection of the tender areas. It remains uncertain whether hyperalgesia is the result of referred pain with reflex muscle contraction or whether muscles are a primary source of headache.

Autonomic disturbance

Gotoh et al. (1984) investigated autonomic function in 21 migraine patients (10 with aura, 11 without) between headaches and compared their responses with 30 age-matched controls. Blood pressure changes with the Valsalva manoeuvre were dimin-ished, postural hypotension was present and the pupils dilated excessively after dilute (1.25 per cent) adrenaline eye drops, more so on the habitual headache side. In accord with these indications of sympathetic hypofunction, the plasma level of noradrenaline was lower than controls and failed to rise 30 minutes after head-up tilting, unlike the normal subjects.

Fanciullacci (1979) showed that the pupils of migrainous patients dilated poorly in response to fenfluramine (which releases noradrenaline from nerve terminals), con-stricted more than controls after the application of guanethidine (which depletes axonal transmitter stores) and dilated excessively in response to a dilute phenyleph-rine (1 per cent) eye drop. These tests indicate reduced stores of noradrenaline with receptor supersensitivity. Drummond (1987) found that the mean pupil diameter in migraine patients was smaller during headache than that of normal controls and was significantly smaller on the affected side in patients with unilateral headache. Pupil-lary asymmetry was greater in darkness than in light, suggesting an acquired sympa-thetic deficit, similar but milder than that frequently observed in cluster headache and attributed originally by Kunkle and Anderson (1961) to involvement of the sympathetic plexus in the wall of the internal carotid artery.

Because of the tendency to postural hypotension, faintness or fainting is not uncommon in migraine. Some 10 per cent of patients had fainted on at least one occasion during the headache in the series of Selby and Lance (1960). One must be aware of interpreting the nonspecific symptom of 'dizziness' as 'faintness' because anxiety overbreathing is common during migraine headache (Blau and Dexter, 1980) and may cause lightheadedness and bilateral paraesthesiae, which might be thought incorrectly to be part of the aura. Some patients feel cold during headache, although others sweat excessively and body temperature may increase (Sacks, 1992). Sometimes areas in the mouth or scalp may swell, resembling large hives.

Sodium and fluid retention

Increase in weight, with or without signs of generalized oedema, is noted by about half of migraine patients before the migraine attack. Oliguria is common before the attack and roughly 30 per cent of patients notice polyuria as the headache subsides. The blood sodium level has been shown to increase before and during headache while serum protein concentration falls (Campbell, Hay and Tonks, 1951). The urinary output of sodium in migraine subjects between attacks after being given a water load of 1000–1500 ml is almost double that of controls. There is therefore evidence that sodium and fluid retention is associated with migraine but it is unlikely to be a cause of migraine, because the administration of diuretics, which minimizes weight fluctuations, does not prevent the regular recurrence of migraine headache. Stanford and Greene (1970) suggested that aldosterone might be responsible for the sodium and fluid retention in migraine patients and reported the cure of premenstrual migraine by the surgical treatment of Conn's syndrome.

Precipitating factors

Migraine headache often recurs regularly or in cycles without any obvious precipitating factors. It is probable that some internal mechanism or 'biological clock' determines the pattern of the disorder in such patients.

Friedman (1970) told of one of his patients who 'has an occupation that takes him through the world from the Himalayas in Tibet to Somaliland, indeed from the highest altitudes to the lowest, from the wettest to the driest – experiencing climatic, food and culture changes. But his migraine remains, for he carries his personal environment with him'.

As well as the pattern of recurrence, the time of onset may depend on an internal clock or circadian rhythm, for example those patients who are awakened from sleep by headache.

On occasions, excessive input to the nervous system may induce migraine symptoms with such rapidity that it is difficult to imagine any other than a neural mechanism being responsible. Perhaps a sudden jar to the head may also evoke a neural discharge or may initiate changes directly in the cerebral cortex ('spreading depression of Leão') or in cranial blood vessels by a vibratory stimulus to their walls. The mechanism by which emotional disturbance or relaxation after a hard week's work induces migraine presumably involves neural and humoral mechanisms, although the precise sequence of events remains obscure. The careful listing of trigger factors while taking the history is an important step in treatment because their avoidance may lessen the frequency and severity of migraine headache.

Stress and relaxation after stress

A stressful event is probably the most commonly recognized precipitant of migraine (Henryk-Gutt and Rees, 1973) and the frequency of headache usually increases if the patient is worried by some protracted problem, such as an impending divorce or financial difficulties. The record diaries of 33 patients studied by Levor et al. (1986) showed a significant increase in stressful events and a decline in physical activity for the 4 days leading up to and including each headache day. At times of real emergency, when patients have to summon up all their internal resources, they usually remain free of headache, which tends to occur as soon as the crisis is resolved. The same principle underlies 'weekend headache'. Patients remain free while under the sustained stress of a working week but suffer from headache at the moment of 'letdown' or relaxation. On some occasions, an emotional shock may be followed by the symptoms of classical migraine within seconds or minutes.

Sleep

Migraine not uncommonly awakens a patient from sleep. Dexter and Riley (1975) found that the onset of headache was related to the onset of rapid eye movement (REM) phase in 11 of 19 instances. Blood levels of 5-HT and noradrenaline fall at this time in association with headache. Sleeping later than the normal hour of rising ('sleeping in') is particularly liable to bring on a headache.

Sleep-walking is more common in migrainous children (30 per cent) compared with control subjects (about 5 per cent) (Barabas, Ferrari and Matthews, 1983).

Trauma

A sudden jar or blow to the head may induce symptoms of classical migraine, particularly in children. Matthews (1972) reported that soccer players who 'head' the ball may experience blurring of vision within minutes, followed by headache ('footballer's migraine'). Other types of football are not exempt. Bennett et al. (1980) described three members of an American university football team who had each experienced a number of episodes of scintillating scotomas, paraesthesiae and amnesia, not always followed by headache, after a comparatively minor blow to the head. It is not uncommon for children to develop similar migrainous symptoms after bumping their head while playing, falling off a chair or similar accidents (Haas, Pineda and Lourie, 1975). The child may develop complete cortical blindness for 30 minutes or so, which is very worrying for one not familiar with the syndrome, and may lead to fears of serious intracranial damage.

Migraine may also be brought on by painful compression of the head, for example, the wearing of tight goggles during swimming training (Pestronk and Pestronk, 1983).

Afferent stimulation

Glare, flickering light, noise and smells are common trigger factors. Marcus and Soso (1989) found that 82 per cent of migraine patients experienced visual discomfort while looking at a black and white striped pattern, compared with only 6.2 per cent of non-migraine subjects. The latent period between exposure to an afferent stimulus and the development of migraine is so brief at times that it suggests a central reflex response. Psychophysical tests such as the reaction of migrainous patients to visual stimuli indicate hypersensitivity of the visual cortex (Chronicle and Mulleners, 1996). Moreover, the nature of the induced aura may resemble the precipitating stimulus. Lord (1982) cites from his personal experiences auras of central visual disturbance after exposure to a flash bulb, of visual disorientation after driving on a winding road, and of paraesthesiae in one arm after using that arm vigorously to sandpaper an object.

Food and eating habits

Missing a meal often induces a migraine attack, possibly as the result of hypoglycaemia. About 25 per cent of patients consider that their attacks are provoked by eating certain foods, particularly fatty foods, chocolate and oranges (Selby and Lance, 1960). There is some doubt whether this is a delayed hypersensitivity reaction to the chemical content of these foods, or whether it depends on a conditioned reflex. Wolff (1963) quotes experiments in which incriminated foods were ingested by patients without their knowledge and without a headache ensuing.

There is contentious literature on tyramine-containing foods, described in the fourth edition of this book. It can be summarized by stating that there is no firm evidence that tyramine or abnormalities of its metabolism play any part in the genesis of migraine. Similarly, there have been contradictory reports on whether chocolate is a precipitating factor. The most recent study by Gibb et al. (1991) tested 20 patients who considered that their attacks followed the consumption of chocolate by administering a 40 g chocolate bar or a placebo bar, the flavour of each being disguised by carob, in double blind fashion. Five of the 12 patients challenged with chocolate and none of the eight given placebo developed a migraine headache within 24 hours.

A similar trial involved patients susceptible to headache after drinking red wine being given chilled red wine or vodka, the colour being concealed by a brown glass bottle from which the participants drank with a straw. A typical migraine attack developed in nine of 11 of the red wine drinkers but none of the eight who drank vodka (Littlewood et al., 1988).

Whether certain foodstuffs can precipitate migraine remains controversial since the results of elimination diets have been reported as positive (Monro et al., 1980) and negative (Medina and Diamond, 1978). In our own trial (McQueen et al., 1989),

95 migraine patients suffering 4–12 headaches each month were entered but 36 dropped out during the first 6 weeks. The elimination diet was followed for 4–6 weeks by 59 patients, of whom 22 did not improve and 37 became free of headache for at least 2 weeks. Of the latter group, only 19 completed the challenge phase, and were given an appropriate diet for 1 month and an inappropriate diet for 1 month in random fashion, separated by a washout period. On the appropriate diet, nine patients improved, nine were unchanged and four were worse when compared with their period on the inappropriate diet. It may be concluded that the dietary management of migraine is of little if any value, at least in adults, but it is obviously prudent for patients to avoid any food that they are convinced provokes an attack.

Vasodilators

Vasodilator agents such as nitroglycerin (which releases nitric oxide), histamine and prostaglandin E_1 may precipitate migraine. The application of nitroglycerin ointment to the temple of migrainous patients who usually experienced pain in that site was found to induce headache within 30 minutes in seven out of 10 patients whereas application of the ointment to another bodily site caused only a delayed headache after about 7 hours in three of 10 patients (Bonuso et al., 1989). Exposure to excessive heat or strenuous exercise will sometimes trigger migraine, presumably from dilatation of cerebral and extracranial vessels.

Changes in barometric pressure and weather conditions

Normal subjects have developed migrainous phenomena for the first time when subjected to rapid changes in barometric pressure in compression or decompression chambers. The precipitation of migraine by flying at high altitudes and the significance of a migrainous history in aircrew is considered by Appenzeller, Feldman and Friedman (1979).

Many patients attribute migraine attacks to changes in the weather, particularly an approaching thunderstorm. Cull (1981) correlated the incidence of migraine with changes in barometric pressure on the day of headache and for the preceding 48 hours. Curiously, the mean barometric pressure was found to be significantly higher on migraine days than headache-free days. A fall in barometric pressure over a 24-hour period was not associated with an increased incidence of migraine the following day, but a rise in pressure of more than 15 mbar correlated with a reduction in the attack rate the next day. Cull concluded that the minor changes in attack rate may be explained more easily by indirect factors, such as the lack of glare on cool, cloudy days, than by any direct effect of barometric pressure.

Sulman et al. (1970) pointed out that hot, dry winds 'of ill repute' are notorious for causing irritability and headache. They include the Shirav of Israel, the Santa Ana of Southern California, Arizona desert winds, the Argentine Zonda, the Sirocco of the Mediterranean, the Maltese Xlokk, the Chamsin of Arab countries, the Foehn of Switzerland and the North Winds of Melbourne. They attributed the symptoms of nervous tension and headache to the increased ionization of the air which precedes the arrival of the hot, dry wind and correlated this with excessive urinary excretion of serotonin.

Hormonal changes

Johannis van der Linden in *De Hemicrania Menstrua* (1660) described a unilateral headache accompanied by nausea and vomiting, recurring in the Marchioness of Brandenburg each month 'during the menstrual flux'.

The periodicity of migraine is related to the menstrual cycle in about 60 per cent of women patients, the headaches appearing or becoming more severe just before menses. Migraine is relieved by pregnancy in about 60 per cent of women, but this does not depend upon a previous association with menstruation, although there is a positive correlation. Of women whose migraine was linked with menses, 64 per cent lost their headache during pregnancy, compared with 48 per cent of those in whom this relationship was absent (Lance and Anthony, 1966). There is no link between relief during pregnancy and the sex of the fetus. Some women may experience migraine for the first time during pregnancy, which may cease to be a problem after the child is born (Chancellor, Wroe and Cull, 1990).

Somerville (1972b) undertook a survey of 200 women attending an antenatal clinic during the last 4 weeks of pregnancy. He found that 31 patients had been subject to migraine headache in the 12 months before becoming pregnant, giving a prevalence of 15 per cent of women in the reproductive years. Of the 31 patients, 24 improved during pregnancy, seven becoming completely free of headache. Only seven patients had developed migraine for the first time in the current pregnancy, mostly in the first trimester. Somerville found that there was no significant difference in the plasma progesterone of those women whose migraine had improved (98.4 ng/ml), those women whose migraine continued during pregnancy (101.2 ng/ml) and the non-migrainous control patients (119.4 ng/ml).

Somerville (1971, 1972a) clarified the relationship of migraine to the hormonal changes of the menstrual cycle. Normal and migrainous women were found to have a similar fluctuation of hormone levels. Plasma oestradiol rose to an early pre-ovulatory peak, followed by a rapid fall, then a secondary rise during the luteal phase with a final fall before menstruation. Plasma progesterone remained low during menstruation and the follicular phase, then increased at or just after mid-cycle to a plateau during the luteal phase, before declining premenstrually. There were no significant differences between the peak progesterone concentrations in migrainous and non-migrainous women.

Premenstrual migraine occurred regularly during or after the time at which plasma oestradiol and progesterone fell to their lowest levels. To determine which of these hormones was the more influential in triggering migraine headache, Somerville treated six women with progesterone and six women with oestradiol in the pre-menstrual phase while measuring their hormone levels daily. He found that the administration of progesterone to maintain artificially high blood levels postponed uterine bleeding, but that the migraine attack occurred in five out of the six women at the expected time in the cycle. On the other hand, the injection of oestradiol did not postpone menstruation but delayed the onset of migraine headache in all patients

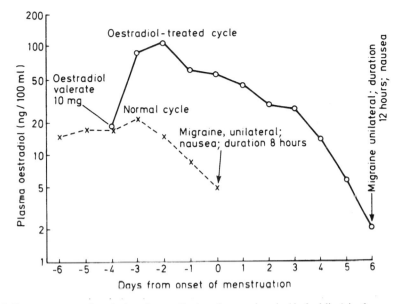

Figure 7.2 Oestrogen-treated cycle (continuous line) and normal cycle (dashed line) in the same patient. The onset of migraine is postponed until the oestrogen level falls. (From Somerville, 1972a, by permission of the editor of *Neurology*)

by 3–9 days (Figure 7.2). Migraine began after the oestradiol level fell below 20 ng/ 100 ml and could not be postponed further if another injection of oestradiol was given at this time. Two other women had consistently low levels of progesterone, indicating the absence of ovulation. One developed migraine 10 days after an injection of oestradiol, followed on the 11th day by oestrogen-withdrawal bleeding. The second patient, who was menopausal, suffered a typical episode of migraine as the oestrogen level fell 9 days after injection, without any withdrawal bleeding.

It is therefore apparent that the withdrawal of oestrogen, rather than progesterone, sets in motion a series of changes that culminate in the onset of migraine. This could account for the mid-cycle headache which afflicts some women in addition to their menstrual migraine. There is probably some intermediary between oestrogen withdrawal and the sequelae of menstruation and migraine. The prostaglandins are possible contenders because of their actions on the uterus, and the known effect of PGE_1 in precipitating migraine when infused into normal subjects (Carlson, Ekelund and Oro, 1968). Alternatively, the hypothalamopituitary axis may be responsible for hormonal changes and migraine occurring together.

The use of oral contraceptive tablets containing a high dose of oestrogen commonly exacerbates migraine. Dalton (1975) found that 34 per cent of women taking contraceptive pills and 60 per cent of those who had ceased to take them considered that their migraine was worse while on the pill. Permanent neurological deficit has been reported in patients whose phase of intracranial vasoconstriction was prolonged while taking oral contraceptives (Gardner, Van den Noort and Horenstein, 1967).

The relationship of migraine headache to hormonal changes in the menstrual cycle was reviewed by Silberstein and Merriam (1991) who conclude that the adverse reports concerning the exacerbation of migraine by the oral contraceptive pill refer mainly to the high-dose oestrogen pill used in earlier days and cite double-blind trials showing no increase in frequency on low-dose oestrogen pills. Oral contraceptives as a risk factor for stroke is discussed in Chapter 6.

Radiotherapy

Migraine-like headaches with prominent aura symptoms have been reported in children after cranial irradiation and chemotherapy (Parker, Vezina and Stacy Nicholson, 1994). We have had an adult patient who developed similar features years after cranial radiotherapy.

Associated diseases

Migraine may be aggravated by hypertension, aldosteronism (Stanford and Greene, 1970) and hyperthyroidism (Thomas et al., 1996). It has been reported as a symptom of hyper-pre-beta-lipoproteinaemia, possibly because of changes in plasma viscosity or red cell aggregation, and it disappears with restoration of serum lipids to normal (Leviton and Camenga, 1969). Migraine has been recorded during episodes of thrombocytopenia (Damasio and Beck, 1978) and there are instances reported of migraine with aura being precipitated or aggrevated by dissection or obstruction of cerebral arteries (Welch and Levine, 1990). It is probable that viral meningoencephalitis can precipitate a series of migraine attacks, but this is not always a convincing explanation for migraine-like episodes associated with CSF abnormalities. Fifty patients with headache, transient neurological symptoms and a lymphocytic reaction in the CSF were described as having 'pseudo-migraine' by Gomez-Aranta et al. (1977) who considered that an immune reaction following a viral infection was the most likely explanation.

Watkins and Espir (1969) found that 27 per cent of 100 patients with multiple sclerosis (MS) suffered from migraine, compared with 12 per cent of a control group matched for age and sex. Surprisingly, a family history of migraine was present in 20 per cent of the MS patients and only 10 per cent of the controls. Rolak (1985) confirmed that headache was more common in MS patients than controls but could find no correlation with the signs or symptoms of MS. Acute demyelination of the pons can give rise to a unilateral headache associated with brain stem and cerebellar symptoms (Nager, Lanska and Daroff, 1989) and MS may present with severe headache (Galer et al., 1990), probably caused by a midbrain plaque of demyelination (Haas, Kent and Friedman, 1993) (Figure 7.3).

It is doubtful whether arteriovenous malformations are associated with migraine more than would be expected by chance, although they may determine the nature of aura symptoms since the cortical disturbance is more likely to begin in a region of marginal perfusion. Haas (1991) concluded that there was a relationship but the two cases he reported argue against this proposition.

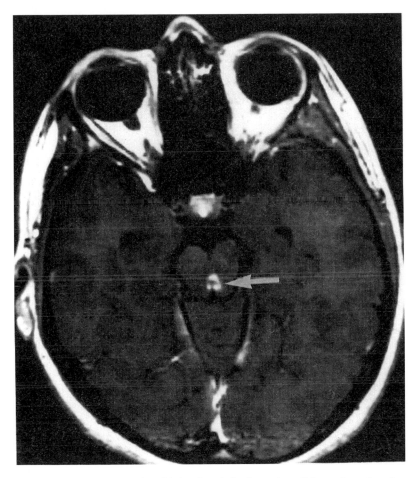

Figure 7.3 A demyelinated plaque of multiple sclerosis in the region of the periaqueductal grey matter associated with the acute onset of headache. (From Haas, Kent and Friedman, 1993, with permission)

Litman and Friedman (1978) reported that 64 (28 per cent) of 230 patients with prolapsed mitral valves suffered from migraine but Pfaffenrath el al. (1991) found that the prevalence of mitral valve prolapse or other risk factors for stroke was no greater in 44 migraine patients than in 32 controls. Raynaud's phenomenon has been reported to occur more often in migraine patients than would be expected by chance (Zahavi *et al.*, 1984) but the vascular response to cold is in fact normal in the digital arteries (Corbin and Martyn, 1985).

Migraine is associated with mitochondrial abnormalities in the MELAS syndrome, mentioned in Chapter 6.

Physical examination

There are no physical signs of migraine detectable between attacks. Hearing a bruit over the skull or orbits may give rise to concern and warrant carotid angiography to exclude the presence of an intracranial angioma or vascular tumour. In one series of 500 patients, 10 were found to have an audible cranial bruit (Selby and Lance, 1960). Two were children under 10 years of age in whom skull bruits are usually not of any significance. In four adult patients the bruit was heard over both eyes and in four it was unilateral. Carotid angiograms in three of the latter were completely normal.

In the above-mentioned series, a blood pressure of more than 150 mmHg systolic and 100 mmHg diastolic was found in 13 per cent of patients. Hypertension is said to be significantly more common over 50 years of age in migraine patients than in the general population (see Chapter 14).

While a migraine headache is in progress, excessive pulsation of temporal arteries may be noted and veins are often prominent on the forehead and temple. The face and scalp are commonly pale and sweaty in severe attacks. The patient may be mentally confused, stuporose or even lose consciousness for a brief time. Speech may be slurred (dysarthria) or there may be inability to choose the correct word or phrase (dysphasia). There may be a transient Horner's syndrome or dilated pupil on the side of the headache and, very rarely, paresis of extra-ocular muscles (ophthalmoplegic migraine). Weakness of upper motor neurone type may be observed (hemiparetic migraine) or, uncommonly, dystonic postures or involuntary movements.

Differential diagnosis and investigation

Since the differential diagnosis of migraine includes almost every cause of intermittent focal neurological symptoms and every cause of recurrent headache, the list of conditions to be considered could be extensive. In practice, the recurrent pattern of migraine is so characteristic that it is rarely necessary to undertake any investigations. The first attack of classical migraine in the absence of a family history can be worrying and, if there is any doubt about the diagnosis, the appropriate tests can be carried out as outlined in Chapter 18.

Episodes of cerebral embolism, as in subacute bacterial endocarditis, can sometimes mimic migraine. The focal neurological symptoms of classical migraine may also suggest a viral meningoencephalitis at times, particularly if the episode is accompanied by a fever. Lumbar puncture may indeed disclose a mononuclear pleocytosis in the CSF at the height of such a migraine attack (Gomez-Aranda et al., 1997). The point must be stressed that there is no indication for lumbar puncture, or indeed any other investigation, in typical uncomplicated migraine.

Electroencephalography

The EEG is not usually helpful in the diagnosis or management of migraine. There have been many reports of uncontrolled observations in the past which have suggested that EEG abnormalities may be more common in migrainous patients. Focal slow-wave changes have been described in patients with severe and prolonged attacks, in hemiplegic migraine for example, but Lauritzen Trojaborg and Olesen (1981) could find no abnormality in a study of 21 patients during common or classical migraine attacks, including three patients examined while they were experiencing photopsia. Bille (1962) did not find any significant difference between the EEGs of migrainous children and those of a control group. There are certain patients with vertebrobasilar migraine, discussed earlier in this chapter, with EEG abnormalities, including some with an almost continuous pattern of occipital spike-wave discharges (Camfield, Metrakos and Andermann, 1978; Panayiotopoulos. 1980). There is a tendency towards synchronization of the rhythms in the visual cortex of migrainous patients and EEG abnormalities may appear in association with severe neurological symptoms in migraine, and a minority of patients do show epileptiform abnormalities, although the relationship of these to migraine is uncertain. There does not appear to be any basis for the concept of 'dysrhythmic migraine' (Winter, 1987).

Visual evoked potentials (VEPs)

Visual evoked potentials are attenuated during a migraine attack when it is accompanied by visual symptoms. Between attacks, with flash stimulation the positive wave, which appears at a latency of about 100 ms (P100), is not delayed but the trough between P100 and the ensuing negative wave (N120) is enhanced in migrainous subjects when compared with a control group (Connolly, Gawel and Clifford Rose, 1982). The increase in amplitude of this primary response in the visual cortex to an afferent volley could underlie the sensitivity of the migraine patient to glare and flickering light. Winter (1987) summarized the extensive literature on visual evoked responses in migraine. In his own study, the latency in pattern reversal VEPs of P100 and N140 components was longer in female migraine patients. The reported changes are not sufficiently consistent or specific to be useful as a clinical tool.

Brain imaging and cerebral angiography

Computerized tomography (CT) scanning has demonstrated cerebral oedema, cortical infarction and areas of cortical atrophy in migraine patients (Hungerford, du Boulay and Zilkha, 1976; Mathew et al., 1977; Dorfman, Marshall and Enzmann, 1979). Magnetic resonance imaging (MRI) was reported to show punctate white matter abnormalities in seven of 17 patients suffering from migraine and, in four of seven patients with associated neurologic deficits, a cerebral or cerebellar infarct was demonstrated (Soges et al., 1988). Ziegler et al. (1991) compared the MRI scans of 18 patients subject to migraine with aura and those of 15 headache-free controls. A cortical infarction was noted in one migraine patient but small white matter lesions were found in two controls as well as in three of the patients. However, Igarashi et al. (1991) found a significant difference between 91 migraine subjects and 98 controls. Small white matter lesions were found in 30 per cent of patients of less than 40 years of age, compared with 11 per cent of age-matched controls, and the prevalence of abnormalities over the whole age range was 40 per cent. Lesions were no more frequent in patients with than without aura and their cause remains to be determined.

Cerebral angiography is indicated only if there is some doubt about the diagnosis, and aneurysm or other vascular abnormalities have to be excluded. There has always been some reluctance to perform angiography in migraine patients but Shuaib and Hachinski (1988) found that focal cerebral events followed the procedure in only 2.6 per cent of migraine patients compared with 2.8 per cent in a prospective study of 1002 patients undergoing angiography for different reasons. MR angiography provides a non-invasive alternative and is often sufficient.

Natural history and prognosis

The prognosis of migraine may be deduced from the little we know about its natural history. A migrainous child has a 60 per cent chance of remission in adolescence. Of the patients who remit, one-third will start to have attacks again, so that 60 per cent of affected children will still be subject to migraine at 30 years of age (Bille, 1981). Migraine seems to run a more benign course in boys as, at 30 years of age, 52 per cent of males and only 30 per cent of females were free of migraine. Between 37 and 43 years of age, 53 per cent still suffered from migraine (Bille, 1989). One-third of the original cohort of 73 children had suffered from migraine ever since childhood. In half the cases, the adult attacks were less severe and less frequent than those in childhood. The latest follow-up at 40 years disclosed that over 50 per cent of patients were still subject to migraine in the age group 47–53 years (Bille, 1997). Of patients with migraine in adult life, 70 per cent lose their headaches or improve over a period of 14 years, although 50 per cent may still be liable to occasional attacks at 65 years of age (Whitty and Hockaday, 1968).

References

Andermann, F. (1987). Migraine and epilepsy: an overview. In *Migraine and Epilepsy*, Eds F. Andermann and E. Lugaresi. pp. 405–422. Boston, Butterworths

Appenzeller, O., Feldman, R. G. and Friedman, A. P. (1979). Neurological and neurosurgical conditions associated with aviation safety. Migraine, headache and related conditions. *Arch. Neurol.* **36**, 784–805

Arregui, A., Cabrera, J., LeonVelarde, F., Parades, S., Viscarra, D. and Arbaiza, D. (1991). High prevalence of migraine in a high altitude population. *Neurology* **41**, 1668–1670

Bakal, D. A. and Kaganov, I. A. (1977). Muscle contraction and migraine headache: psychophysiologic comparison. *Headache* **17**, 208–215

Baker, C. H. B. and Bernat, J. L. (1985). The neuroanatomy of vomiting in man: association of projectile vomiting with a solitary metastasis in the lateral tegmentum of the pons and the middle cerebellar peduncle. *J. Neurol. Neurosurg. Psychiat.* **48**, 1165–1168

Barabas, G., Ferrari, M. and Matthews, W. S. (1983). Childhood migraine and somnambulism. *Neurology* **33**, 948–949

Benassi, G., D'Alessandro, R., Lenzi, P. L., Manzaroli, D., Baldrati, A. and Lugaresi. E. (1986). The economic burden of headache: an epidemiological study in the Republic of San Marino. *Headache* **26**, 457–459

Bennett, D. R., Fuenning, S. I., Sullivan, G. and Weber, J. (1980). Migraine precipitated by head trauma in athletes. *Am. J. Sports Med.* **8**, 202–205

Bille, B. (1962). Migraine in schoolchildren. *Acta Paediat. Stockh.* **51** (Suppl. 136), 1–151

Bille, B. (1981). Migraine in childhood and its prognosis. *Cephalalgia* **1**, 71–75

Bille, B. (1989). Migraine in childhood: a 30-year follow-up. In *Headache in Children and Adolescents*, Eds G. Lanzi, V. Balottin and A. Cernibori. pp. 19–26. Amsterdam, Elsevier

Bille, B. (1997). A 40-year follow-up of school children with migraine. *Cephalalgia* **17**, 488–491

Bladin, P. F. (1987). The association of benign Rolandic epilepsy with migraine. In *Migraine and Epilepsy*, Eds F. Andermann and E. Lugaresi. pp. 145–152. Boston, Butterworths

Blau, J. N. and Dexter, S. L. (1980). Hyperventilation during migraine attacks. *Br. Med. J.* **280**, 1254

Blau, I. N. and Drummond, M. F. (1991). *Migraine.* London, Office of Health Economics

Bonuso, S., Marano, E., Di Stasio, E., Sorge, F., Barbieri, F. and Ullucci, E. (1989). Source of pain and primitive dysfunction in migraine: an identical site? *J. Neurol. Neurosurg. Psychiat.* **52**, 1351–1354

Breslau, N. and Andreski, P. (1995). Migraine, personality and psychiatric comorbidity. *Headache* **35**, 382–386

Breslau, N. and Davis, G.C. (1992). Migraine, major depression and panic disorder: a prospective epidemiologic study of young adults. *Cephalalgia* **12**, 85–90

Camfield, P. R., Metrakos, K. and Andermann, F. (1978). Basilar migraine, seizures and severe epileptiform EEG abnormalities. *Neurology* **28**, 584–588

Campbell, D. A., Hay, K. M. and Tonks, E. M. (1951). An investigation of salt and water balance in migraine. *Br. Med. J.* **2**, 1424–1429

Carlson, L. A., Ekelund, L.G. and Orö, L. (1968). Clinical and metabolic effects of different doses of prostaglandin E in man. *Acta Med. Scand.* **183**, 423–430

Chancellor, A. M., Wroe, S. J. and Cull, R. E. (1990). Migraine occurring for the first time in pregnancy. *Headache* **30**, 224–227

Chronicle, E. P. and Mulleners, W. M. (1996). Visual system dysfunction in migraine: a review of clinical and pathophysiological findings. *Cephalalgia* **16**, 525–535

Connolly, F. J., Gawel, M. and Clifford Rose, F. (1982). Migraine patients exhibit abnormalities in the visual-evoked potential. *J. Neurol. Neurosurg. Psychiat.* **45**, 464–467

Corbin, D and Martyn, C. (1985). Migraine is not a manifestation of a generalized vasospastic disorder. *Cephalalgia* **5** (Suppl. 3), 458–459

Cull, R. E. (1981). Barometric pressure and other factors in migraine. *Headache* **21**, 102–104

Cummings, J. L. and Gittinger, J. W. (1981). Central dazzle. A thalamic syndrome? *Arch. Neurol.* **38**, 372–374

Cunningham, S. J., McGrath, P. J., Ferguson. H. B., Humphreys, P., D'Astous, J., Latter, J., Goodman, J. T. and Firestone, P. (1987). Personality and behavioural characteristics in pediatric migraine. *Headache* **27**, 16–20

Dalsgaard-Nielsen, J. (1970). Some aspects of the epidemiology of migraine in Denmark. In *Kliniske Aspekter i Migraeneforskningen.* pp. 18–30. Copenhagen, Nordlundes Bogtrykkeri

Dalton, K. (1975). Migraine and oral contraceptives. *Headache* **15**, 247–251

Damasio, H. and Beck. D. (1978). Migraine, thrombocytopenia and serotonin metabolism. *Lancet* **i**, 240 242

D'Amico, D., Leone, M., Macciardi, F., Valentini, S. and Bussone, G. (1991). Genetic transmission of migraine without aura: a study of 68 families. *Ital. J. Neurol. Sci.* **12**, 581–584

Dexter, J. D. and Riley, T. L. (1975). Studies in nocturnal migraine. *Headache* **15**, 51–62

Dorfman, L. J., Marshall, W. H. and Enzmann, D. R. (1979). Cerebral infarction and migraine: clinical and radiologic correlations. *Neurology* **29**, 317–322

Drummond, P. D. (1986). A quantitative assessment of photophobia in migraine and tension headache. *Headache* **26**, 465–469

Drummond, P. D. (1987). Pupil diameter in migraine and tension headache. *J. Neurol. Neurosurg. Psychiat.* **50**, 228–230

Essink-Bot, M L., van Royen, L., Krabbe, P., Donsel, G. J. and Rutten, F. F. H. (1995). The impact of migraine on health status. *Headache* **35**, 200–206

Fanciullacci, M. (1979). Iris adrenergic impairment in idiopathic headache. *Headache* **19**, 8–13

Fisher, C. M. (1980). Late-life migraine accompaniments as a cause of unexplained transient ischemic attacks. *Can. J. Neurol. Sci.* **7**, 917

Friedman, A. P. (1970). The (infinite) variety of migraine. In *Background to Migraine. Third Migraine Symposium*, Ed. A. L. Cochrane. pp. 165–180. London, Heinemann

Galer, B. S., Lipton, R. B., Weinstein, S., Bello, L. and Solomon, S. (1990). Apoplectic headache and oculomotor nerve palsy: an unusual presentation of multiple sclerosis. *Neurology* **40**, 1465–1466

Gardner, J. H., Van den Noort, S. and Horenstein, S. (1967). Cerebrovascular disease in young women taking oral contraceptives. *Neurology* **17**, 297–298

Gibb, C. M., Davies, P. T. G., Glover, V., Steiner, T. J., Clifford Rose, F. and Sandler, M. (1991). Chocolate is a migraine-provoking agent. *Cephalalgia* **11**, 93–95

Gomez-Aranda, F., Canadillas, F., Marti-Masso, J. F., Diez-Tejedor, E., Serano, P. J., Leira, R., Gracia, M. and Pascual, J. (1997). Pseudo-migraine with temporary neurological symptoms and lymphocytic pleocytosis. A report of 50 cases. *Brain* **120**, 1105–1113

Gotoh, F., Komatsumoto, S., Araki, N. and Gomi, S. (1984). Noradrenergic nervous activity in migraine. *Arch. Neurol.* **41**, 951–955

Green, J. E. (1977). A survey of migraine in England 1975–1976. *Headache* **17**, 67–68

Guidetti, V., Fornara, R., Ottaviano, S., Petrilli, A., Seri, S. and Cortesi, F. (1987). Personality inventory for children and childhood migraine. *Cephalalgia* **7**, 225–230

Haas, D. C., Kent, P. F. and Friedman, D. I. (1993). Headache caused by a single lesion of multiple sclerosis in the periaqueductal grey area. *Headache* **33**, 452–455

Haas, D. C., Pineda, G. S. and Lourie, H. (1975). Juvenile head trauma syndromes and their relationship to migraine. *Arch. Neurol.* **32**, 727–737

Haas, D. H. (1991). Arteriovenous malformations and migraine: case reports and an analysis of the relationship. *Headache* **31**, 509–513

Henry, P., Michel, P., Brochet, B., Dartigues, J. F., Tison, S., Salamon, R. and the GRIM (1992). A nationwide survey of migraine in France: prevalence and clinical features in adults. *Cephalalgia* **12**, 229–237

Henryk-Gutt, R. and Rees, W. L. (1973). Psychological aspects of migraine. *J. Psychosom. Res.* **17**, 141–153

Hungerford, G. D., du Boulay, G. H. and Zilkha, K. J. (1976). Computerized axial tomography in patients with severe migraine: a preliminary report. *J. Neurol. Neurosurg. Psychiat.* **39**, 990–994

Igarashi, H., Sakai, F., Kan, S., Okada, J. and Tazaki, Y. (1991). Magnetic resonance imaging of the brain in patients with migraine. *Cephalalgia* **11**, 69–74

Kayan, A. and Hood, J. D. (1984). Neuro-otological manifestations of migraine. *Brain* **107**, 1123–1142

Kunkle, E. C. and Anderson, W. B. (1961). Significance of minor eye signs in headache of migraine type. *Arch. Ophthalmol.* **65**, 504–508

Lance, J. W. and Anthony, M. (1966). Some clinical aspects of migraine: A prospective survey of 500 patients. *Arch. Neurol.* **15**, 356–361

Larsson, B., Bille, B. and Pederson, N. L. (1995). Genetic influence in headaches: a Swedish twin study. *Headache* **35**, 513–519

Laurence, K. M. (1987). Genetics of migraine. In *Migraine. Clinical and Research Aspects*, Ed. J. N. Blau. pp. 479–484. Baltimore, Johns Hopkins University Press

Lauritzen, M., Trojaborg, W. and Olesen, J. (1981). EEG during attacks of common and classical migraine. *Cephalalgia* **1**, 63–66

Leviton, A. and Camenga, D. (1969). Migraine associated with hyper-pre-beta-lipoproteinemia. *Neurology* **19**, 963–966

Levor, R. M., Cohen, M. J., Naliboff, B. D. and McArthur, D. (1986). Psychosocial precursors and correlates of migraine headache. *J. Consult. Clin. Psychol.* **54**, 347–353

Linet, M. S., Stewart, W. F., Celentano, D. D., Ziegler, D. and Sprechner, M. (1989). An epidemiologic study of headache among adolescents and young adults. *JAMA* **261**, 2211–2216

Lipton, R. B., Silberstein, D. S. and Stewart, W. F. (1994). An update on the epidemiology of migraine. *Headache* **34**, 319–328

Litman, G. I. and Friedman, H. M. (1978). Migraine and the mitral valve prolapse syndrome. *Am. Heart J.* **96**, 610–614

Littlewood, J. T., Gibb, C., Glover, V., Sandler, M., Davies, P. T. G. and Clifford Rose, F. (1988). Red wine as a cause of migraine. *Lancet* **i**, 558–559

Lord, G. D. A. (1982). A study of premonitory focal neurological symptoms in migraine. In *Advances in Migraine Research and Therapy.*, Ed. F. Clifford Rose. pp. 45–48. New York, Raven Press

Marcus, D. A. and Soso, M. J. (1989). Migraine and stripe-induced visual discomfort. *Arch. Neurol.* **46**, 1129–1132

Mathew, N. T., Meyer, J. S., Welch, K. M. A. and Neblett, C. R. (1977). Abnormal CT scans in migraine. *Headache* **16**, 272–279

Matthews, W. B. (1972). Footballer's migraine. *Br. Med. J.* **1**, 326–327

McQueen, J., Loblay, R. H., Swain, A. R., Anthony, M. and Lance, J. W. (1989). A controlled trial of dietary modification in migraine. In *New Advances in Headache Research*, Ed. F. Clifford Rose. pp. 235–242. London, Smith-Gordon

Medina, J. L. and Diamond, S. (1976). Migraine and atopy. *Headache* **15**, 271–274

Medina, J. L. and Diamond, S. (1978). The role of diet in migraine. *Headache* **18**, 31–34

Merikangas, K.R. (1996). Sources of genetic complexity in migraine. In *Migraine, Pharmacology and Genetics*, Eds M. Sandler, M. Ferraris and S. Harnett, pp 254–281. London, Chapman and Hall

Merikangas, K. R. and Angst, J. (1990). Depression and migraine. In *Migraine, A Spectrum of Ideas*, Eds M. Sandler and G. Collins, pp 248–258. Oxford, Oxford University Press

Merrett, J., Peatfield, R. C., Clifford Rose, F. and Merrett, T. G. (1983). Food-related antibodies in headache patients. *J. Neurol. Neurosurg. Psychiat.* **46**, 738–742

Monro, J., Brostoff, J., Carini, C. and Zilkha, K. (1980). Food allergy in migraine: study of dietary exclusion and RAST. *Lancet* **ii**, 1–4

Nager, B. J., Lanska, D. J. and Daroff, R. B. (1989). Acute demyelination mimicking vascular hemicrania. *Neurology* **29**, 423–424

Nikiforow, R. and Hokkanen, E. (1979). Effects of headache on working ability: a survey of an urban and a rural population in Northern Finland. *Headache* **19**, 214–218

Osuntokun, B. O., Bademosi, O. and Osuntokun, O. (1982). Migraine in Nigeria. In *Advances in Migraine Research and Therapy*, Ed. F. Clifford Rose. pp. 25–38. New York, Raven Press

Osuntokun, B. O. and Osuntokun, O. (1972). Complicated migraine and haemoglobin AS in Nigerians. *Br. Med. J.* **2**, 621–622

Ottman, R. and Lipton R. B. (1994). Comorbidity of migraine and epilepsy. *Neurology* **44**, 2105–2110

Ottman, R. and Lipton, R. B. (1996). Is the comorbidity of epilepsy and migraine due to a shared genetic susceptibility? *Neurology* **47**, 918–924

Panayiotopoulos, C. P. (1987). Difficulties in differentiating migraine and epilepsy based on clinical and EEG findings. In *Migraine and Epilepsy*, Eds. A. Andermann and E. Lugaresi. pp. 31–46. Boston, Butterworths

Panayiotopoulos, C. P. (1996). Elementary visual hallucinations in migraine and epilepsy. *J. Neurol. Neurosurg. Psychiat.* **60**, 117

Parker, R. J., Vezina, G. and Stacy Nicholson, H. (1994). Complicated 'migraine-like' headaches in children following cranial irradiation and chemotherapy. *Ann. Neurol.* **36**, 509–510

Pestronk, A. and Pestronk, S. (1983). Goggle migraine. *New Engl. J. Med.* **308**, 226–227

Pfaffenrath, V., Kommissari, I., Pöllman, W., Kaube, H. and Rath, M. (1991). Cerebrovascular risk factors in migraine with prolonged aura and without aura. *Cephalalgia* **11**, 257–261

Rasmussen, B. K., Jensen, R. and Olesen, J. (1992). Impact of headache on sickness absence and utilisation of medical services: A Danish population study. *J. Epidemiol. Community Health* **46**, 443–446

Rasmussen, B. K., Jensen, R., Schroll, M. and Olesen, J. (1991). Epidemiology of headache in a general population: a prevalence study. *J. Clin. Epidemiol.* **44**, 1147–1157

Rolak, L. A. (1985). Headache in patients with multiple sclerosis. *Neurology* **35** (Suppl. 1), 267

Rowat, B. M. T., Merrill, C. F., Davis, A. and South, V. (1991). A double-blind comparison of granisetron and placebo for the treatment of acute migraine in the emergency department. *Cephalalgia* **11**, 207–213

Russell, M. B. and Olesen, J. (1995). Increased familial risk and evidence of genetic factor in migraine. *Brit. Med. J.* **311**, 541–544

Sacks, O. W. (1992). *Migraine*. pp 37–38. Berkeley, University of California Press

Scobie, B. A. (1983). Recurrent vomiting in adults. A syndrome? *Med. J. Aust.* **1**, 329–331

Selby, G. and Lance, J. W. (1960). Observations on 500 cases of migraine and allied vascular headache. *J. Neurol. Neurosurg. Psychiat.* **23**, 23–32

Septien, L., Pelletier, J. L., Brunotte, F., Giroud, M. and Dumas, R. (1991). Migraine in patients with history of centro-temporal epilepsy in childhood. *Cephalalgia* **11**, 281–284

Shuaib, A. and Hachinski, V. C. (1988). Migraine and the risks from angiography. *Arch. Neurol.* **45**, 911–912

Silberstein, S. D., Lipton, R. B. and Breslau, N. (1995). Migraine: association with personality characteristics and psychopathology. *Cephalalgia* **15**, 358–369

Silberstein, S. D. and Merriam, G. R. (1991). Estrogens, progestins, and headache. *Neurology* **41**, 786–793

Soges, L. J., Cacayorin, E. D., Petro, G. R. and Ramachandran, T. S. (1988). Migraine: evaluation by MR. *Am. J. Neuroradiol.* **9**, 425–429

Somerville, B. W. (1971). The role of progesterone in menstrual migraine. *Neurology, Minneap.* **21**, 853–859

Somerville, B. W. (1972a). The role of oestradiol withdrawal in the etiology of menstrual migraine. *Neurology, Minneap.* **22**, 355–365

Somerville, B. W. (1972b). A study of migraine in pregnancy. *Neurology, Minneap.* **22**, 824–828

Stanford, E. and Green, R. (1970). A case of migraine cured by treatment of Conn's syndrome. In *Background to Migraine. Third British Migraine Symposium.* pp. 53–57. London, Heinemann

Stewart, W. F., Lipton, R. B., Celentano, D. D. and Reed, M. L. (1992). Prevalence of migraine headache in the United States. Relation to age, income, race and other sociodemographic factors. *JAMA* **267**, 64–69

Stewart, W. F., Lipton, R. B. and Liberman, J. (1996). Variation in migraine prevalence by race. *Neurology* **47**, 52–59

Stewart, W. F., Lipton, R. B. and Simon, D. (1996). Work-related disability: results from the American Migraine Study. *Cephalalgia* **16**, 231–238

Sulman, F. G, Danon, A., Pfeifer, Y., Tal, E. and Weller, C. P. (1970). Urinalysis of patients suffering from climatic heat stress. *Int. J. Biomet.* **14**, 45–53

Tfelt-Hansen, P., Lous, I. and Olesen, J. (1981). Prevalence and significance of muscle tenderness during migraine attacks. *Headache* **21**, 49–54

Thomas, D. J., Robinson, S., Robinson, A. and Johnson, D. G. (1996). Migraine threshold is altered in hyperthyroidism. *J. Neurol. Neurosurg. Psychiat.* **61**, 222

van der Linden, J. A. (1660). *De Hemicrania Menstrua.* Amsterdam, Elsevier

Watkins, S. M. and Espir, M. (1969). Migraine and multiple sclerosis. *J. Neurol. Neurosurg. Psychiat.* **32**, 35–37

Webster, I. W., Waddy, N., Jenkins, L. V. and Lai, Y. C. L. (1977). Health status of a group of narcotic addicts in a methadone treatment programme. *Med. J. Aust.* **2**, 485–491

Welch, K. M. A. and Levine, S. R. (1990). Migraine-related stroke in the context of the International Headache Society classification of head pain. *Arch. Neurol.* **47**, 458–462

Whitty, C. W. M. and Hockaday, J. M. (1968). Migraine. A follow-up study of 92 patients. *Br. Med. J.* **1**, 735–736

Winter, A. L. (1987). Neurophysiology and migraine. In *Migraine. Clinical and Research Aspects*, Ed. J. N. Blau. pp. 485–510. Baltimore, Johns Hopkins University Press

Wolff, H. G. (1963). *Headache and Other Head Pain.* p. 327. New York, Oxford University Press

Woodhouse, A. and Drummond, P. D. (1993). Mechanisms of increased sensitivity to noise and light in migraine headache. *Cephalalgia* **13**, 417–421

Zahavi. I., Chagnac, A., Hering, R., Davidovich, S. and Kuritzky, A. (1984). Prevalence of Raynaud's phenomenon in patients with migraine. *Arch. Intern. Med.* **144**, 742–744

Ziegler, D. K., Batnitzky, S., Barter, R. and McMillan, J. H. (1991). Magnetic Resonance Image abnormality in migraine with aura. *Cephalalgia* **11**, 147–150

Chapter 8

Migraine: pathophysiology

Migraine may be regarded as an hereditary tendency to have headache that is characterized by certain associated signature symptoms, such as nausea or sensitivity to light, sound or to head movement. The basis of this predisposition is instability in the control of pain and other sensory information coming from the pain-producing intracranial structures and a sensitivity to cyclic changes in the central nervous system. The frequency of migraine headache varies from once in a lifetime to almost daily, so that there may be no clear dividing line between a migrainous and non-migrainous brain although the degree of predisposition may vary. Our present concept is one of a threshold of susceptibility determined by some of the factors mentioned below.

The predisposition – a migrainous brain

What are the factors that may play a part in setting the migrainous threshold?

Genetic factors

Perhaps among the most important recent developments in understanding migraine pathophysiology have been advances in understanding the possible basis for the hereditary aspects of the disease. It has been long speculated and most clearly demonstrated from twin studies that there is an important hereditary component to migraine. It has been shown that a rare form of migraine that is clearly autosomal dominant, familial hemiplegic migraine, can be due to mis-sense mutations in the α_1 subunit of the P/Q type voltage-gated calcium channel on chromosome 19 (Ophoff et al., 1996). This mutation explains about 55 per cent of cases with a further 15 per cent being recently localized to another locus on chromosome 1 (Ducros et al., 1997) and the final 30 per cent being unaccounted for at present. This finding in this rare form of migraine has an important biological implication. Neurological disorders due to abnormalities in channels, so called channelopathies (Griggs and Nutt, 1995), often have the characteristic of episodicity which is so much a part of migraine.

Abnormalities on chromosome 19 may account in part for the genetic suscepti-bility to other types of migraine in some patients (May et al., 1995) but much work needs to be done to sort out the molecular basis of migraine. Other recent data have suggested the involvement of various parts of the dopamine receptor and synthesis pathways (Peroutka, 1997) and more data are eagerly awaited.

Magnesium deficiency

The measurement of brain phosphates by nuclear magnetic resonance imaging after the intravenous injection of ^{31}P has enabled the indirect assay of magnesium content by examining the chemical shift properties of the ^{31}P resonance signals. By using this non-invasive technique Welch's group (Ramadan et al., 1989) found that magnesium ion concentration was lower during migraine headache. Magnesium ion concentration gates and blocks the N-methyl-D-aspartate (NMDA)-subtype glutamate receptor so that this preliminary result suggests a basis for cerebral hyperexcitability via increased activity at NMDA receptors (Welch and Ramadan, 1995). Given that NMDA-mediated activation is essential for spreading depression (Lauritzen, 1994), a relative reduction in brain magnesium may make the brain more susceptible to triggering of spreading depression.

Excitatory amino acids

D'Andrea et al. (1989a) reported that the platelet content of glutamate and aspartate was increased in patients subject to migraine with aura, during headache-free periods, when compared with normal controls and migraine patients without aura. The glutamate level rose further during headache. Ferrari et al. (1990) measured these amino acids in plasma and found the level to be elevated in migraine patients between attacks, more so in those patients whose migraine was accompanied by an aura, and to increase further during headache. If a similar elevation of excitatory amino acids were shown to exist in the cortex, this would also increase its excitability.

Neurophysiological changes

The contingent negative variation, a slow event-related potential which is thought to be mediated by noradrenergic pathways, is enhanced in migraine patients and is reduced by the administration of beta-blockers (Maertens de Noordhout, Timsit-Berthier and Schoenen, 1985). The amplitude difference between the primary positive and negative waves of the visual evoked response is increased in migrainous subjects (Gawel, Connolly and Clifford Rose, 1983). Variations in the visual evoked responses are not related to the duration or severity of migraine attacks and probably reflect a predisposition to migraine (Winter, 1987). Migraine sufferers do not show the same habituation of visual evoked potentials over time as normal controls (Schoenen et al., 1995). Consistent with this increased level of activation the intensity dependence of the auditory cortical evoked potential is increased in migraine sufferers (Wang, Timsit-Berthier and Schoenen, 1996).

The hypothalamo-pituitary axis and dopaminergic transmission

There is some interesting evidence for a role of dopaminergic transmission in the pathophysiology of migraine (Peroutka, 1997). About 25 per cent of patients report symptoms of elation, irritability, depression, hunger, thirst or drowsiness during the 24 hours preceding headache. Most of these manifestations can arise in the hypothalamus (Kupfermann, 1985) and this, along with circadian functions in the region of the suprachiasmatic nucleus (Swaab et al., 1993), suggests a central site for their evolution. A substantial proportion of migraine patients report yawning (Russell et al., 1996) which, of all the premonitory symptoms, is most distinctively dopaminergic. Yawning can be activated in experimental animals by dopamine-2 receptor activation (Serra, Collu and Gessa, 1986) but is blocked by dopamine-1 receptor blockers although not by peripherally acting drugs like domperidone (Serra, Collu and Gessa, 1987). Similarly, in humans the potent dopamine receptor agonist apomorphine induces yawning in a greater number of migraineurs than controls (Bene, Poggonioni and de Tommasi, 1994; Blin et al., 1991) and may induce headache (Bene, Poggonioni and de Tommasi, 1994). Migraine is uncommon in patients with Parkinson's disease yet apomorphine can induce migraine in patients with a past history of the condition (Sabatini et al., 1990).

Suppression of prolactin secretion by dopaminergic agents is diminished in migrainous women (Nappi and Savoldi, 1985) and the control of prolactin secretion varies between control subjects and migraineurs during the menstrual cycle (Murialdo et al., 1986). Prolactin is excreted excessively in response to stimulation of the hypothalamus by hormones (Awaki et al., 1989) or, in the case of migraine patients with aura, by a levodopa loading test (Vardi et al., 1981). These data suggest dominance of excitatory 5-hydroxytryptamine (5-HT) mechanisms over dopaminergic inhibition. Glover et al. (1996) reported that the administration of fenfluramine, which releases 5-HT, caused a significantly higher prolactin level in eight migraineurs and than in six controls, suggesting supersensitivity of hypothalamic 5-HT receptors. Five patients developed migraine headache 1 hour after fenfluramine, at which time the prolactin level started to rise. It peaked at 3 hours and returned to baseline level at about 5 hours. Previous studies had not shown any prolactin increase with unprovoked migraine headache.

The thyrotropin response to TRH (thyrotropin releasing hormone) is also diminished in some migraine patients (Daras et al., 1987). Patients with 'essential headache', including migraine, are more responsive to hallucinogenic agents such as LSD and psilocybin than control subjects (Fanciullacci, Franchi and Sicuteri, 1974). Migraine patients are unusually sensitive to the emetic effects of apomorphine (Sicuteri, 1977) and become hypotensive more readily when given bromocriptine (Fanciullacci et al., 1980). Information presently available therefore suggests a dopamine deficiency in migraine with supersensitivity of dopamine receptors.

Opioids and the endogenous pain control system

Endogenous opioids have been implicated as inhibitory neurotransmitters liberated from interneurones in the central regulation of pain pathways. They comprise β-

endorphin, enkephalins and dynorphins. There have been conflicting reports on plasma β-endorphin levels in migraine. Bach *et al.* (1985) could not detect any difference between plasma levels in and out of attacks. Plasma methionine-metenke-phalin levels are higher in migraine patients than in normal controls and increase further during headache (Ferrari *et al.*, 1987; Mosnaim *et al.*, 1985). The extent to which blood and CSF levels reflect central opioid function remains uncertain. It is interesting that the intramuscular injection of naloxone 0.8 mg shortened the migrainous aura in most patients but, when the aura followed its usual course, the ensuing headache was of normal severity (Sicuteri *et al.*, 1983).

Pain control mechanisms must be partially defective in migraine patients because spontaneous jabs of pain in the head ('ice-pick pains') and headaches induced by eating ice-cream are more common in migraine patients than in control subjects. Drummond and Lance (1984) found that both of these pains were felt in the part of the head habitually affected by migraine headache in about one-third of patients, indicating a latent defect in that part of the endogenous pain control system.

Vascular reactivity

The cerebral vasodilator response to carbon dioxide is greater in migraine patients than in normal controls (Sakai and Meyer, 1979) and the reaction of extracranial arteries to exercise (Drummond and Lance, 1981) and stress (Drummond, 1982) is greater on the side of their usual migraine headache.

The trigger – initiation of the migraine attack

Given that the brain of susceptible subjects has a low 'migraine threshold' as outlined above, what is responsible for triggering each episode? For many patients, no external factor can be identified. Episodes may recur regularly as though determined by some internal clock. It is probable that the relevant biological clock involves the hypothalamus (Figure 8.1) because premonitory symptoms, such as elation, a craving for sweet foods, thirst or drowsiness, may precede headache by some 24 hours (Blau, 1980; Drummond and Lance, 1984). In other cases, the attack originates in the nervous system in response to stress or excessive afferent stimulation such as flickering light, noise or the smell of strong perfumes.

Some trigger factors appear to act primarily on the cranial blood vessels (Figure 8.1). For example, the injection of a contrast medium into the carotid or vertebro-basilar circulations or the ingestion of vasodilator agents. Nitrates cause vasodilatation by conversion to nitric oxide. Headaches may be caused by vascular distension, particularly if the wall is sensitized by a perivascular reaction caused, for example, by antidromic release of peptides from the trigeminovascular system (Buzzi and Moskowitz, 1990; Moskowitz, 1984; Moskowitz and Buzzi, 1991). Craniovascular afferents may then excite central pathways (Figure 8.2, 8.3). The migraine attack clearly depends upon interaction between the brain and the cranial circulation.

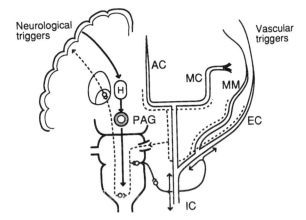

Figure 8.1 The mechanism of migraine headache. Migraine can be initiated by a central generator, probably in the vicinity of the hypothalamus (H) or triggered by afferent stimulation such as flickering light, noise or strong smells. Descending fibres influence the processing of head pain and originate in the upper brain-stem, periaqueductal grey matter (PAG) and dorsolateral pontine tegmentum. Migraine can also be triggered by stimulation of vascular afferents (vasodilator drugs, arteriography) which induce excessive neural activity in central pathways released from modulation by the pain control system as well as increasing vasodilatation by the trigeminovascular reflex illustrated in Figure 8.2. Arteries: middle meningeal (MM), external carotid (EC), others as in Figure 8.2

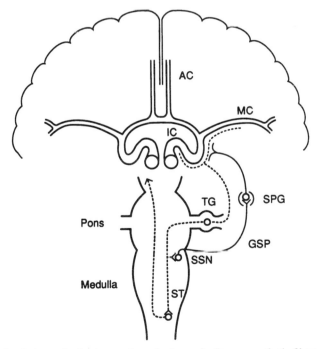

Figure 8.2 Interaction between brain stem and cerebral vessels. Parasympathetic fibres arising from the superior salivatory nucleus (SSN) pass in the greater superficial petrosal (GSP) nerve, synapse in the sphenopalatine ganglion (SPG) and supply the cerebral arteries with vasodilator fibres. Afferent fibres from the vessels traverse the trigeminal ganglion (TG), descend in the spinal tract (ST) and send collaterals to the SSN, completing the trigeminovascular reflex. Arteries: internal carotid (IC), anterior cerebral (AC), middle cerebral (MC)

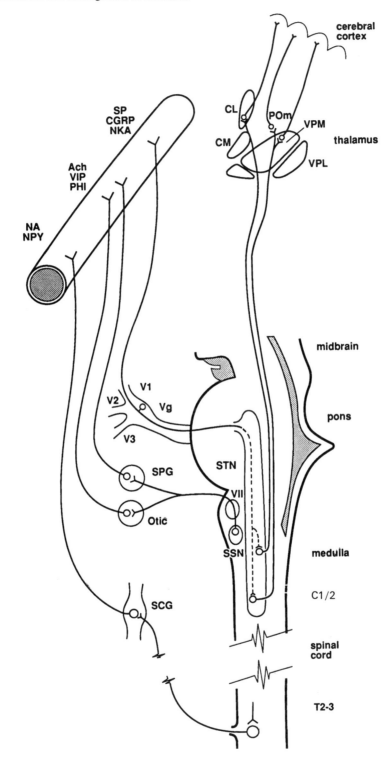

The migrainous aura – is it spreading depression?

Attention has been lavished on the migrainous aura because of the spectacular and often frightening nature of the symptoms, although most migraine patients will never have an aura. The classical 'slow march' of symptoms such as fortification spectra is experienced by only 10 per cent of patients, whereas less specific disturbances of 'spots in front of the eyes' or 'shimmering vision' cover the whole visual field simultaneously in about 25 per cent (Lance and Anthony, 1966).

Human observation of aura

Lashley (1941) plotted the expansion of his own visual scotoma in migraine and calculated that the visual cortex was being compromised by some process advancing at about 3 mm each minute. A similar conclusion was reached by Lauritzen et al. (1983a) who demonstrated by blood flow studies that oligaemia spread from the occipital lobe forwards over the cortex with much the same speed, between 2 and 6 mm each minute (Figure 8.4).

In some patients with migrainous aura (Olesen, Larsen and Lauritzen, 1981) or hemiplegic migraine (Friberg et al., 1987), patchy areas of increased blood flow have been seen before cerebral blood flow diminished. Diminution of the flow starts in the occipital region or watershed area at the occipito-parietal junction and extends forward as a 'spreading oligaemia' (Olesen, Larsen and Lauritzen, 1981). The wave of oligaemia progresses over the cortex at about 2–3 mm per minute, irrespective of arterial territories, stopping short at the central and lateral sulci, although the frontal lobes also become oligaemic independently in some patients (Lauritzen et al., 1983a). Spreading oligaemia typically begins before the patient notices focal neurological symptoms and reaches the sensorimotor area only after the appropriate symptoms have started and outlasts these symptoms. Oligaemia lasts for several hours and is followed by delayed hyperaemia (Andersen et al., 1988). The headache usually starts while cerebral blood flow is still diminished (Olesen et al., 1990) (Figure 8.5). From these studies, the authors concluded that cortical oligaemia was a reflection of cortical spreading depression (CSD), which was responsible for

---

Figure 8.3 Peptide neurotransmitters associated with afferent and efferent pathways in the trigeminovascular system. (From Goadsby, Zagami and Lambert, 1991, by permission of the editor of *Headache*)

Vascular afferent fibres have their cell bodies in the Gasserian ganglion (Vg) and descend in the spinal tract of the trigeminal nerve before synapsing in the nucleus caudalis and the upper cervical (C1/2) segments of the spinal cord, the trigeminocervical complex. The second-order neurones project to the ventroposteromedial (VPM), the intralaminar or centrolateral (CL) nuclei of the thalamus and the medial nucleus of the posterior complex (POm). The centromedian (CM) and ventroposterolateral (VPL) nuclei are also marked on the diagram. Other structures that take part in migraine are: the trigeminovascular system, marked by the neuropeptides substance P (SP), calcitonin gene-related peptide (CGRP) and neurokinin A (NKA); sympathetic fibres originating in the superior cervical ganglion (SCG) marked by noradrenaline (NA), peptide YY (PYY) and neuropeptide Y (NPY); and parasympathetic fibres arising in the superior salivatory nucleus (SSN) that emerge in the seventh cranial nerve (VII) and traverse the sphenopalatine ganglion (SPG) and otic ganglion, being marked by vasoactive intestinal polypeptide (VIP), peptide histidine isoleucine (PHI) and acetylcholine (ACh).

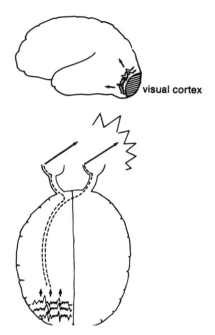

Figure 8.4 Mechanism of fortification spectra. A wave of excitation followed by inhibition moves slowly over the visual cortex, causing scintillations and scotomas in the contralateral half of the visual field. (From Lance, 1986, by permission of the publishers, Charles Scribner's Sons, New York)

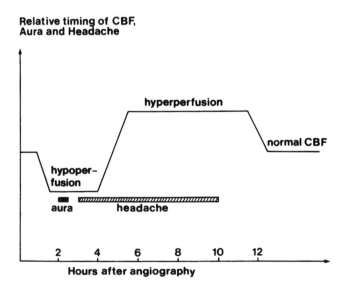

Figure 8.5 Relationship of aura and headache to changes in regional cerebral blood flow (CBF). (From Olesen *et al.*, 1990, by permission of the editor of *Annals of Neurology*)

the slow march of fortification spectra and other neurological symptoms as Leão had predicted (Lauritzen, 1994).

The description of a patient with migraine without aura who had an attack during a positron emission tomography (PET) study (Woods, Iacoboni and Mazziotta, 1994) placed beyond doubt the existence of the phenomenon of spreading oligaemia. When this is considered with the earlier observation of Herold *et al.* (1985) that a migrainous aura was not accompanied by hypoxia, the arguments ventured that the spreading oligaemia is due to Compton scatter and ischaemia (Friberg *et al.*, 1987; Skyhøj-Olsen, Friberg and Lassen, 1987) can be discarded. Similarly, studies have now emerged using functional MRI (fMRI) blood flow methods, such as BOLD (blood oxygenation level detection), to demonstrate spreading flow changes in aura (Cutrer *et al.*, 1998) which again have been argued to be not ischaemic in nature (Cao *et al.*, 1997).

The PET study of Woods and colleagues (1994) did, however, open a more interesting question. The patient studied did *not* have aura in any traditional sense, indeed she only had some transient visual blurring. These data open up the exciting possibility that blood flow changes may occur in both migraine with and without aura. Indeed it is remarkable that a spreading oligaemia can traverse cortex usually considered clinically eloquent and have little clinical sequelae. Perhaps remarks by patients of impaired concentration and memory should be viewed in the context of subtle pathophysiological changes that may be taking place.

Animal studies of spreading depression

Leão (1944) described a progressive shutdown of cortical function, known as 'spreading depression', in animal brain and speculated that it may be related to the fortification spectra of migraine. Waves of inhibition (often preceded by transient excitation) move slowly over the cerebral cortex, suppressing normal activity, at a speed of 2–3 mm each minute and lasting for 5–60 minutes before recovery takes place. Spreading depression may be preceded or followed by a phase of vasoconstriction and is associated with dilatation of the pial arteries and cerebral oedema. Lauritzen *et al.* (1982) showed that induced spreading depression in the rat was accompanied by a transient hyperaemia for some 3 minutes followed by a 20–25 per cent depression of cerebral blood flow for 60 minutes or more. Comparable changes have been found in the gyrencephalic cortex of the cat (Goadsby, 1992; Piper, Lambert and Duckworth, 1991) and in the brain stem of the rat (Mraovitch *et al.*, 1992). Spreading depression has been described in the human hippocampus and caudate nucleus during stereotactic surgery by Sramka *et al.* (1977). Piper *et al.* (1991) have looked for signs of spreading depression during neurosurgical operations, with suggestive changes in cortical blood flow found in only two of nine patients studied.

Gloor (1986) reported in a letter that he had not observed EEG changes consistent with spreading depression during human neurosurgery while others have not observed the electrical changes when directly studied in human cortex (McLachlan and Girvin, 1994). Barkley *et al.* (1990), using magnetoencephalography, have demonstrated long-duration decrements in EEG amplitude and large amplitude DC shifts in migraine patients during headache (14 migraine with aura, three migraine without aura). The latter two changes are similar to those seen during CSD in animals and suggest that these findings may represent evidence of CSD in humans.

Correlating aura and spreading depression

The neurological changes during aura parallel what is seen when the brain is directly stimulated (Brindley and Lewin, 1968; Penfield and Perot, 1963) and resemble what might be predicted if ocular dominance columns (Hubel and Weisel, 1968) were serially activated. Cerebrovascular reactivity is altered in the low-flow areas observed during the aura. Olesen, Larsen and Lauritzen (1981) demonstrated impairment of the usual increase in cortical flow accompanying cortical activation. Three groups using xenon-133 clearance have found that reactivity to hypercapnia is impaired during the aura of migraine (Lauritzen et al., 1983b; Sakai and Meyer, 1979; Simard and Paulson, 1973). Sakai and Meyer (1979) considered that autoregulation was impaired, whereas Lauritzen (1994) found that it was not disturbed. As loss of CO_2 reactivity and reduced cortical blood flow during functional activation with preservation of autoregulation are characteristics of spreading depression (Lauritzen, 1984; Piper et al., 1991), their convincing demonstration during the migrainous aura would help to define a pathophysiological role for CSD in humans.

An interesting pharmacotherapeutic correlate between experimental work and aura is that in some species the cerebral blood flow changes associated with spreading depression can be attenuated or eliminated by blockade of nitric oxide synthase (NOS) (Goadsby, Kaube and Hoskin, 1992), while Olesen's group has recently demonstrated that NOS blockade can abort acute migraine attacks including headache and other symptoms (Lassen et al., 1997). When these various observations are taken together, spreading depression or the human equivalent, made somewhat different by the cytoarchitecture of the human brain, is the most likely explanation for the migrainous aura.

The relationship of the aura to migraine headache

Although auras may occur without an ensuing headache and migraine headache usually occurs without any aura, it is tempting to seek some connection between the two phenomena. Is it possible that the cortical events responsible for the aura also set in train the neurovascular disturbance that causes headache?

Moskowitz and his colleagues (1993) have shown that the intravenous injection of capsaicin or stimulation of the trigeminal nerve for 5 minutes induces plasma extravasation from dural vessels in rats, neurogenic plasma protein extravasation (PPE; see below). Moskowitz (1984) suggested that his experimental findings showed how the trigeminal nerve, or the central nervous system via the trigeminal nerve, could provoke unilateral vascular changes, and that the antidromic release of vasodilator peptides from the nerve could induce a sterile inflammatory reaction responsible for headache. Moskowitz thought that spreading depression of the cortex during the aura phase of migraine might depolarize trigeminal nerve fibres surrounding the pial arteries and thus initiate the headache phase of migraine (Moskowitz, Nozaki and

Kraig, 1993). If this were the case, headache would always develop on the side of the head responsible for the cerebral symptoms, i.e. a left visual field aura would be followed by a right-sided headache. Most authors agree that the headache may appear on the inappropriate side (Peatfield and Rose, 1991).

Olesen el al. (1990) have also sought to link the phenomena underlying the aura phase with the development of headache. They found that the majority of patients studied did have their headache on the side relevant to the production of the aura but, even so, three of their 38 patients experienced their unilateral headache on the 'wrong' side. Of 19 patients with bilateral headache, aura symptoms were bilateral in six and unilateral in 13. Of 10 patients with bilateral aura, six developed bilateral and four unilateral headache. An earlier prospective study of the Copenhagen group had found that aura symptoms were ipsilateral to the headache in 19 patients and contralateral in 18 (Jensen *et al.*, 1986).

The correlation between the site of the cortical process responsible for the aura (constriction of the cortical microcirculation, cerebral oligaemia and spreading depression) and the site of the headache which may follow is by no means invariable. There is no evidence that ischaemia alone or the metabolic change accompanying spreading depression is sufficient to cause headache. We have to account for the large number of patients who experience migraine headache without aura or, less commonly, aura without headache. To do this we have to consider the following possibilities:

1. That the process causing the aura is an intrinsic property of cerebral cortex, which may trigger pain on either side of the head by central connections.
2. That projections from brain stem to cortex may play a part in initiating the aura and the vascular changes of migraine. In this way brain stem activity could account for the dissociation between aura and headache, and for the switching of headache from one side to the other during a migraine attack.

The source of pain in migraine

Migraine headache often starts as a dull pain in the frontotemporal region, upper neck or occipital area and becomes pulsatile in character only as the severity of the attack increases. Because of the throbbing quality of the pain, the conspicuous dilatation of extracranial arteries in some instances and the known pain sensitivity of cranial blood vessels, migraine has long been considered as a 'vascular headache'.

Pain-producing structures

Our knowledge of pain-producing structures in the human head owes much to the work of Harold G. Wolff and his colleagues who studied the reaction of conscious subjects to the probing, stimulation or distension of the brain, meninges and blood vessels (Wolff, 1963). Direct stimulation of the cerebral cortex, the ependymal lining of the ventricles, choroid plexuses and much of the dura and pia-arachnoid does not cause pain, although selective stimulation of certain areas in the brain may augment

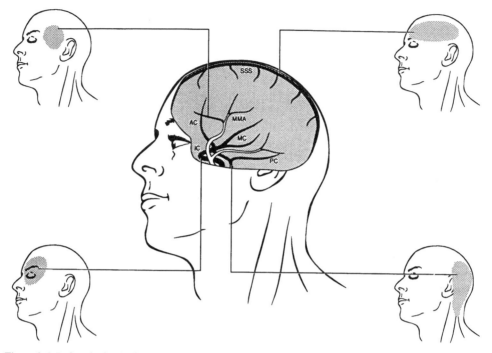

Figure 8.6 Referral of pain from intracranial vessels. (Fields of referral are based on the observations of Wolff, 1963)

Internal carotid artery (IC), anterior cerebral artery (AC), middle cerebral artery (MC), posterior cerebral artery (PC), middle meningeal artery (MMA) and superior sagittal sinus (SSS).

or diminish the perception of pain. The floor of the anterior and posterior fossa gives rise to pain but the middle cranial fossa is sensitive only in the vicinity of the middle cerebral artery. The most important structures that register pain are the blood vessels, particularly the proximal part of the cerebral and dural arteries, and the large veins and venous sinuses (Ray and Wolff, 1940).

Cranial bone is insensitive but pain is experienced when the periosteum is stretched (Wolff, 1963). Distension of the middle meningeal artery causes referred pain to the back of the eye as well as the overlying area (Figure 8.6). Stimulation of the intracranial segment of the internal carotid artery and the proximal 2 cm of the middle cerebral and anterior cerebral arteries causes referred pain to the area in and around the eye, including forehead and temple. The vertebral artery causes referred pain to the occiput. Pain elicited from the superior sagittal sinus is less intense than that evoked from cerebral arteries and is felt in the frontoparietal area on the side stimulated (Wolff, 1963) (Figure 8.6). Inflation of a balloon in the internal carotid and middle cerebral arteries (Nichols *et al.*, 1993) during embolization of arteriovenous malformations has given additional localizing information. The distal internal carotid artery and proximal part of the middle cerebral artery causes discomfort or pain in an area lateral to the eye, whereas the middle third causes retro-orbital pain and the distal third of the middle cerebral artery causes referred pain above the ipsilateral

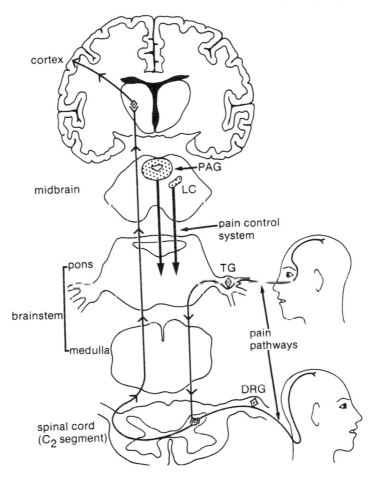

Figure 8.7 Pathways serving head pain. (From Lance, 1986, by permission of the publishers, Charles Scribner's Sons, New York)

The main afferent pathway for the anterior two-thirds of the head is the ophthalmic division of the trigeminal nerve. The central axon of the cell body in the trigeminal ganglion (TG) descends in the spinal tract of the trigeminal nerve to the second cervical cord segment where fibres from the occipital region traverse the dorsal root ganglion (DRG) to converge on second-order neurones. Transmission at this synapse is controlled by the endogenous pain control system descending from the periaqueductal grey matter (PAG) and the region of the locus coeruleus (LC).

eye. In general terms, pain arising from the anterior and middle fossae is felt anterior to a line drawn vertically above the ear, whereas pain from the posterior fossa or neck is felt behind that line, although referral of pain from one to the other region is common (Figure 8.7).

Nociceptive pathways from dural and intracranial vessels

Pain from the upper surface of the tentorium and the anterior and middle cranial fossae is transmitted by the trigeminal nerve. In 1851, Arnold described the tentorial

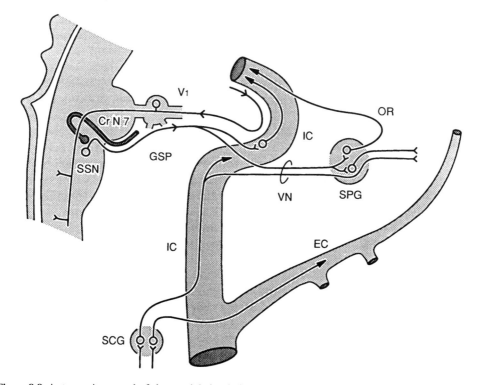

Figure 8.8 Autonomic control of the cranial circulation

Parasympathetic fibres arise in the superior salivatory nucleus (SSN) and accompany the facial nerve (CrN7) before branching off as the greater superficial petrosal (GSP) nerve to synapse on cells in the wall of the internal carotid (IC) artery while other fibres pass on with sympathetic fibres in the Vidian nerve (VN) to the sphenopalatine ganglion (SPG). Post-ganglionic neurones innervate branches of the external carotid (EC) artery as well as looping back to the internal carotid artery, via orbital rami (OR).
   Sympathetic fibres from the superior cervical ganglion (SCG) form a plexus in the walls of both internal and external carotid arteries. Afferent fibres from the internal carotid circulation traverse the first division of the trigeminal nerve (V_1).

nerve, which supplies the superior surface of the tentorium, falx and venous sinuses. Most of its fibres originate from the ophthalmic division (McNaughton, 1938), so that pain from these structures is referred to the eye and frontoparietal area (Figure 8.6). In monkeys, trigeminal and sympathetic fibres from the superior cervical ganglion mingle in the wall of the cavernous sinus, forming the cavernous plexus from which the tentorial nerve arises (Ruskell, 1988).

   Some parasympathetic fibres from the pterygopalatine (sphenopalatine) ganglion as well as some fibres from the second trigeminal division join the plexus anteriorly. Horse-radish peroxidase (HRP) tracer studies in cats have shown that the recurrent parasympathetic fibres are distributed to the middle cerebral artery (Walters, Gillespie and Moskowitz 1986). Application of HRP to the proximal segment of the middle cerebral artery in cats labelled cell bodies in that part of the trigeminal ganglion receiving afferents from the ophthalmic division (Mayberg *et al.*, 1981) (see Figure 8.8). The internal carotid artery and the anterior part of the circle of

Willis in monkeys is innervated by branches of the cavernous plexus containing trigeminal and autonomic fibres (Ruskell and Simons, 1987). Other branches of the cavernous plexus pass back with the sixth cranial (abducens) nerve to its origin from the pons where they join the basilar artery to be distributed to the posterior half of the circle of Willis and vertebral arteries. It is probable that branches of the vagal and glossopharyngeal nerves contribute to the innervation of the posterior circulation.

Afferent fibres from the middle meningeal artery are of trigeminal origin, mainly from the second and third divisions (McNaughton, 1938). The tentorium is the watershed for dural innervation because its superior surface is supplied by the trigeminal nerve and refers pain to the eye and forehead, whereas its inferior surface and the posterior fossa are supplied primarily by the upper three cervical roots and so refer pain to the occiput and upper neck (Figure 8.7). The glossopharyngeal and vagal nerves make a small contribution to the dura of the posterior fossa so that pain may sometimes be referred to the back of the throat or ear.

Neurogenic plasma protein extravasation (PPE)

Moskowitz (1984) has provided an elegant series of experiments to suggest that the pain of migraine may be a form of sterile neurogenic inflammation. Neurogenic plasma extravasation can be seen during electrical stimulation of the trigeminal ganglion in the rat (Markowitz, Saito and Moskowitz, 1987). Plasma extravasation can be blocked by ergot alkaloids (Markowitz, Saito and Moskowitz, 1988), indomethacin, acetylsalicylic acid (Buzzi, Sakas and Moskowitz 1989), the serotonin (5-HT)-1-like agonist, sumatriptan (Buzzi and Moskowitz, 1990), GABA agonists, such as valproate and benzodiazepines (Lee et al., 1995), neurosteroids (Limmroth et al., 1995) and substance P antagonists (Cutrer et al., 1995; Lee, Moussaoui and Moskowitz, 1994). PPE is a plausible explanation for the aggravation of migraine pain by movement but does not explain the entire syndrome. It is unlikely to be the fundamental element of dysfunction nor does it explain all aspects of the syndrome. The phenomenon has not been observed in humans and has been sought with sensitive MRI techniques (Nissila et al., 1996). Furthermore, although bosentan, a potent endothelin antagonist (Clozel et al., 1994) blocks PPE (Brandli et al., 1995), it was ineffective in double-blind placebo-controlled studies in migraine patients (May et al., 1996). Similarly, there are two negative studies of neurokinin-1 (substance P) antagonists which despite being potent inhibitors of PPE are ineffective as acute antimigraine agents (Diener, 1996; Goldstein and Wang, 1997).

Perhaps most difficult to reconcile in terms of an important role for PPE in migraine is the fact that the highly potent blocker of PPE (Lee and Moskowitz, 1993), the conformationally restricted analogue of sumatriptan, CP122,288 (Gupta et al., 1995), is also ineffective in treating acute migraine attacks (Roon et al., 1997). It may be of relevance that both substance P antagonists (Hoskin and Goadsby, 1997) and CP122,288 (Knight, Edvinsson and Goadsby, 1997) are ineffective inhibitors of trigeminocervical complex activation in experimental conditions designed to activate intracranial pain-producing nerves. Further studies of other compounds active in the PPE model, such as a neurosteroid currently in phase II, will better clarify the role of this process in migraine.

Pain and the intracranial vessels

Headache does not depend on increased cortical perfusion, because migraine without aura (common migraine) is not usually associated with alteration of regional cerebral blood flow (Olesen *et al.*, 1981) and the headache of migraine with aura (classical migraine) usually starts while blood flow is still reduced (Lauritzen *et al.*, 1983a; Olesen *et al.*, 1990) (Figure 8.5). Kobari *et al.* (1989) found that cerebral blood flow was increased during migraine headache but this increase was not related to the side on which headache was experienced. Géraud *et al.* (1989) described areas of hypo-perfusion (clinically silent oligaemic areas) as well as regions of hyperperfusion coexisting in patients with migraine without aura. Migrainous headache may be relieved by ergotamine (Norris *et al.*, 1975) or codeine (Sakai and Meyer, 1978), although cerebral perfusion remains increased.

Transcranial Doppler sonography has been used to assess the velocity of flow in proximal branches of the internal carotid artery. Friberg *et al.* (1991) found that flow in the middle cerebral artery was reduced on the side affected by headache. Since regional cerebral blood flow in the territory supplied by that artery was unaltered, they deduced that the lower velocity was caused by dilatation of the middle cerebral artery. Following the intravenous infusion of 2 mg of the 5-HT agonist, sumatriptan, the headache was relieved within 30 minutes while the velocity of flow in the middle cerebral artery returned to normal. These observations are reminiscent of those made by Graham and Wolff (1938) concerning the effect of ergotamine on extra-cranial arteries. They indicate that vascular dilatation accompanies some migraine attacks, but it does not follow necessarily that the distended vessels are entirely responsible for headache. Diener *et al.* (1991) could not demonstrate any change of blood flow velocity in the extracranial portions of the internal or external carotid arteries, or in the middle cerebral or basilar arteries, after the injection of suma-triptan 4 mg subcutaneously.

Moskowitz (1992) has pointed out that sumatriptan and the ergot alkaloids attenuate the release of neuropeptides from trigeminovascular fibres and may thus play a wider role than vasoconstriction by reducing the 'sterile inflammatory re-sponse' of migraine headache. The level of the vasodilator substance calcitonin gene-related peptide (CGRP) in the jugular venous blood, which is elevated during migraine headache, returns to baseline after the headache is relieved by sumatriptan (Goadsby and Edvinsson, 1993). The observations of Goltman (1935/36) on a migraine patient with a cranial bone defect are interesting in this context. The skull defect was depressed before the headache started and bulged during the head-ache phase. The latter has also been reported by Lance (1995).

Pain from extracranial arteries

Pain from the supra-orbital, frontal and superficial temporal arteries is mediated by the trigeminal nerve. Afferent fibres from extracranial arteries pursue their course to the trigeminal ganglion separate from the intracranial innervation and are not col-laterals of intracranial fibres (Borges and Moskowitz, 1983), so that referred pain must depend upon their convergence centrally on second-order neurones. Pain may be referred to the temple in the distribution of the zygomaticotemporal nerve, a branch of the second division of the trigeminal nerve, and the auriculotemporal nerve, which derives from the third division. Pain from the post-auricular and occi-pital arteries is mediated by the upper cervical roots.

Graham and Wolff (1938) recorded the pulsation of branches of the superficial temporal artery during migraine headache and observed that the amplitude of the pulse wave declined as the intensity of headache diminished after the injection of ergotamine tartrate. The concept of migraine being an 'extracranial vascular head-ache' appeared to be strengthened by the studies of Tunis and Wolff (1953) who reported that the mean amplitude of temporal artery pulsations was greater during headache than in periods of freedom. This conclusion may have been biased by the fact that they selected 10 patients for analysis after examining 5000 recordings from 75 patients. In any event, vascular dilatation by itself would not cause headache. In periarterial fluid sampled during migraine headache Chapman et al. (1960) found a substance similar to the polypeptide found in blister fluid, which they named 'neu-rokinin'. This bradykinin-like substance was postulated to set up a sterile inflamma-tory response in the vessel, which thus became pain-producing.

Sakai and Meyer (1978) found that extracranial blood flow increased by about 20 per cent on the side affected by headache. Elkind, Friedman and Grossman (1964) observed increased clearance of sodium-24 from the skin of the frontotemporal region during migraine attacks. Jensen and Olesen (1985) reported that temporal muscle blood flow increased by about one-third during headache but this did not reach statistical significance and there was no difference between headache and non-headache sides. Nevertheless, arteries and veins do become prominent in the temple during migraine, and pressure over them eases the pain. Blau and Dexter (1981) assessed the contribution of extracranial arteries to migraine headache by inflating a sphygmomanometer cuff around the patient's head. Of 47 patients, only 21 experi-enced relief from headache after inflation of the pericranial cuff whereas the majority complained that their headaches were aggravated by coughing, jolting or holding their breath, indicating an intracranial component to head pain. Drummond and Lance (1983) compared the pulse amplitude of the superficial temporal artery and its main frontotemporal branch with the intensity of pain felt in the temple while the ipsilateral common carotid and temporal arteries were compressed alternately. Of 62 patients, selected only by the presence of a unilateral migrainous headache, the pain appeared to be of extracranial vascular origin in about one-third, was of mainly intracranial vascular origin in one-third, and had no detectable vascular component in the remaining one-third. In the subgroup with increased arterial pulsation in the frontotemporal region, thermography demonstrated increased heat loss from this area, and temporal artery compression eased the headache briefly. Although the frontal branches of the temporal artery were found to dilate in one-third of patients, Drummond and Lance (1983) could not detect any change in the pulsation of the superficial temporal artery itself. Iversen et al. (1990) have since demonstrated by Doppler studies that the lumen of the temporal artery is increased during ipsilateral migraine headache relative to that of the opposite side and the lumen of peripheral arteries. They interpreted this as a generalized vasoconstriction, sparing the temporal artery on the headache side. These studies make it clear that the extracranial circulation contributes to the pain of migraine headache in only a minority of patients.

Neuropeptides and headache: linking experimental and human observations
(see Figure 8.3)

Studies of cranial venous neuropeptide levels have proved valuable in elucidating some of the mechanisms involved in primary headaches. Stimulation of the trigeminal ganglion in the cat leads to an increase in cranial venous levels of both substance P (SP) and calcitonin gene-related peptide (CGRP). Similarly, stimulation of the trigeminal ganglion in humans undergoing thermocoagulation for trigeminal neuralgia leads to elevation in the cranial venous outflow of both peptides (Goadsby, Edvinsson and Ekman, 1988). More specific stimulation of pain-producing intracranial structures, such as the superior sagittal sinus, also results in cranial venous release of CGRP and not substance P (Zagami, Goadsby and Edvinsson, 1990). During migraine CGRP is elevated in the external jugular vein blood whereas substance P is not in both adults (Goadsby, Edvinsson and Ekman, 1990) and in adolescents (Gallai et al., 1995).

These data clearly demonstrate activation of trigeminovascular neurones during migraine with or without aura. Similarly, CGRP but not substance P is elevated during acute attacks of cluster headache, both spontaneous (Goadsby and Edvinsson, 1994) and provoked (Fanciullacci et al., 1995), and during the pain of chronic paroxsymal hemicrania (Goadsby and Edvinsson, 1996). It is important to note in terms of understanding the pathophysiology of cluster headache that vasoactive intestinal polypeptide (VIP), a marker for cranial parasympathetic nerve activation, is also elevated in cluster headache and paroxysmal hemicrania (Goadsby and Edvinsson, 1994; Goadsby and Edvinsson, 1996). Moreover, treatment with sumatriptan reduces CGRP levels in humans as their migraine subsides and in experimental animals during trigeminal ganglion stimulation (Goadsby and Edvinsson, 1993). Similarly, treatment with avitriptan, a potent clinically effective $5\text{-HT}_{1B/1D}$ agonist (Couch, Saper and Meloche, 1996; Ryan, Elkind and Goldstein, 1997), blocks CGRP release in experimental animals while administration of the potent blocker of neurogenic plasma protein extravasation (PPE), CP122,288, is not effective at doses specific for PPE (Knight, Edvinsson and Goadsby, 1997). The release of these peptides offers the prospect of a marker for migraine that can be measured in a venous blood sample and seems highly predictive of migraine activity in humans.

Pain from other extracranial structures

Disorders of the upper cervical spine refer pain to the occiput related to the distribution of the second and third cervical roots. Pain may also be felt behind the eye of the same side (Kerr, 1961) because pain fibres from the upper cervical roots converge with those in the spinal tract of the trigeminal nerve on neurones in the dorsolateral quadrant of the upper cervical cord (Goadsby and Hoskin, 1997; Goadsby, Hoskin and Knight, 1997; Kerr and Olafson, 1961).

There is much greater overlap between the trigeminal and cervical distribution than was previously realized. Denny-Brown and Yanagisawa (1973) sectioned the sensory root of one trigeminal nerve in a monkey and found the expected sensory loss over the anterior two-thirds of the face and scalp. When the animal was given a subconvulsive dose of strychnine, the area of anaesthesia receded until the only unresponsive region was around the eye, cheek and upper lip, apparently the only area innervated exclusively by the fifth cranial nerve. Conversely, section of the second, third and fourth cervical dorsal roots produced a sensory loss over the occipital region and upper neck, which shrank to a thin band around the neck after administration of strychnine. When trigeminal and cervical inflow were both destroyed, there was still an area of innervation by the vagus and facial nerves around the ear, which spread in a wedge shape to supply the posterior half of the scalp under the influence of strychnine. It has not been appreciated that the vagus nerve, through its communication with auriculotemporal and posterior temporal branches, supplies the ear and a large part of the scalp. It remains to be seen whether this can be applied to the patient with headache.

Muscle contraction

Pain from muscle contraction may add a non-vascular component to migraine headache. Excessive contraction of the temporal, masseter and neck muscles is common in migraine patients (Lous and Olsen, 1982), more so than in patients with 'tension headache', and becomes evident just before the headache reaches its maximum (Bakke *et al.*, 1982). Tfelt-Hansen, Lous and Olesen (1981) found that infiltration of tender muscle areas with local anaesthetic or normal saline relieved migraine headaches within 70 min in 28 of 48 patients. Serotonin (5-HT) and bradykinin potentiated the pain-producing effects of one another when injected into the temporal muscle of normal volunteers but did not evoke headache (Jensen *et al.*, 1990). The sites of muscle contraction in migraine correlate with the spatial distribution of pain and tenderness, suggesting that it is a secondary phenomenon but one that nonetheless contributes to headache.

Central trigeminal pain pathways

The sites within the brain stem that are responsible for craniovascular pain have now begun to be mapped. Using c-*Fos*-immunocytochemistry, a method for looking at activated cells, after meningeal irritation with blood, expression is reported in the trigeminal nucleus caudalis (Nozaki, Boccalini and Moskowitz, 1992). After stimulation of the superior sagittal sinus *Fos*-like immunoreactivity is seen in monkey (Goadsby and Hoskin, 1997), cat (Kaube *et al.*, 1993) and rat (Strassman, Mineta and Vos, 1994) in the trigeminal nucleus caudalis and in the dorsal horn at the C_1 and C_2 levels. These latter findings are in accord with similar data using 2-deoxyglucose measurements with superior sagittal sinus stimulation (Goadsby and Zagami,

1991) and more recent studies demonstrating a similar organization in the monkey (Goadsby and Hoskin, 1997).

These data contribute to our view of the trigeminal nucleus extending beyond the traditional nucleus caudalis to the dorsal horn of the high cervical region in a functional continuum that includes a cervical extension that could be regarded as a *trigeminal nucleus cervicalis*. The entire group of cells may be usefully regarded as the trigeminocervical complex to place emphasis upon the integrative role that these neurones have in head pain. The data clearly demonstrate that a substantial portion of the trigeminovascular nociceptive information comes by way of the most caudal cells. The rather diffuse activation of neurones in the trigeminal nucleus in visceral pain, such as that arising from intracranial vessels, is to be contrasted with what is seen when pain stimuli are applied to discrete facial structures. Neuronal activation is more restricted (Strassman and Vos, 1993; Strassman *et al.*, 1993) in line with the relatively good spatial localization of more superficial pain. This concept provides an anatomical explanation for the referral of pain to the back of the head in migraine.

Further direct evidence for the trigeminocervical complex as the site of referred pain comes from an animal study in which the greater occipital nerve, a branch of C_2, was directly stimulated and 2-deoxyglucose activation observed in the entire complex including the trigeminal nucleus caudalis (Goadsby, Hoskin and Knight, 1997). Moreover, experimental pharmacological evidence suggests that some abortive antimigraine drugs, such as ergots (Goadsby and Gundlach, 1991; Hoskin, Kaube and Goadsby, 1996), acetylsalicylic acid (Kaube, Hoskin and Goadsby, 1993a), naratriptan (Goadsby and Knight, 1997b), sumatriptan (after blood–brain barrier disruption) (Kaube, Hoskin and Goadsby, 1993b), rizatriptan (Cumberbatch, Hill and Hargreaves, 1997) and zolmitriptan (Goadsby and Hoskin, 1996), can have actions at these second-order neurones to reduce cell activity. Using autoradiographic studies it has been shown that $5\text{-HT}_{1B/1D/1F}$ receptors are all present in the trigeminocervical complex (Castro *et al.*, 1997; Goadsby and Knight, 1997a; Mills and Martin, 1995; Pascual *et al.*, 1996), although which of these receptor subtypes dominates is unclear since both zolmitriptan and sumatriptan when iontophoresed on trigeminal neurones inhibit their firing (Storer and Goadsby, 1997). Taken together these data suggest trigeminocervical complex neurones as an additional possible site for the action of brain-penetrant antimigraine drugs (Goadsby, 1997).

Following transmission in the caudal brain stem and high cervical spinal cord, information is relayed in a group of fibres (the quintothalamic tract) to the thalamus (Figure 8.3). Processing of vascular pain in the thalamus occurs in the ventroposteromedial thalamus, medial nucleus of the posterior complex and in the intralaminar thalamus (Zagami and Goadsby, 1991; Zagami and Lambert, 1990). Zagami and Lambert (1991) have shown by application of capsaicin to the superior sagittal sinus that trigeminal projections with a high degree of nociceptive input are processed in neurones particularly in the ventroposteromedial thalamus and in its ventral periphery. The properties and further higher centre connections of these neurones are the subject of ongoing studies which will allow us to build up a more complete picture of the trigeminovascular pain pathways.

The role of central nervous system modulation in migraine pain

Even in periods of freedom from migraine, migrainous subjects carry with them susceptibility to head pain. Raskin and Knittle (1976) found that cold drinks or ice-cream evoked headache in 93 per cent of migraine patients compared with only 31 per cent of control subjects. One-third of patients with ice-cream headache state that this pain involves precisely the same part of the head as their habitual migraine headaches (Drummond and Lance, 1984). Moreover, 42 per cent of migraine patients are prone to sudden jabs of pain in the head ('ice-pick pains'), compared with 3 per cent of non-headache controls (Raskin and Schwartz, 1980). Drummond and Lance (1984) found that ice-pick pains coincided with the site of the customary headache in 40 per cent of patients. The trigeminal pathways may thus become activated spontaneously in paroxysms lasting a fraction of a second (ice-pick pains) or may be activated reflexly for seconds or minutes by sudden cooling of the pharynx (ice-cream headache). This indicates a persisting disinhibition of a segment of the trigeminal pathways in migraine patients, suggesting that the trigeminal system could also discharge excessively for hours or days to provide a neural origin for migraine headache. During headache, sensitivity to pressure is increased over the areas where pain is felt but can be normal or increased in the fingers (Drummond, 1987), so that any defect in pain control mechanisms appears to be localized to the affected areas.

Stimulation of the periaqueductal grey matter by indwelling electrodes is used in the control of otherwise intractable bodily pain (Baskin et al., 1986). Raskin, Hosobuchi and Lamb (1987) reported that 15 of 175 patients developed migraine-like headaches after the electrode insertion. This observation was confirmed by Veloso and Kumer (1996) who found that 15 of 64 patients implanted had developed unilateral headaches for the first time. It thus appears that the endogenous pain control system can be switched on or off from the periaqueductal grey matter (see Figure 8.9) and that switching off can permit the development of headache with the characteristics of migraine.

Neural control of the cranial circulation and endogenous pain control systems

The brain stem nuclei innervating the cerebral circulation are in a unique position to influence brain blood flow while also involved in nociceptive processing from pain-producing craniovascular structures. This dual role provides a focus for special attention to neurovascular anatomy and physiology in the context of *vascular headache*.

Brain stem influences
Cerebral vascular resistance increases (i.e. blood flow falls) by about 20 per cent with low frequency stimulation of the locus coeruleus (LC) in the monkey (Goadsby, Lambert and Lance, 1982). Regional cerebral blood flow was shown to diminish in the cat, particularly in the occipital cortex (Goadsby and Duckworth, 1987). On the other hand, external carotid resistance diminishes (i.e. blood flow increases) as the frequency of LC stimulation increases. The extracranial vasodilator effect was

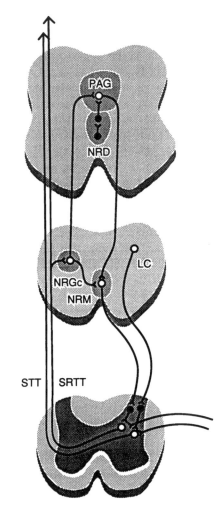

Figure 8.9 Simplified version of the endogenous pain control system

The descending pathway from the periaqueductal grey matter (PAG) excites the nucleus raphe magnus (NRM), which projects together with descending fibres from the region of the locus coeruleus (LC), to inhibitory interneurones in the spinal trigeminal nucleus and dorsal horn of the upper cervical spinal cord.

The pain suppression system is activated by ascending fibres in the spinoreticulothalamic tract (SRTT), which accompanies the spinothalamic tract (STT) and synapses in the nucleus reticularis gigantocellularis (NRGc), and is inhibited by neurones from the nucleus raphe dorsalis (NRD) and adjacent reticular formation. ○ = exciting neurones; ● = inhibitory neurones.

later shown to be mediated by the greater superficial petrosal (GSP) branch of the facial nerve (Goadsby, Lambert and Lance, 1983). These changes, which were predominantly ipsilateral, bear a striking resemblance to the vascular changes accompanying migraine with aura. This effect of LC stimulation is presumably exerted on the microcirculation because it does not produce any consistent change in the discharge frequency of cells in the cat occipital cortex (Adams, Lambert and Lance, 1989). In contrast, stimulation of the nucleus raphe dorsalis increases cerebral blood

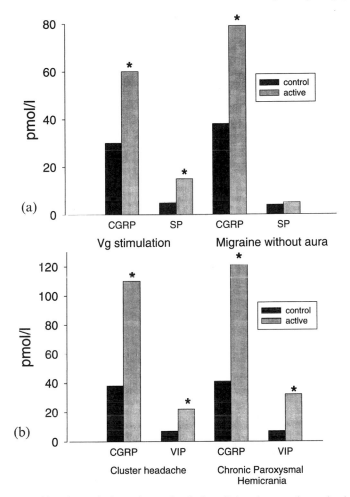

Figure 8.10 Neuropeptide release during primary headaches. Trigeminovascular activation with direct stimulation of the trigeminal ganglion and (a) in migraine and (b) cluster headache and chronic paroxysmal hemicrania, as reflected in elevations in calcitonin gene-related peptide (CGRP) but not substance P (SP) compared to elevation of both peptides during trigeminal ganglion (Vg) stimulation in humans

flow in the monkey; in the cat and monkey it dilates both internal and external carotid circulation through connections with the facial (GSP) nerve (Goadsby *et al.*, 1985a, 1985b) (see Figures 8.8 and 8.11). The degree of extracranial vasodilatation is comparable with the reflex effects of LC stimulation.

Extrinsic (autonomic) influences
Thermocoagulation of the Gasserian ganglion for tic douloureux, a procedure that would be very painful if the patient was not anaesthetized, produces a facial flush in the distribution of the division or divisions coagulated (Drummond, Gonski and Lance, 1983). Lambert *et al.* (1984) showed that electrical stimulation of the Gas-

serian ganglion in cats diminished carotid resistance and increased blood flow and facial temperature by a reflex pathway traversing the trigeminal root, as its afferent limb, and the GSP branch of the facial nerve, as its efferent limb, the 'trigeminovascular reflex' (Figure 8.2). A minor component of the response, particularly that elicited from the third division, persisted after section of the trigeminal root, almost certainly caused by the liberation of vasoactive peptides from antidromic activation of trigeminal nerve terminals (Moskowitz, 1984). The main reflex vasodilator response to stimulation of the locus coeruleus, raphe nuclei or the trigeminal nerve is mediated by the sphenopalatine and otic ganglia (Goadsby, Lambert and Lance, 1984), and employs vasoactive intestinal polypeptide (VIP) as its neurovascular transmitter (Goadsby and Macdonald, 1985).

A pathway has therefore been established that can account for extracranial vascular dilatation accompanying a primary pain-producing excitation of trigeminal pathways, a mechanism that may prove relevant to the vascular changes of migraine.

Interrelationship between intrinsic and extrinsic craniovascular innervation
Activation of the trigeminal nerve, nucleus raphe dorsalis or high frequency stimulation of the locus coeruleus increases cerebral and extracranial blood flow through their connections with the greater superficial petrosal (GSP) nerve (Goadsby and Lance, 1988; Lance *et al.*, 1983) (Figures 8.1 and 8.2). Trigeminal nerve terminals can also release vasodilator peptides antidromically to increase cerebral blood flow in cats (Lambert *et al.*, 1984) and promote the leakage of plasma protein from blood vessels in the rat dura mater (Markowitz, Saito and Moskowitz, 1987).

There are thus two ways in which pain-mediating trigeminal pathways can cause cerebral, dural and extracranial blood flow to increase: reflexly via the parasympathetic outflow in the GSP nerve, and directly by the antidromic release of vasodilator peptides (Goadsby and Edvinsson, 1993; Goadsby and Edvinsson, 1994; Goadsby, Edvinsson and Ekman, 1988, 1990).

The vascular effects evoked from the locus coeruleus and nucleus raphe dorsalis, which are predominantly unilateral, simulate flow changes reported in patients with migraine headache, which could therefore be secondary to neural changes in the brain stem. The locus coeruleus appears to exert an inhibitory influence on the contralateral locus (Buda *et al.*, 1975), which could be the basis for unilateral cerebral changes alternating from hemisphere to hemisphere in migraine. The identification using PET of areas of activation in humans during migraine in regions of the periaqueductal grey matter and dorsolateral pontine tegmentum (Weiller *et al.*, 1995), which contain the nucleus raphe dorsalis and locus coeruleus, respectively, is consistent with an aminergic dysmodulation in the brain stem accounting for many features of the migraine syndrome (see Figures 8.9, 8.11).

The implication of 5-hydroxytryptamine (5-HT, serotonin) in the migraine syndrome

5-Hydroxytryptamine has long been considered as a possible mediator of the migraine syndrome because of its action on blood vessels, renal function and the gastrointestinal tract. It became a serious contender when Sicuteri (1959) reported that methysergide, a known 5-HT antagonist, was of value in preventing migraine. Kimball, Friedman and Vallejo (1960) in a brief but influential paper noted that the intramuscular injection of 2.5 mg of reserpine, which releases 5-HT from body stores, induced a typical headache in 10 out of 15 migraine patients. They also found that the intravenous injection of 5-HT 5 mg relieved migraine headache in five patients with spontaneous attacks but caused transient dyspnoea, faintness, flushing and paraesthesiae.

The urinary output of the principal catabolite of 5-HT, 5-hydroxyindoleacetic acid (5-HIAA) was shown to be increased during migraine headache by Sicuteri, Testi and Anselmi (1961) with the mean daily excretion rising from 4 mg to 10.6 mg. This was confirmed by Curran, Hinterberger and Lance (1965) who found that 5 HIAA excretion increased in 15 of 22 headaches and also reported that the content of 5-HT in platelets fell at the onset of migraine headache. Anthony, Hinterberger and Lance (1967) followed this up in 15 patients, finding that the 5-HT level dropped in 20 of 21 headaches studied, by an average of 45 per cent. No change was found in patients with headache following pneumoencephalography or in those undergoing stressful procedures such as angiography. The content of 5-HT in platelets fell, as would be expected, in nine out of 10 patients after the intravenous injection of reserpine 2.5 mg which caused a typical headache in migraine patients but only a dull ache in subjects not prone to migraine. The intravenous injection of 5-HT 2–7.5 mg eased both spontaneous and reserpine-induced migraine. Anthony, Hinterberger and Lance (1969) went on to show that the incubation of platelets with platelet-free plasma taken during headache caused 5-HT to be released, but this did not occur when platelets were incubated with post-headache plasma. This observation, that a 5-HT releasing factor was present in the plasma during migraine headache, was supported by findings from other laboratories (Dvilansky et al., 1976; Launay and Pradalier, 1985; Mück-Želer, Deanović and Dupelj, 1979) but could not be replicated by Ferrari et al. (1987). The latter group reported that platelet 5-HT content fell only in migraine without aura but that the level of free 5-HT in plasma increased by more than 100 per cent during migraine headache whether it was preceded by an aura or not (Ferrari et al., 1989). Platelet dense bodies, the storage organelles for 5-HT, are increased in migraine with aura (D'Andrea et al., 1989b). The 5-HT releasing factor in migraine has not been identified but is of molecular weight less than 50,000. Free fatty acids are possible contenders (Anthony, 1978).

An attempted synthesis

The cardinal features of migraine are recurrent headache and its association with transient neurological symptoms. The headache, usually felt in the region of distribution of the trigeminal nerve and upper cervical roots, implies unrestrained firing of cells in the spinal trigeminal nucleus and its extension into the upper cervical cord. On occasions, migrainous pain may spread to the shoulder, arm and even to the lower limb (Figure 8.12), suggesting that cells in the basal nuclei of the thalamus may also be involved. The frequency of 'ice-pick pains' and ice-cream headache' in migraine patients indicates that this part of their pain control system is defective, permitting a high frequency neuronal discharge spontaneously or in response to a cold stimulus. Such an unstable system may then respond by a continuous discharge when subjected to stimulation from higher centres (cortex, hypothalamus) as the result of stress or by excessive afferent input from the special senses or from cerebral or extracranial vessels.

The aura phase of migraine may take the form of a slow advance of neurological symptoms, explicable by a phenomenon similar to the spreading cortical depression of Leão, or may affect cortical function more diffusely without any step-wise progression of symptoms being apparent. If spreading depression is responsible for fortification spectra in migraine, the way in which it is produced remains uncertain. Does it arise in the cortex or is it induced by subcortical structures?

An animal model (illustrated in Figure 8.11) is available for the reported vascular changes of migraine (Goadsby and Lance, 1988). As outlined above, the locus coeruleus can induce cerebral vasoconstriction and extracranial vasodilatation in monkeys and the nucleus raphe dorsalis can dilate both circulations. It is conceivable that a similar mechanism in human patients could account for the vascular changes of migraine being secondary to brain stem activity. Once the trigeminal system is activated centrally or peripherally it may promote the leakage of plasma protein from dural vessels and increase blood flow intra- and extracranially by antidromic discharge and by a reflex connection with the parasympathetic outflow through the GSP nerve (Figures 8.8 and 8.11).

It is conceivable that constriction of the cortical microcirculation induced by discharge of locus coeruleus or other brain stem nuclei could induce focal cortical oligaemia, which in turn could provoke spreading depression. The caudal projection of the locus coeruleus to the thoracic sympathetic outflow could cause the release of noradrenaline into the systemic circulation, which sets in motion the platelet release of 5-HT (Figure 8.11). Following a phase of monoaminergic excitation, a phase of depletion could follow, thus reducing the activity of the endogenous pain control system, removing the remaining restraint on the discharge of neurones in the spinal tract of the trigeminal nerve. The resulting headache could be aggravated by afferent impulses from dilated cerebral and extracranial arteries.

This explanation of the interaction between the brain and its vascular supply in the causation of migraine is speculative but even in the light of newer human functional imaging studies remains plausible and consistent with clinical observations and the information gained from animal experimentation.

Summary

Migraine is a neurovascular reaction in response to sudden changes in the internal or external environment. Each individual has an hereditary 'migrainous threshold', with the degree of susceptibility depending on the balance between excitation and inhibition at various levels of the nervous system. Such a balance may be influenced by magnesium deficiency, excitatory amino acids, monoamines, opioids and other factors outlined above. Neural and vascular elements both contribute to headache.

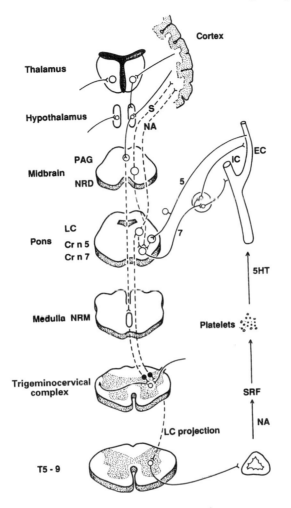

Figure 8.11 The neurovascular hypothesis for migraine. (From Lance *et al.*, 1989, by permission of the editors of *Migraine: A Spectrum of Ideas*)

Brain stem mechanisms are triggered by descending pathways from the cerebral cortex (in response to emotion or stress), from the thalamus (in response to excessive afferent stimulation, light, noise. or smells), or from the hypothalamus (in response to changes in the internal environment or 'internal clocks'). The nucleus raphe dorsalis (NRD) and locus coeruleus (LC) project diffusely to the cerebral cortex, employing serotonin (S) and noradrenaline (NA), respectively as transmitter agents. LC causes constriction of the ipsilateral cortical microcirculation through this direct pathway. Stimulation of NRD, LC or the trigeminal nerve (5) induces dilatation of the extracranial circulation (EC) by connections with the parasympathetic component of the facial nerve (7) (the greater superficial petrosal nerve) and the sphenopalatine and otic ganglia, and releases vasoactive intestinal peptide as a peripheral transmitter agent ('the trigeminovascular reflex'). NRD causes dilatation in the internal carotid circulation (IC) through the same direct pathway. Stimulation of the LC area causes release of NA from the adrenal gland by its connection with the intermediolateral cell column of the thoracic cord (LC projection). NA, or a serotonin (5-HT) releasing factor (SRF) liberated by NA, causes a platelet release reaction. Free serotonin released from platelets increases the sensitivity of vascular receptors, thus augmenting the afferent inflow through the trigeminal nerve (5). The spinal tract of the trigeminal nerve (not illustrated) descends to the second cervical segment of the spinal cord (C2) where it converges with fibres from the second cervical root on to second-order neurones in the pain pathway ('trigeminocervical complex'). Transmission at this synapse is regulated by inhibitory neurones (black circles) which, in turn, are modulated by the endogenous pain control pathway descending from the periaqueductal grey matter (PAG) through the nucleus raphe magnus (NRM), and from LC. Activity in brain stem monoaminergic pathways is thus able to replicate the vascular changes of migraine as well as to regulate the perception of pain arising from cranial vessels.

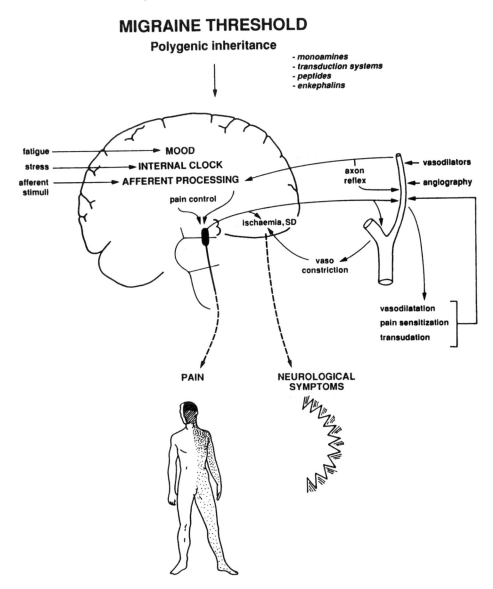

Figure 8.12 A schema for the neurovascular basis of migraine. (From Lance *et al.*, 1989, by permission of the editors of *Migraine: A Spectrum of Ideas*)

An inherited 'migraine threshold' renders the subject susceptible to fluctuations in hypothalamic function (signalled by alteration of mood or craving for sweet foods), environmental changes, fatigue, stress or excessive afferent stimulation (including input from cranial vessels). Brain stem monoaminergic nuclei influence cerebral and extracranial blood flow by direct and indirect projections. Cortical ischaemia, often accompanied by spreading depression (SD), is associated with focal neurological symptoms. The release of 5-hydroxytryptamine (5-HT, serotonin) and vasodilator peptides induces a sterile inflammatory response in blood vessels, which feeds pain-producing impulses back to the nervous system and may produce further vascular responses by an axon reflex or a central reflex pathway. Depression of the endogenous pain control system may be an additional factor in increasing the discharge frequency of trigeminothalamic (and sometimes spinothalamic) neurones so that migrainous pain is experienced in the head with radiation to the neck (often), shoulder and arm (occasionally). or leg (rarely). Pharmacotherapy is aimed at interrupting this vicious circle in the central nervous system, or peripherally in the nerves innervating the cranial vasculature and by direct vasoconstriction of those vessels.

The mechanism of migraine has been presented as an unstable trigeminovascular reflex with a segmental defect in the pain control pathway, thus permitting excessive discharge of part of the spinal nucleus of the trigeminal nerve and its thalamic connections in response to excessive afferent input or corticobulbar drive. The end result is interaction between brain stem and cranial blood vessels (Figures 8.1, 8.2 and 8.11) with the afferent impulses from the latter intensifying pain perception through the trigeminovascular reflex. Diffuse projections from the locus coeruleus to the cerebral cortex could initiate cortical oligaemia and possibly spreading depression. Activity in this system could account for the migrainous aura, which may occur quite independently of the headache, although one commonly follows the other. The headache phase may be interrupted by therapy aimed at either the central or peripheral end of the trigeminovascular reflex.

There is strong evidence that 5-HT plays an important part in the genesis of migraine. Whether the place of 5-HT lies in central pain control pathways, in the serotonergic projection to the cerebral cortex, in a direct action on the cranial blood vessels or in its action at all three sites remains uncertain. It seems probable that the primary action of specific anti-migraine treatments, such as sumatriptan or ergotamine in terminating migraine headache is exerted on the cerebral and extracranial vascular and dural structures and their trigeminal innervation, whereas medications employed in prophylaxis may act centrally.

References

Adams, R. W., Lambert, G. A. and Lance, J. W. (1989). Stimulation of brain stem nuclei in the cat: effect on neuronal activity in the primary visual cortex of relevance to cerebral blood flow and migraine. *Cephalalgia* **9**, 107-118

Andersen, A. R., Friberg, L., Skyhøj-Olsen, T. and Olesen, J. (1988). SPECT demonstration of delayed hyperemia following hypoperfusion in classic migraine. *Arch. Neurol.* **45**, 154-159

Anthony, M. (1978). Role of individual free fatty acids in migraine. *Res. Clin. Study Headache* **6**, 110–116

Anthony, M., Hinterberger, H. and Lance, J. W. (1967). Plasma serotonin in migraine and stress. *Arch. Neurol.* **16**, 544–552

Anthony, M., Hinterberger, H. and Lance, J. W. (1969). The possible relationship of serotonin to the migraine syndrome. In *Research and Clinical Studies in Headache*, Vol. 2, Ed. A. P. Friedman. pp. 29–59. Basel, Karger

Awaki, E., Takeshima, T., Nishikawa, S. and Takabashi, K. (1989). A neuroendocrinological study in female migraineurs: prolactin and thyroid stimulating hormone responses. *Cephalalgia* **9** (Suppl. 10), 53–54

Bach, F. W., Jensen, K., Blegvad, N., Fenger, M., Jordal, R. and Olesen, J. (1985). β-Endorphin and ACTH in plasma during attacks of common and classic migraine. *Cephalalgia* **5**, 177–182

Bakke, M., Tfelt-Hansen, P., Olesen, J. and Møller, E. (1982). Action of some pericranial muscles during provoked attacks of common migraine. *Pain* **14**, 121–135

Barkley, G. L., Tepley, N., Nagel-Leiby, S., Moran, J. E., Simkins, R. T. and Welsh, K. M. A. (1990). Magnetoencephalographic studies of migraine. *Headache* **30**, 428–434

Baskin, D. S., Mehler, W. R., Hosobuchi, Y., Richardson, D. E., Adams, J. E. and Flitter, M. A. (1986). Autopsy analysis of the safety, efficacy and cartography of electrical stimulation of the central gray in humans. *Brain Res.* **371**, 231–236

Bene, Ed., Poggonioni, M. and de Tommasi, F. (1994). Video assessment of yawning induced by sublingual apomorphine in migraine. *Headache* **34**, 536–538

Blau, J. N. (1980). Migraine prodromes separated from the aura; complete migraine. *Br. Med. J.* **21**, 658–660

Blau, J. N. and Dexter, S. L. (1981). The site of pain origin during migraine attacks. *Cephalalgia* 1, 143–147

Blin, O., Azulay, J., Masson, G., Aubrespey, G. and Serratrice, G. (1991). Apomorphine-induced yawning in migraine patients: enhanced responsiveness. *Clin. Neuropharmacol.* 14, 91–95.

Borges, L. F. and Moskowitz, M. A. (1983). Do intracranial and extracranial trigeminal afferents represent divergent axon collaterals? *Neurosci. Lett.* 35, 265–70

Brandli, P., Loffler, B.-M., Breu, V., Osterwalder, R., Maire, J.-P. and Clozel, M. (1995). Role of endothelin in mediating neurogenic plasma extravasation in rat dura mater. *Pain* 64, 315–322

Brindley, G. S. and Lewin, W. S. (1968). The sensations produced by electrical stimulation of the visual cortex. *J. Physiol.* 196, 479–493

Buda, M., Roussel, B., Renard, B. and Pujol, J.-F. (1975). Increase in tyrosine hydroxylase activity in the locus coeruleus of the rat brain after contralateral lesioning. *Brain Res.* 93, 564–569

Buzzi, M. G. and Moskowitz, M. A. (1990). The antimigraine drug, sumatriptan (GR43175), selectively blocks neurogenic plasma extravasation from blood vessels in dura mater. *Br. J. Pharmacol.* 99, 202–206

Buzzi, M. G., Sakas, D. E. and Moskowitz, M. A. (1989). Indomethacin and acetylsalicylic acid block neurogenic plasma protein extravasation in rat dura mater. *Eur. J. Pharmacol.* 165, 251–258

Cao, Y., Welch, K. M. A., Aurora, S. K. and Vikingstad, E. (1997). Functional MRI (BOLD) of visually triggered headache in migraine patients. *Cephalalgia* 17, 254

Castro, M. E., Pascual, J., Romon, T., Arco, Cd., Olmo, Ed. and Pazos, A. (1997). Differential distribution of [^{3}H]sumatriptan binding sites (5-HT$_{1B}$, 5-HT$_{1D}$ and 5-HT$_{1F}$ receptors) in human brain: focus on brainstem and spinal cord. *Neuropharmacol.* 36, 535–542

Chapman, L. F., Ramos, A. O., Goodell, H., Silverman, G. and Wolff, H. G. (1960). A humoral agent implicated in vascular headache of the migrainous type. *Arch. Neurol.* 3, 223–229

Clozel, M., Breu, V., Gray, A. G. *et al.* (1994). Pharmacological characterisation of bosentan, a new potent orally active nonpeptide endothelin receptor antagonist. *J. Pharmacol. Exp. Ther.* 270, 228–235

Couch, J. R., Saper, J. and Meloche, J. P. (1986). Treatment of migraine with BMS180048: response at 2 hours. *Headache* 36, 523–530

Cumberbatch, M. J., Hill, R. G. and Hargreaves, R. J. (1997). Rizatriptan has central antinociceptive effects against durally evoked responses. *Eur. J. Pharmacol.* 328, 37–40

Curran, D. A., Hinterberger, H. and Lance, J. W. (1965). Total plasma serotonin, 5-hydroxyindoleacetic acid and p-hydroxy-m-methoxymandelic acid excretion in normal and migrainous subjects. *Brain* 88, 997–1010

Cutrer, F. M., Garret, C., Moussaoui, S. M. and Moskowitz, M. A. (1995). The non-peptide neurokinin-1 antagonist, RPR 100893, decreases c-fos expression in trigeminal nucleus caudalis following noxious chemical meningeal stimulation. *Neuroscience* 64, 741–750

Cutrer, F. M., Sorensen, A. G., Weisskoff, R. M., Ostergaard, L., Sanchez del Ria, M., Lee, J., Rosen, B. R. and Moskowitz, M. A. (1998). Perfusion-weighted imaging defects during spontaneous migrainous aura. *Ann. Neurol.* 43, 25–31

D'Andrea, G., Cananzi, A. R., Joseph, R. *et al.* (1989a). Platelet excitatory amino acids in migraine. *Cephalalgia* 9 (Suppl. 10), 105–106

D'Andrea, G. K., Welch, K. M. A., Riddle, J. M., Grunfled, S. and Joseph, R. (1989b). Platelet serotonin metabolism and ultrastructure in migraine. *Arch. Neurol.* 46, 1187–1189

Daras, M., Papkostas, T., Markianos, M. and Stefanis, C. (1987). Neuroendocrine approach to migraine. The TRH test. In *Current Problems in Neurology. Volume 4: Advances in Headache Research*, Ed. F. Clifford Rose. pp. 59–64. London, John Libbey

Denny-Brown, D. and Yanagisawa, N. (1973). The function of the descending root of the fifth nerve. *Brain* 96, 783–814

Diener, H. C. (1996). Substance-P antagonist RPR100893-201 is not effective in human migraine attacks. In *Proceedings of the VIth International Headache Seminar*, Copenhagen, Eds J. Olesen and P. Tfelt-Hansen. New York, Lippincott-Raven

Diener, H. C., Haab, J., Peters, C., Ried, S., Dichgans, J. and Pilgrim, A. (1991). Subcutaneous sumatriptan in the treatment of headache during withdrawal from drug-induced headache. *Headache* 31, 205–209

Drummond, P. D. (1982). Extracranial and cardiovascular reactivity in migrainous subjects. *J. Psychosom. Res.* 26, 317–331

Drummond, P. D. (1987). Scalp tenderness and sensitivity to pain in migraine and tension headache. *Headache* **27**, 45–50

Drummond, P. D., Gonski, A. and Lance, J. W. (1983). Facial flushing after thermocoagulation of the Gasserian ganglion. *J. Neurol. Neurosurg. Psychiat.* **46**, 611–616

Drummond, P. D and Lance, J. W. (1981). Extracranial vascular reactivity in migraine and tension headache. *Cephalalgia* **1**, 149–155

Drummond, P. D. and Lance, J. W. (1983). Extracranial vascular changes and the source of pain in migraine headache. *Ann. Neurol.* **13**, 32–37

Drummond, P. D. and Lance, J. W. (1984). Neurovascular disturbances in headache patients. *Clin. Exp. Neurol.* **20**, 93–99

Ducros, A., Joutel, A., Vahedi, K., *et al.* (1997). Familial hemiplegic migraine: mapping of the second gene and evidence for a third locus. *Cephalalgia* **17**, 232

Dvilansky. A., Rishpon, S., Nathan, I., Zolorow, Z. and Korczyn, A. D. (1976). Release of platelet 5-hydroxytryptamine by plasma taken from patients during and between migraine attacks. *Pain* **2**, 315–318

Elkind, A. H, Friedman, A. P and Grossman, J. (1964). Cutaneous blood flow in vascular headache of the migrainous type. *Neurology,Minneapolis* **14**, 24–30

Fanciullacci, M., Alessandri, M., Figini, M., Geppetti, P. and Michelacci, S. (1995). Increases in plasma calcitonin gene-related peptide from extracerebral circulation during nitroglycerin-induced cluster headache attack. *Pain* **60**, 119–123

Fanciullacci, M., Franchi, G. and Sicuteri, F. (1974). Hypersensitivity to lysergic acid diethylamide (LSD-25) and psilocybin in essential headache. *Experentia* **30**, 1441–1442

Fanciullacci, M., Michelacci, S., Curradi, C. and Sicuteri, F. (1980). Hyper-responsiveness of migraine patients to the hypotensive action of bromocriptine. *Headache* **20**, 99–102

Ferrari, M. D, Frolich, M., Odink, J., Tapparelli, C., Portielje, J. E. A. and Bruyn, G. W. (1987). Methionine-enkephalin and serotonin in migraine and tension headache. In *Current Problems in Neurology. Volume 4: Advances in Headache Research*, Ed. F. Clifford Rose. pp. 227–234. London, John Libbcy

Ferrari, M. D., Odink, J., Box, K. D., Malessy, M. J. A. and Bruyn, G. W. (1990). Neuroexcitatory plasma amino acids are elevated in migraine. *Neurology* **40**, 1582–1586

Ferrari, M. D., Odink, J., Tapparelli, C., Kempen, G. M. J. V., Pennings, E. J. M. and Bruyn, G. W. (1989). Serotonin metabolism in migraine. *Neurology* **39**, 1239–1242

Friberg, L., Olesen, J., Iversen, H. K. and Sperling, B. (1991). Migraine pain associated with middle cerebral artery dilatation–reversal by sumatriptan. *Lancet* **338**, 13–17

Friberg, L., Skyhøj-Olsen, T., Roland, P. E. and Lassen, N. A. (1987). Focal ischaemia caused by instability of cerebrovascular tone during attacks of hemiplegic migraine. *Brain* **110**, 917–934

Gallai, V., Sarchielli, P., Floridi, A., *et al.* (1995). Vasoactive peptides levels in the plasma of young migraine patients with and without aura assessed both interictally and ictally. *Cephalalgia* **15**, 384–390

Gawel, M., Connolly, J. F and Rose, F. C. (1983). Migraine patients exhibit abnormalities in the visual evoked potential. *Headache* **23**, 49–52

Géraud, G., Besson, M., Fabre, N., Danet, B. and Bès, A. (1989). Heterogenous cerebral blood flow during spontaneous attacks of migraine with and without aura: a Tc-99m HMPAO SPECT study. *Cephalalgia* **9** (Suppl. 10), 31–32

Gloor, P. (1986). Migraine and regional cerebral blood flow. *Trends Neurosci.* **2**, 21

Glover, V., Ahmed, F., Hussein, N., Jarman, J. and Peatfield, R. C. (1996). Central 5-hydroxytryptamine supersensitivity in migraine. In *Migraine Pharmacology and Genetics*, Eds M. Sandler, M. Ferrari and S. Harnett. pp. 117–126. London, Chapman and Hall

Goadsby, P. J. (1992). The oligemic phase of cortical spreading depression is not blocked by tirilazad mesylate (U-74006F). *Brain Res.* **588**, 140–143

Goadsby, P. J. (1997). Bench to bedside: what have we learnt recently about headache? *Curr. Opin. Neurol.* **10**, 215–220

Goadsby, P. J. and Duckworth, J. W. (1987). Locus coeruleus stimulation leads to reductions in regional cerebral blood flow in the cat. *J. Cereb. Blood Flow Metabol.* **7**, S221

Goadsby, P. J. and Edvinsson, L. (1993). The trigeminovascular system and migraine: studies characterising cerebrovascular and neuropeptide changes seen in man and cat. *Ann. Neurol.* **33**, 48–56

Goadsby, P. J. and Edvinsson, L. (1994). Human *in vivo* evidence for trigeminovascular activation in cluster headache. *Brain* **117**, 427–434

Goadsby, P. J. and Edvinsson, L. (1996). Neuropeptide changes in a case of chronic paroxysmal hemicrania – evidence for trigemino-parasympathetic activation. *Cephalalgia* **16**, 448–450

Goadsby, P. J., Edvinsson, L. and Ekman, R. (1988). Release of vasoactive peptides in the extracerebral circulation of man and the cat during activation of the trigeminovascular system. *Ann. Neurol.* **23**, 193–196

Goadsby, P. J., Edvinsson, L. and Ekman, R. (1990). Vasoactive peptide release in the extracerebral circulation of humans during migraine headache. *Ann. Neurol.* **28**, 183–187

Goadsby, P. J. and Gundlach, A. L. (1991). Localization of [^{3}H]-dihydroergotamine binding sites in the cat central nervous system: relevance to migraine. *Ann. Neurol.* **29**, 91–94

Goadsby, P. J. and Hoskin, K. L. (1996). Inhibition of trigeminal neurons by intravenous administration of the serotonin (5HT)-1-D receptor agonist zolmitriptan (311C90): are brain stem sites a therapeutic target in migraine? *Pain* **67**, 355–359

Goadsby, P. J. and Hoskin, K. L. (1997). The distribution of trigeminovascular afferents in the non-human primate brain *Macaca nemestrina*: a c-fos immunocytochemical study. *J. Anatomy* **190**, 367–375

Goadsby, P. J., Hoskin, K. L. and Knight, Y. E. (1997). Stimulation of the greater occipital nerve increases metabolic activity in the trigeminal nucleus caudalis and cervical dorsal horn of the cat. *Pain* **73**, 23–28

Goadsby, P. J., Kaube, H. and Hoskin, K. (1992). Nitric oxide synthesis couples cerebral blood flow and metabolism. *Brain Res.* **595**, 167–170

Goadsby, P. J. and Knight, Y. E. (1997a). Direct evidence for central sites of action of zolmitriptan (311C90): an autoradiographic study in cat. *Cephalalgia* **17**, 153–158

Goadsby, P. J. and Knight, Y. E. (1997b). Naratriptan inhibits trigeminal neurons after intravenous administration through an action at the serotonin (5HT$_{1B/1D}$) receptors. *Br. J. Pharmacol.* **122**, 918–922

Goadsby, P. J., Lambert, G. A. and Lance, J. W. (1982). Differential effects on the internal and external carotid circulation of the monkey evoked by locus coeruleus stimulation. *Brain Res.* **249**, 247–254

Goadsby, P. J., Lambert, G. A. and Lance, J. W. (1983). Effects of locus coeruleus stimulation on carotid vascular resistance in the cat. *Brain Res.* **278**, 175–183

Goadsby, P. J., Lambert, G. A. and Lance, J. W. (1984). The peripheral pathway for extracranial vasodilatation in the cat. *J. Auto. Nerv. Syst.* **10**, 145–155

Goadsby, P. J. and Lance, J. W. (1988). Brainstem effects on intra- and extracerebral circulations. Relation to migraine and cluster headache. In *Basic Mechanisms of Headache*, Eds J. Olesen and L. Edvinsson. pp. 413–427. Amsterdam, Elsevier Science Publishers

Goadsby, P. J. and Macdonald, G. J. (1988). Extracranial vasodilatation mediated by VIP (Vasoactive Intestinal Polypeptide). *Brain Res.* **329**, 285–288

Goadsby, P. J., Piper, R. D., Lambert, G. A. and Lance, J. W. (1985a). The effect of activation of the nucleus raphe dorsalis (DRN) on carotid blood flow. I. The Monkey. *Am. J. Physiol.* **248**, R257–R262

Goadsby, P. J., Piper, R. D., Lambert, G. A. and Lance, J. W. (1985b). The effect of activation of the nucleus raphe dorsalis (DRN) on carotid blood flow. II. The Cat. *Am. J. Physiol.* **248**, R263–R269

Goadsby, P. J. and Zagami, A. S. (1991). Stimulation of the superior sagittal sinus increases metabolic activity and blood flow in certain regions of the brainstem and upper cervical spinal cord of the cat. *Brain* **114**, 1001–1011

Goadsby, P. J., Zagami, A. S. and Lambert, G. A. (1991). Neural processing of craniovascular pain: a synthesis of the central structures involved in migraine. *Headache* **31**, 365–371

Goldstein, D. J. and Wang, O. (1997). Ineffectiveness of neurokinin-1 antagonist in acute migraine: a crossover study. *Cephalalgia* **17**, 245

Goltman, A. M. (1935/36). The mechanism of migraine. *J. Allergy* **7**, 351–355

Graham, J. R. and Wolff, H. G. (1938). Mechanism of migraine headache and action of ergotamine tartrate. *Arch. Neurol. Psychiatry* **39**, 737–763

Griggs, R. C. and Nutt, J. G. (1995). Episodic ataxias as channelopathies. *Ann. Neurol.* **37**, 285–287

Gupta, P., Brown, D., Butler, P. *et al.* (1995). The *in vivo* pharmacological profile of a 5-HT1 receptor agonist, CP122,288, a selective inhibitor of neurogenic inflammation. *Br. J. Pharmacol.* **116**, 2385–2390

Herold, S., Gibbs, J. M., Jones, A. K. P., Brooks, D. J., Frackowiak, R. S. J. and Legg, N. J. (1985). Oxygen metabolism in migraine. *J. Cereb. Blood Flow Metabol.* **5** (Suppl.), S445–S446

Hoskin, K. L. and Goadsby, P. J. (1997). The substance P antagonist, GR205171, does not inhibit trigeminal neurons activated by stimulation of the sagittal sinus: does NK1 blockade have a role in migraine? *Cephalalgia* **17**, 347

Hoskin, K. L., Kaube, H. and Goadsby, P. J. (1996). Central activation of the trigeminovascular pathway in the cat is inhibited by dihydroergotamine: a c-*Fos* and electrophysiology study. *Brain* **119**, 249–256

Hubel, D. H. and Weisel, T. N. (1968). Receptive fields and functional architecture of monkey striate cortex. *J. Physiol.* **195**, 215–243

Iversen, H. K., Nielsen, T. H., Olesen, J. and Tfelt-Hansen, P. (1990). Arterial responses during migraine headache. *Lancet* **336**, 837–839

Jensen, K. and Olesen, J. (1985). Temporal muscle blood flow in common migraine. *Acta Neurol. Scand.* **71**, 561–570

Jensen, K., Pedersen-Bjergaard, U., Tuxen, C., Jansen, I., Edvinsson, L. and Olesen, J. (1990). Pain and tenderness in human temporal muscle induced by bradykinin and 5-hydroxytryptamine. *Peptides* **11**, 1127–1132

Jensen, K., Tfelt-Hansen, P., Lauritzen, M. and Olesen, J. (1986). Classic migraine. A prospective reporting of symptoms. *Acta Neurol. Scand.* **73**, 359–362

Kaube, H., Hoskin, K. L. and Goadsby, P. J. (1993a). Intravenous acetylsalicylic acid inhibits central trigeminal neurons in the dorsal horn of the upper cervical spinal cord in the cat. *Headache* **33**, 541–550

Kaube, H., Hoskin, K. L. and Goadsby, P. J. (1993b). Sumatriptan inhibits central trigeminal neurons only after blood-brain barrier disruption. *Br. J. Pharmacol.* **109**, 788–792

Kaube, H., Keay, K., Hoskin, K. L., Bandler, R. and Goadsby, P. J. (1993). Expression of c-fos-like immunoreactivity in the trigeminal nucleus caudalis and high cervical cord following stimulation of the sagittal sinus in the cat. *Brain Res.* **629**, 95–102

Kerr, F. W. L. (1961). A mechanism to account for frontal headache in cases of posterior fossa tumours. *J. Neurosurg.* **18**, 605–609

Kerr, F. W. L. and Olafson, R. A. (1961). Trigeminal and cervical volleys. *Arch. Neurol.* **5**, 69–76

Kimball, R. W., Friedman, A. P. and Vallejo, E. (1960). Effect of serotonin in migraine patients. *Neurology, Minneap.* **10**, 107–111

Knight, Y. E., Edvinsson, L. and Goadsby, P. J. (1997). Blockade of release of CGRP after superior sagittal sinus stimulation in cat: a comparison of avitriptan and CP122,288. *Cephalalgia* **17**, 248

Kobari, M., Meyer, J. S., Ichjo, M., Imai, K. and Oravez, W. T. (1989). Hyperperfusion of cerebral cortex, thalamus and basal ganglia during spontaneously occurring migraine headaches. *Headache* **29**, 282–289

Kupfermann, I. (1985). Hypothalamus and limbic system II: motivation. In *Principles of Neural Science*, Eds E. R. Kandel and J. H. Schwartz. pp. 626–635. Elsevier, Amsterdam Science Publishers

Lambert, G. A., Bogduk, N., Goadsby, P. J., Duckworth, J. W. and Lance, J. W. (1984). Decreased carotid arterial resistance in cats in response to trigeminal stimulation. *J. Neurosurg.* **61**, 307–315

Lance, J. W. (1986). *Migraine and Other Headaches*. New York, Charles Scribner and Sons

Lance, J. W. (1995). Swelling at the site of a skull defect during migraine headache. *J. Neurol. Neurosurg. Psychiat.* **59**, 641

Lance, J. W. and Anthony, M. (1966). Some clinical aspects of migraine: a prospective survey of 500 patients. *Arch. Neurol.* **15**, 356–361

Lance, J. W., Lambert, G. A., Goadsby, P. J. and Duckworth, J. W. (1983). Brainstem influences on cephalic circulation: experimental data from cat and monkey of relevance to the mechanism of migraine. *Headache* **23**, 258–265

Lance, J. W., Lambert, G. A., Goadsby, P. J. and Zagami, A. S. (1989). Contribution of experimental studies to understanding the pathophysiology of migraine. In *Migraine: A Spectrum of Ideas*, Eds M. Sandler and G. M. Collins. pp. 21–39. Oxford, Oxford University Press

Lashley, K. S. (1941). Patterns of cerebral integration indicated by the scotomas of migraine. *Arch. Neurol. Psychiat.* **46**, 331–339

Lassen, L. H., Ashina, M., Christiansen, I., Ulrich, V. and Olesen, J. (1997). Nitric oxide synthesis inhibition in migraine. *Lancet* **349**, 401–402

Launay, J. M. and Pradalier, A. (1985). Common migraine attack: platelet modifications are mainly due to plasma factor(s). *Headache* **25**, 262–268

Lauritzen, M. (1984). Long-lasting reduction of cortical blood flow of the rat brain after spreading depression with preserved autoregulation and impaired CO_2 response. *J. Cereb. Blood Flow Metabol.* **4**, 546–554

Lauritzen, M. (1994). Pathophysiology of the migraine aura. The spreading depression theory. *Brain* **117**, 199–210

Lauritzen, M., Jorgensen, M. B., Diemer, N. H., Gjedde, A. and Hansen, A. J. (1982). Persistent oligaemia of rat cerebral cortex in the wake of spreading depression. *Ann. Neurol.* **12**, 469–474

Lauritzen, M., Skyhøj-Olsen, T., Lassen, N. A. and Paulson, O. B. (1983a). The changes of regional cerebral blood flow during the course of classical migraine attacks. *Ann. Neurol.* **13**, 633–641

Lauritzen, M., Skyhøj-Olsen, T., Lassen, N. A. and Paulson, O. B. (1983b). Regulation of regional cerebral blood flow during and between migraine attacks. *Ann. Neurol.* **14**, 569–572

Leão, A. A. P. (1944). Spreading depression of activity in cerebral cortex. *J. Neurophysiol.* **7**, 359–390

Lee, W. K., Limmroth, V., Ayata, C. *et al.* (1995). Peripheral GABA-A receptor mediated effects of sodium valproate on dural plasma protein extravasation to substance P and trigeminal stimulation. *Br. J. Pharmacol.* **116**, 1661–1667

Lee, W. S. and Moskowitz, M. A. (1993). Conformationally restricted sumatriptan analogues, CP-122,288 and CP-122,638, exhibit enhanced potency against neurogenic inflammation in dura mater. *Brain Res.* **626**, 303–305

Lee, W. S., Moussaoui, S. M. and Moskowitz, M. A. (1994). Blockade by oral or parenteral RPR100893 (a non-peptide NK1 receptor antagonist) of neurogenic plasma protein extravsation in guinea-pig dura mater and conjunctiva. *Br. J. Pharmacol.* **112**, 920–924

Limmroth, V., Lee, W. S., Cutrer, F. M., Waeber, C. and Moskowitz, M. A. (1995). Progesterone and its ring-A-reduced metabolites suppress dural plasma protein extravasation by activation of peripheral $GABA_A$ receptors. *Cephalalgia* **15** (Suppl. 14), 98

Lous, I. and Olsen, J. (1982). Evaluation of pericranial tenderness and oral function in patients with common migraine, muscle contraction headache and 'combination headache'. *Pain* **12**, 385–393

Maertens de Noordhout, A., Timsit-Berthier, M. and Schoenen, J. (1985). Contingent negative variation (CNV) in migraineurs before and during prophylactic treatment with beta-blockers. *Cephalalgia* **5** (Suppl. 3), 34–35

Markowitz, S., Saito, K. and Moskowitz, M. A. (1987). Neurogenically mediated leakage of plasma proteins occurs from blood vessels in dura mater but not brain. *J. Neurosci.* **7**, 4129–4136

Markowitz, S., Saito, K. and Moskowitz, M. A. (1988). Neurogenically mediated plasma extravasation in dura mater: effect of ergot alkaloids. A possible mechanism of action in vascular headache. *Cephalalgia* **8**, 83–91

May, A., Gijsman, H. J., Wallnoefer, A., Jones, R., Diener, H. C. and Ferrari, M. D. (1996). Endothelin antagonist bosentan blocks neurogenic inflammation, but is not effective in aborting migraine attacks. *Pain* **67**, 375–378

May, A., Ophoff, R. A., Terwindt, G. M. *et al.* (1995). Familial hemiplegic migraine locus on chromosome 19p13 is involved in common forms of migraine with and without aura. *Human Genet.* **96**, 604–608

Mayberg, M., Langer, R. S., Zervas, N. T. and Moskowitz, M. A. (1981). Perivascular meningeal projections from cat trigeminal ganglia: possible pathway for vascular headaches in man. *Science* **213**, 228–230

McLachlan, R. S. and Girvin, J. P. (1994). Spreading depression of Leão in rodent and human cortex. *Brain Res.* **666**, 133–136

McNaughton, F. L. (1938). The innervation of the intracranial blood vessels and dural sinuses. *Proc. Assoc. Res. Nervous Mental Dis.* **18**, 178–200

Mills, A. and Martin, G. R. (1995). Autoradiographic mapping of [^{3}H]sumatriptan binding in cat brain stem and spinal cord. *Eur. J. Pharmacol.* **280**, 175–178

Moskowitz, M. A. (1984). The neurobiology of vascular head pain. *Ann. Neurol.* **16**, 157–168

Moskowitz, M. A. (1992). Neurogenic versus vascular mechanisms of sumatriptan and ergot alkaloids in migraine. *Trends Pharmacol. Sci.* **13**, 307–311

Moskowitz, M. A. and Buzzi, M. G. (1991). Neuroeffector functions of sensory fibres: implications for headache mechanisms and drug actions. *J. Neurol.* **238**, S18–S22

Moskowitz, M. A. and Cutrer, F. M. (1993). Sumatriptan: a receptor-targeted treatment for migraine. *Ann. Rev. Med.* **44**, 145–154

Moskowitz, M. A., Nozaki, K. and Kraig, R. P. (1993). Neocortical spreading depression provokes the expression of c-fos protein-like immunoreactivity within the trigeminal nucleus caudalis via trigemino-vascular mechanisms. *J. Neurosci.* **13**, 1167–1177

Mosnaim, A. D., Wolf, M. E., Chevesich, J., Callaghan, O. H. and Diamond, S. (1985). Plasma methionine enkephalin levels. A biological marker for migraine? *Headache* **25**, 259–261

Mraovitch, S., Calando, Y., Goadsby, P. J. and Seylaz, J. (1992). Subcortical cerebral blood flow and metabolic changes elicited by cortical spreading depression in rat. *Cephalalgia* **12**, 137–141

Mück-Šěler, D., Deanović, Ž. and Dupelj, M. (1979). Platelet serotonin (5-HT) and 5-HT releasing factor in plasma of migrainous patients. *Headache* **19**, 14–17

Murialdo, G., Martignoni, E., Maria, D. *et al.* (1986). Changes in the dopaminergic control of prolactin secretion and in ovarian steriods in migraine. *Cephalalgia* **6**, 43–49

Nappi, G. and Savoldi, F. (1985). *Headache: Diagnostic System and Taxonomic Criteria.* pp. 53–59. London, John Libbey

Nichols, F. T., Mawad, M., Mohr, J. P., Hilal, S. and Adams, R. J. (1993). Focal headache during balloon inflation in the vertebral and basilar arteries. *Headache* **33**, 87–89

Nissila, M., Parkkola, R., Sonninen, P. and Salonen, R. (1996). Intracerebral arteries and gadolinium enhancement in migraine without aura. *Cephalalgia* **16**, 363

Norris, J. W., Hachinski, V. C. and Cooper, P. W. (1975). Changes in cerebral blood flow during a migraine attack. *Br. Med. J.* **3**, 676–677

Nozaki, K., Boccalini, P. and Moskowitz, M. A. (1992). Expression of c-fos-like immunoreactivity in brainstem after meningeal irritation by blood in the subarachnoid space. *Neuroscience* **49**, 669–680

Olesen, J., Friberg, L., Skyhøj-Olsen, T. *et al.* (1990). Timing and topography of cerebral blood flow, aura and headache during migraine attacks. *Ann. Neurol.* **28**, 791–798

Olesen, J., Larsen, B. and Lauritzen, M. (1981). Focal hyperemia followed by spreading oligemia and impaired activation of rCBF in classic migraine. *Ann. Neurol.* **9**, 344–352

Olesen, J., Tfelt-Hansen, P., Henriksen, L. and Larsen, B. (1981). The common migraine attack may not be initiated by cerebral ischemia. *Lancet* **II**, 438–440

Ophoff, R. A., Terwindt, G. M., Vergouwe, M. N. *et al.* (1996). Familial hemiplegic migraine and episodic ataxia type-2 are caused by mutations in the Ca^{2+} channel gene CACNLA4. *Cell* **87**, 543–552

Pascual, J., Arco, Cd., Romon, T., Olmo, Cd. and Pazos, A. (1996). [^{3}H] Sumatriptan binding sites in human brain: regional-dependent labelling of 5-HT1D and 5-HT1F receptors. *Eur. J. Pharmacol.* **295**, 271–274

Peatfield, R. C. and Clifford Rose, F. (1991). Prospective study of unilateral classical migraine. In *New Advances in Headache Research: 2*, Ed. F. Clifford Rose. London, Smith-Gordon and Co. Ltd

Penfield, W. and Perot, P. (1963). The brain's record of auditory and visual experience. *Brain* **86**, 595–696

Peroutka, S. J. (1997). Dopamine and migraine. *Neurology* **49**, 650–656

Piper, R. D., Lambert, G. A. and Duckworth, J. W. (1991). Cortical blood flow changes during spreading depression in cats. *Am. J. Physiol.* **261**, H96–H102

Piper, R. D., Matheson, J. M., Hellier, M. *et al.* (1991). Cortical spreading depression is not seen intraoperatively during temporal lobectomy in humans. *Cephalalgia* **11** (Suppl. 11), 1

Ramadan, N. M., Halvorson, H., Vande-Linde, A., Levine, S. R., Helpern, J. A. and Welch, K. M. A. (1989). Low brain magnesium in migraine. *Headache* **29**, 416–419

Raskin, N. H., Hosobuchi, Y. and Lamb, S. (1987). Headache may arise from perturbation of brain. *Headache* **27**, 416–420

Raskin, N. H. and Knittle, S. C. (1976) Ice cream headache and orthostatic symptoms in patients with migraine headache. *Headache* **16**, 222–225

Raskin, N. H. and Schwartz, R.K. (1980). Icepick-like pain. *Neurology* **30**, 203–205

Ray, B. S. and Wolff, H. G. (1940). Experimental studies on headache. Pain sensitive structures of the head and their significance in headache. *Arch. Surg.* **41**, 813–856

Roon, K., Diener, H. C., Ellis, P. *et al.* (1997). CP-122,288 blocks neurogenic inflammation, but is not effective in aborting migraine attacks: results of two controlled clinical studies. *Cephalalgia* **17**, 245

Ruskell, G. L. (1988) The tentorial nerve in monkeys is a branch of the cavernous plexus. *J. Anatomy* **157**, 67–77

Ruskell, G. L. and Simons, T. (1987). Trigeminal nerve pathways to the cerebral arteries in monkeys. *J. Anatomy* **155**, 23–37

Russell, M. B., Rassmussen, B. K., Fenger, K. and Olesen, J. (1996). Migraine without aura and migraine with aura are distinct clinical entities: a study of four hundred and eight-four male and female migraineurs from the general population. *Cephalalgia* **16**, 239–245

Ryan, R. E., Elkind, A. and Goldstein, J. (1997). Twenty-four hour effectiveness of BMS 180048 in the acute treatment of migraine headaches. *Headache* **37**, 245–248

Sabatini, U., Rascol, O., Rascol, A. and Montastruc, J. (1990). Migraine attacks induced by subcutaneous apomorphine in two migrainous Parkinsonian patients. *Clin. Neuropharmacol.* **13**, 264–267

Sakai, F. and Meyer, J. S. (1978). Regional cerebral hemodynamics during migraine and cluster headaches measured by the ^{133}Xe inhalation method. *Headache* **18**, 122–132

Sakai, F. and Meyer, J. S. (1979). Abnormal cerebrovascular reactivity in patients with migraine and cluster headache. *Headache* **19**, 257–266

Schoenen, J., Wang, W., Albert, A. and Delwaide, P. J. (1995). Potentiation instead of habituation characterizes visual evoked potentials in migraine patients between attacks. *Eur. J. Neurol.* **2**, 115–122

Serra, G., Collu, M. and Gessa, G. L. (1986). Dopamine receptors mediating yawning: are they autoreceptors? *Eur. J. Pharmacol.* **120**, 187–192

Serra, G., Collu, M. and Gessa, G. L. (1987). Yawning is elicited by D2 dopamine agonists but is blocked by the D1 antagonist, SCH23390. *Psychopharmacol.* **91**, 330–333

Sicuteri, F. (1959). Prophylactic and therapeutic properties of UML-491 in migraine. *Int. Arch. Allergy* **15**, 300–307

Sicuteri, F. (1977). Dopamine, the second putative protagonist in headache. *Headache* **17**, 129–131

Sicuteri, F., Boccuni, M., Fanciullacci, M. and Gatto, G. (1983). Naloxone effectiveness on spontaneous and induced perceptive disorders in migraine. *Headache* **23**, 179–183

Sicuteri, F., Testi, A. and Anselmi, B. (1961). Biochemical investigations in headache: increase in hydroxyindoleacetic acid excretion during migraine attacks. *Int. Arch. Allergy* **19**, 55–58

Simard, D. and Paulson, O. B. (1973). Cerebral vasomotor paralysis during migraine attack. *Arch. Neurol.* **29**, 207–209

Skyhøj-Olsen, T., Friberg, L. and Lassen, N. A. (1987). Ischemia may be the primary cause of the neurological deficits in classic migraine. *Arch. Neurol.* **44**, 156–161

Sramka, M., Brozek, G., Bures, J. and Nadvornik, P. (1977). Functional ablation by spreading depression: possible use in human stereotactic neurosurgery. *Appl. Neurophysiol.* **40**, 48–61

Storer, R. J. and Goadsby, P. J. (1997). Microiontophoretic application of serotonin (5-HT)-1B/1D agonists inhibits trigeminal cell firing in the cat. *Brain* **120**, 2171–2177

Strassman, A. M., Mineta, Y. and Vos, B. P. (1994). Distribution of fos-like immunoreactivity in the medullary and upper cervical dorsal horn produced by stimulation of dural blood vessels in the rat. *J. Neurosci.* **14**, 3725–3735

Strassman, A. M. and Vos, B. P. (1993). Somatotopic and laminar organization of fos-like immunoreactivity in the medullary and upper cervical dorsal horn induced by noxious facial stimulation in the rat. *J. Comp. Neurol.* **331**, 495–516

Strassman, A. M., Vos, B. P., Mineta, Y., Naderi, S., Borsook, D. and Burstein, R. (1993). Fos-like immunoreactivity in the superficial medullary dorsal horn induced by noxious and innocuous thermal stimulation of the facial skin in the rat. *J. Neurophysiol.* **70**, 1811–1821

Swaab, D. F., Hofman, M. A., Lucassen, P. J., Purba, J. S., Raadsheer, F. C. and van de Ness, J. A. (1993). Functional neuroanatomy and neuropathology of the hypothalamus. *Anat. Embryol.* **187**, 317–330

Tfelt-Hansen, P., Lous, I. and Olesen, J. (1981). Prevalence and significance of muscle tenderness during common migraine attacks. *Headache* **21**, 49–54

Tunis, M. M. and Wolff, H. G. (1953). Long term observations of the reactivity of the cranial arteries in subjects with vascular headache of the migraine type. *Arch. Neurol. Psychiat.* **70**, 551–557

Vardi, J., Fletcher, S., Ayalon, D., Cordova, T. and Oberman, Z. (1981). L-dopa effect on prolactin plasma levels in complicated and common migrainous patients. *Headache* **21**, 14–20

Veloso, F. and Kumar, K. (1996). Deep brain implant migraine. *J. Neurol. Neurosurg. Psychiat.* **46** (Suppl. 7), A168–A169

Walters, D. W., Gillespie, S. A. and Moskowitz, M. (1986). Cerebrovascular projections from the sphenopalatine and otic ganglia to the middle cerebral artery of the cat. *Stroke* **17**, 488–494

Wang, W., Timsit-Berthier, M. and Schoenen, J. (1996). Intensity dependence of the auditory cortical evoked potentials is pronounced in migraine: an indication of cortical potentiation and low serotonergic transmission? *Neurology* **46**, 1404–1409

Weiller, C., May, A., Limmroth, V. *et al.* (1995). Brain stem activation in spontaneous human migraine attacks. *Nat. Medicine* **1**, 658–660

Welch, K. M. and Ramadan, N. M. (1995). Mitochondria, magnesium and migraine. *J. Neurol. Sci.* **134**, 9–14

Winter, A. L. (1987). Neurophysiology in migraine. In *Migraine – Clinical and Research Aspects*, Ed. J. N. Blau. pp. 485–510. Baltimore, Johns Hopkins University Press

Wolff, H. G. (1963). *Headache and Other Head Pain*. New York, Oxford University Press

Woods, R. P., Iacoboni, M. and Mazziotta, J. C. (1994). Bilateral spreading cerebral hypoperfusion during spontaneous migraine headache. *N. Eng. J. Med.* **331**, 1689–1692

Zagami, A. S. and Goadsby, P. J. (1991). Stimulation of the superior sagittal sinus increases metabolic activity in cat thalamus. In *New Advances in Headache Research: 2*, Ed. F. Clifford Rose. pp. 169–171. London, Smith-Gordon and Co. Ltd

Zagami, A. S., Goadsby, P. J. and Edvinsson, L. (1990). Stimulation of the superior sagittal sinus in the cat causes release of vasoactive peptides. *Neuropeptides* **16**, 69–75

Zagami, A. S. and Lambert, G. A. (1990). Stimulation of cranial vessels excites nociceptive neurones in several thalamic nuclei of the cat. *Exp. Brain Res.* **81**, 552–566

Zagami, A. S. and Lambert, G. A. (1991). Craniovascular application of capsaicin activates nociceptive thalamic neurons in the cat. *Neurosci. Lett.* **121**, 187–190

Chapter 9

Migraine: treatment

Migraine is a horrid disability and deserves to be taken seriously. It rarely destroys life but can destroy many of the pleasures of life. It can ruin marriages, families and careers. It is a disorder which warrants full attention from the physician or general practitioner.

At present there is no complete 'cure' for migraine and perhaps there never will be. It is important to explain to patients at the outset that they have been born with a tendency to have headaches that over-reacts to internal changes or external stimuli, and that there is a very good chance that the condition can be brought under control by advice and judicious medication. Many people seek 'natural' methods of treatment and resent the need to take pills. Not unreasonably they want to know the cause of their headaches and the changes in lifestyle necessary to avoid them. Perhaps meditation, manipulation or the removal of some superfluous viscus would do the trick. We all wish that it was as simple as this. Doctors should feel some empathy with their headache patients and take some time to make sure that they understand the principles of management. Most patients are made miserable by their headaches, have done nothing to deserve them and genuinely want to get rid of them.

If the history is typical of migraine headache, patients should be assured that there is no suggestion that a cerebral tumour or other progressive disease is causing their symptoms and therefore no need for extensive and expensive investigations. The history and physical examination may have disclosed precipitating or aggravating factors that require attention. Factors that may increase the frequency and severity of migraine attacks include:

- An anxiety or depressive state.
- The onset of systemic hypertension.
- The use of oral contraceptive pills or vasodilator drugs.
- The excessive consumption of analgesics, caffeine or ergotamine.

General advice includes some guidance on lifestyle which may be given to the patient as follows:

- Try to spread your work load evenly, to avoid peaks and troughs of stress at work or at home.

- Do not sleep in (later than your normal hour of waking) at weekends because this often causes a 'let-down' headache.
- Avoid excessive fatigue.
- Eat at regular times and do not miss meals. Eliminate any article of diet that you believe may bring on an attack. This applies to the intake of alcohol, particularly red wines, in susceptible persons.
- Limit your consumption of tea, coffee and analgesics because these may lead to rebound headaches.
- Watch your posture. Avoid craning your neck forwards. Think tall.
- Keep your muscles as relaxed as possible when not physically active. No frowning or jaw clenching.
- Exercise daily but restrict physical exertion on a hot day.
- Avoid glare or exposure to flickering light, noise or strong smells if these are trigger factors.
- Bear in mind the classic Greek admonition of 'moderation in all things'.

General (non-pharmaceutical) methods of treatment

Psychological management

There is an important role in terms of psychological counselling for the doctor of first contact, very often the family physician or general practitioner, who ideally knows the patient in his or her family setting and is in the best position to give advice. Sometimes patients will discuss embarrassing personal problems more freely with an outsider, such as a consultant physician, neurologist or psychiatrist, than they would with a doctor who knows them and their family socially. Such a discussion takes time and tolerance and may not necessarily find solutions for the problems that emerge. In any event, it gives patients a chance to unburden themselves, the opportunity to gain objective advice, and the knowledge that their problem is not unique and has been overcome by many others. Manipulation of the patient's personality or life pattern is not always possible but the very fact of free discussion helps patients and gives confidence that doctors understand that they are dealing with individuals. It may be possible for patients to rearrange their daily routine to minimize stress and then to adjust happily to those fluctuations which will inevitably remain. The external environment can be stabilized to some extent and then patients must concentrate on themselves and their reactions to change.

Building up resistance to stress from within can use both psychological and physiological techniques. Mitchell and Mitchell (1971) compared two such programmes. In the first programme, relaxation training was followed by the application of this training to the tension-producing situation peculiar to that individual. The second treatment group went on to desensitization procedures, which included making a graded list of anxiety-producing stimuli, evoking these by imagery, and pairing each stimulus with a relaxed state. A further stage was 'assertive therapy' in which the subjects underwent training in acting out their feelings of love, affection or hostility in socially acceptable and appropriate forms. Various difficulties, such as sexual problems, were explained and discussed. While the level of anxiety did not drop appreciably during the 32-week treatment period, the last group with combined relaxation, desensitization and assertive therapy showed significant reduction in the frequency and severity of migraine compared with the other group.

With the object of training patients to increase their stress threshold, Mitchell and White (1976) introduced a programme of 'behavioural self-management', in which patients identify and analyse problems in their personal environment and behaviour, to work out their own management strategy and to apply self-control techniques.

While there is general agreement that psychological factors are important in causing headache, there are few carefully controlled trials to demonstrate the effectiveness of psychological management in general and the comparative merits of the various forms of treatment employed.

Physiological management (relaxation and biofeedback)

Simple relaxation training, as described in Appendix B, can be applied to migraine patients to reduce the frequency and severity of headache. Warner and Lance (1975) found that four sessions of training in conjunction with an outpatient clinic caused improvement that persisted for 6 months.

Relaxation training is often augmented by feedback from an electromyogram (EMG) of the frontal and temporal muscles, from skin temperatures of scalp and hand, or from recordings of the temporal artery pulsations. Spontaneous recovery from migraine headache is associated with an increase in blood flow and skin temperature in the hands. A study of treatment by relaxation and thermal biofeedback demonstrated significant improvement over headache-monitoring control subjects, but the addition of cognitive therapy conferred no further advantage (Blanchard et al., 1990). It must be borne in mind that migraine tends to improve whenever a patient is under supervision in a clinical trial. In our own clinic, placebo results in controlled trials of drug therapy have varied from 20 to 60 per cent improvement, the latter figure being achieved when psychological counselling and relaxation training were part of general management. The results of non-pharmacological treatments of migraine have been summarized by Holroyd and Penzien (1990) who concluded that biofeedback/relaxation therapy was as effective as propranolol in the management of migraine, each yielding a reduction in headache of 43 per cent, whereas placebo produced only a 14 per cent reduction. It is probable that biofeedback achieves no more than relaxation therapy alone but both fulfil the requirements of those patients who demand relief without drugs, and are satisfied with only a modest improvement in their headache pattern.

Transcendental meditation and hypnotherapy

Any means of achieving emotional equilibrium and physical relaxation might be expected to be helpful in migraine, but transcendental meditation was of benefit to only six of 17 patients studied by Benson, Klemchuk and Graham (1974). The results of hypnotherapy are more encouraging. Anderson, Basker and Dalton (1975) compared 23 patients undergoing hypnotherapy with a control group of 24 treated with prochlorperazine. The hypnosis group (in six sessions at intervals of 10–14 days) were given 'ego-strengthening' suggestions that they would have less tension, anxiety and apprehension, as well as specific suggestions about constricting the arteries in their heads. Patients were asked to practise hypnosis daily and to use it to abort a threatened attack of migraine. The trial extended for 12 months, and in the last 3 months of the trial 43.5 per cent of the hypnotherapy group were free of headache, compared with 12.5 per cent of controls. The median number of attacks per month dropped from 4.5 to 0.5 in the patients treated with hypnosis compared with 3.3 to 2.9 in the prochlorperazine group.

Acupuncture

Acupuncture has been practised in China for more than 2000 years and is currently in vogue in the western world. Loh *et al.* (1984) studied the effect of acupuncture in 55 patients with migraine and tension headache who had not responded to 'every kind of drug that had been fashionable at that time'. Of the 41 patients who completed a 3-month course, nine improved greatly, seven moderately, eight slightly and 17 not at all. Baischer (1995) also described the effect of acupuncture, for courses averaging 10 treatments, in 26 patients. An improvement of more than 33 per cent was achieved by 18 patients. Our own impression is that the response to acupuncture is inconsistent and not usually sustained after treatment ceases.

Exercise

Standing on the head improves vasoconstrictor reflexes in scalp arteries (Wolff, 1963) and has a rational basis for the gymnastically adroit, but is of limited application. Strenuous exertion may precipitate migraine in some patients but a gradual increase in exercise, particularly if it is disguised by some agreeable sport or occupation, is usually beneficial.

Prevention of salt and water retention

Fluid retention is common for several days before the menstrual period and is also common immediately before migraine headache. The fact that menstruation and migraine often coincide led to the use of salt restriction and diuretics in the treatment of migraine, whether or not it tended to occur with the menses. Fluid retention may indeed be prevented by such measures but migraine usually continues unabated.

Elimination diets

Dietary factors as possible precipitants of migraine headache were discussed in Chapter 7. This subject was reviewed by McQueen *et al.* (1989) in presenting the results of a controlled trial of dietary modification in 95 patients, of whom 26 considered that their headaches could be precipitated by specific foods, 14 by alcohol and 10 by both. The protocol consisted of an elimination diet for 4–6 weeks (during which time 37 patients improved, 22 did not and 36 dropped out), followed by blinded food challenges and the prescription of diets containing, and diets avoiding, provoking factors in a randomized fashion. Of the 19 patients who completed this rigorous programme, nine had fewer and less severe headaches on the therapeutic diet than on the control diet whereas six were no different and four were worse. It is therefore most unlikely that food allergy plays any part in adult migraine but it is quite possible that simplification of the diet, like other aspects of lifestyle, may exert a benign but non-specific influence on the course of migraine.

Histamine desensitization

Histamine, given by incrementing subcutaneous injections or weekly intravenous infusions, has been used in the treatment of migraine for many years. This is a difficult procedure to adapt to a controlled trial to see whether it is really effective. A follow-up for 8 months after a course of three intravenous infusions at weekly intervals revealed that 21 per cent of patients became headache-free and another 42 per cent were more than half-improved (Selby and Lance, 1960). It is not known whether this treatment has some non-specific effect on vascular reactivity, or whether its action is purely psychological.

Manipulative and surgical procedures

Success has been claimed for manipulation of the neck in the treatment of migraine headache as in many other fields, but objective evidence is lacking. Cyriax (1962) stated that 'an attack of migraine can sometimes be instantly aborted by strong traction on the neck. Half a minute's traction in some cases is regularly successful, in others not. The mechanism is obscure (it may be connected with stretching of the carotid and vertebral arteries) and the phenomenon would clearly repay further study . . . .' Cyriax goes on to say that 'a minority of patients have reported to me, some years after the reduction by manipulation of a cervical disc, that since that time attacks of obvious migraine have ceased'.

Manipulation of the cervical spine has been evaluated by a controlled trial (Parker *et al.*, 1978). Migraine patients were allocated randomly to three groups: one group treated by chiropractic manipulation, a second group in which patients underwent manipulation by a doctor or physiotherapist, and a control group in which subjects had a course of cervical mobilization by a doctor or physiotherapist. Treatment of the last group involved a number of the non-specific therapeutic ingredients common to other groups. Migraine symptoms were reduced by about 28 per cent in all groups but no one group improved significantly more than the other over the 6-month trial, although the severity of headache was less in the chiropractic group. Twenty months after the course of treatment, migraine attacks had diminished by a further 19 per cent, which the authors attributed to the natural history of the disorder (Parker *et al.*, 1980).

Operations on sympathetic or parasympathetic nerve pathways, and ligation of branches of the external carotid or middle meningeal arteries, or both, have not provided any lasting benefit. The painful component of the migraine attack can be reduced or abolished by lesions of the trigeminal ganglion or root or section of the spinal tract and nucleus of the trigeminal nerve (White and Sweet, 1955) but such destructive surgery is rarely, if ever, warranted.

Pharmacotherapy

The pharmacotherapy of migraine falls in to two distinct classes: preventative or prophylactic measures that seek primarily to reduce headache frequency; and abortive or acute attack treatments, whose purpose is to stop attacks when they take place. Some patients who have frequent headache will require a preventative agent and the decision to start must be made after careful consultation and discussion between patient and physician. In general, patients having two or less headaches a month will do reasonably well on acute attack medications alone, while those with more than four attacks a month will often derive benefit from a preventative agent. Decisions for those in the middle will be driven, as will those for the more or less frequent attacks, by the patient's response to acute attack medications including tolerability, efficacy and safety of the acute attack medications. Ultimately, the decision will be an amalgam of the perceptions and views of both the patient and the managing physician, although a golden rule is that it is the patient who suffers and must be involved completely in the decision to commence a preventative medication.

Agents used in the treatment of acute attacks

The development of acute attack treatments over the last decade has been a major advance in the management of migraine sufferers. Acute attack treatments may be divided into two broad categories: non-specific, i.e. analgesics with anti-pain actions that are not specific to migraine; and specific compounds, drugs with antimigraine actions but no general anti-pain actions (Goadsby and Olesen, 1996).

Specific treatments of acute migraine attacks

Current specific antimigraine drugs derive in a broad pharmacological sense from the ergot alkaloids. The *triptans*, first synthesized in the form of sumatriptan, represent a sharpening of pharmacological focus upon certain subclasses of serotonin (5-hydroxytryptamine, 5-HT) receptors. There are currently seven classes of 5-HT receptors (Table 9.1) with the 5-HT1 subclass being the major focus of recent drug development (Table 9.2). A comparison of the pharmacology of dihydroergotamine and sumatriptan (Table 9.3) illustrates that the synthesis of newer compounds has basically been aimed at removal of unwanted effects at receptor sites associated with the side-effects of serotonin administration.

Ergotamine tartrate. Ergotamine has been used in the management of migraine headache for over 50 years and should be given in optimal dosage orally, rectally or by inhalation or injection at the first indication of an attack starting. The effectiveness of ergotamine has been confirmed in a double-blind crossover study

Table 9.1 Classification of serotonin (5-HT) receptors. (Modified from Hoyer *et al.*, 1994)

5-HT receptor class	Second messenger	Antagonist	Function
1	↓ Adenylate cyclase		See Table 9.2 for details
2	↑ Phosphoinositide turnover	Methysergide pizotifen	Contraction of smooth muscle Central nervous system excitation Subtypes: 2_A, 2_B, 2_C
3	$K^+/Ca^{2+}/Na^+$	Ondansetron granisitron	Membrane depolarization
4	↑ Adenylate cyclase	GR113808	Stimulates GI contraction Found in striato-nigral system
5		–	Subclasses A and B
6	↑ Adenylate cyclase	Ro04-6790	Single receptor
7	↑ Adenylate cyclase	SB258719	Role in circadian rhythms; splice varients

Table 9.2 Classification of serotonin (5-HT) subclass 1 receptors. (Modified from Hartig *et al.*, 1996)

Subtype of 5-HT_1 receptor	Agonist	Antagonist	Function
A	8-OH-DPAT† Dihydroergotamine	WAY100, 635	Hypotension Behavioural (satiety)
Rat B	CP-93,129†		Central autoreceptor (rat)
Human B (previously known as $1_{D\beta}$)	Sumatriptan Dihydroergotamine Triptans	SB216641 GR127935†	Craniovascular receptor
D (previously known as $1_{D\alpha}$)	Sumatriptan Dihydroergotamine Triptans	BRL15572 GR127935†	Trigeminal neuronal receptor
E		–	?
F	Sumatriptan Eletriptan Naratriptan Zolmitriptan LY334370*	–	?

† 8-OH-DPAT [8-hydroxy-2-(di-*n*-propylamino)tetralin], WAY100165, BRL15572, SB216641, CP-93,129 and GR127935 are all compounds used in the laboratory for pharmacological purposes and have no current clinical indications.
Triptan: almotriptan, eletriptan, frovatriptan (VML 251), naratriptan, rizatriptan and zolmitriptan.

(Hakkarainen *et al.*, 1979). Ergotamine tartrate is an agonist of 5-HT_1 receptors and a competitive antagonist with partial agonism on α-adrenergic receptors (Muller-Schweinitzer and Fanchamps, 1982). It has a biphasic effect like 5HT itself in that it constricts dilated vessels and dilates constricted vessels, which probably accounts for its ability to shorten the aura phase of migraine. Its action depends on the pre-existing vascular resistance (Aellig and Berde, 1969). The intramuscular injection of 0.25–1.0 mg or the intravenous injection of 0.5 mg ergotamine or 1.0 mg of dihydroergotamine does not alter regional cerebral blood flow in human subjects (Andersen *et al.*, 1987).

Table 9.3 Comparison of the pharmacology of dihydroergotamine and sumatriptan. (Based on receptor affinity data of Berde and Schild, 1978, and Humphrey *et al.*, 1991)

	DHE	*Sumatriptan*
Serotonergic (5-HT):		
1_A	$+++$	$+$
1_B	$++$	$++$
1_D	$++$	$++$
1_E	$++$	$-$
1_F	$+$	$++$
$2_{A/C}$	$+$	$-$
3	$-$	$-$
Adrenergic:		
α_1	$+$	$-$
α_2	$+$	$-$
β	$+/-$	$-$
Dopaminergic:		
D1	$-$	$-$
D2	$+/-$	$-$

There are conflicting reports on the pharmacokinetics of ergotamine, probably because of differing techniques of measurement. By a radio-immunoassay method, therapeutic oral and rectal doses of ergotamine yielded measurable plasma concentrations for about 6 hours, a peak level at 1–2 hours of 0.2 ng/ml being associated with a good clinical response (Hokkanen *et al.*, 1982). In contrast, Tfelt-Hansen, Ibraheem and Paalzow (1982), using high performance liquid chromatography (sensitive to 0.1 ng/ml or more), found that plasma ergotamine did not reach detectable levels after the administration of tablets or suppositories, but did when ergotamine tartrate was inhaled or injected intramuscularly. The discrepancy is probably accounted for by the radio-immunoassay method measuring ergotaminine as well as ergotamine metabolites.

The clinical use of ergotamine is usually restricted to the management of single acute episodes as overdosage causes nausea, vomiting, malaise, rebound headache and peripheral vasoconstriction, which may rarely be severe enough to cause arterial obstruction (Magee, 1991). The excessive use of ergotamine-containing suppositories has been reported to cause anorectal ulceration (Jost *et al.*, 1991). Ergotamine should be avoided in patients with ischaemic or thyrotoxic heart disease (Benedict and Robertson, 1979), or patients with known arterial or venous insufficiency. Patients are generally advised not to exceed an intake of 10 mg weekly but patient tolerance varies widely and each patient must be assessed individually as some may control their migraine without side-effects while using larger amounts whereas others may be unable to tolerate lower doses.

Dihydroergotamine (DHE). DHE constricts venous capacitance vessels more than arteries, has a biological half-life of about 2.5 hours when administered intravenously and poor bioavailability when administered orally because of inadequate absorption and high 'first-pass' metabolism in the liver (Little *et al.*, 1982). It may also have a central effect as it binds to 5-HT receptors in the endogenous pain control system (Goadsby and Gundlach, 1991) and inhibits trigeminocervical neurones when administered peripherally in experimental animals (Hoskin *et al.*, 1996). DHE shares with sumatriptan an affinity for the 5-HT$_{1B/D}$ receptors (Peroutka, 1990). It is used mainly for the management of acute migraine attacks in doses of 0.5–0.75 mg intravenously or 1.0 mg intramuscularly, and has recently become available for intranasal application in some countries (Gallagher, 1996; Massiou, 1996; Touchon *et al.*, 1996).

Raskin (1986) has advocated the use of DHE 0.3–1.0 mg intravenously (the dose depending on patient tolerance, particularly the absence of nausea), in conjunction with metoclopramide 10 mg, 8 hourly in patients with intractable migraine. Of 55 patients treated, 49 became headache-free within 24 hours. In another study, 37 patients seen in an emergency department with acute migraine were all treated with prochlorperazine 5 mg intravenously initially then randomized to receive intravenous DHE 0.75 mg or placebo (Callaham and Raskin, 1986). There was no difference between the result in each group at 30 minutes but pain was significantly less in the first group 60 minutes after DHE. Of patients treated with prochlorperazine and DHE, 13.5 per cent required parenteral narcotics, compared with 45 per cent of patients with migraine headache not enrolled in this study. DHE performs favourably when compared with subcutaneous sumatriptan, with a slower onset of action but many fewer patients having recurrent headache and thus an equal response rate when judged at 24 hours after dosing (Winner *et al.*, 1996).

DHE can be administered by a nasal spray (Ziegler *et al.*, 1994), which gives about 40 per cent bioavailability compared with the intravenous route. In double-blind trials complete relief of pain was achieved by 38 per cent of patients treated with intranasal DHE compared with 17 per cent using placebo (Lataste *et al.*, 1989). DHE nasal spray is inferior to subcutaneous sumatriptan (Touchon *et al.*, 1996), although it gives a lower recurrence rate in patients who respond. When compared with the sumatriptan nasal spray, DHE nasal spray is probably slower in onset but again gives a lower recurrence rate (Massiou, 1996). DHE, like ergotamine tartrate and methysergide, may rarely cause retroperitoneal or pleural fibrosis after repeated usage (Malaquin *et al.*, 1989).

Sumatriptan. Sumatriptan is a specific 5-HT$_1$ agonist (Table 9.2; Figure 9.1) and was the first in its class of *triptans* that bind specifically to the 5-HT$_{1B/1D}$ receptor (Feniuk *et al.*, 1991), thus replicating the beneficial effect of 5-HT in the relief of migraine headache without the severe side-effects that prevented the therapeutic use of the parent substance. Sumatriptan passes the blood–brain barrier poorly (Sleight *et al.*, 1990) and probably acts by constricting cranial blood vessels (Connor *et al.*, 1992) and preventing the release of peptides from trigeminal nerve terminals (Goadsby and Edvinsson, 1993), thus breaking up the neurovascular interaction that characterizes migraine headache. A study using transcranial Doppler (Friberg *et al.*, 1991) showed that the middle cerebral artery dilated during migraine attacks and constricted as the headache was eased by sumatriptan, although Diener *et al.* (1991) did not find any consistent, significant changes in the velocity of blood flow in middle cerebral or basilar arteries after sumatriptan

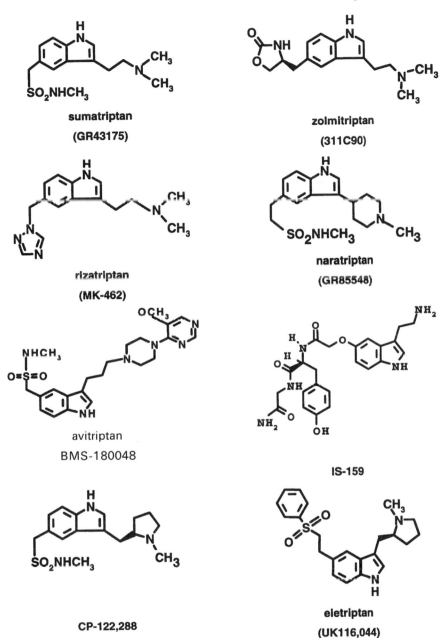

Figure 9.1 Drug structures

administration. Supporting evidence for a vasoconstrictor effect in the internal carotid and middle cerebral arteries of human subjects has been produced by Ferrari
et al. (1991) and for the middle meningeal, and to a lesser extent, cerebral and
temporal arteries, by Edvinsson, Jansen and Olesen (1991). The administration of

sumatriptan 2 mg directly into the middle meningeal artery causes marked vaso-constriction (Henkes *et al.*, 1996). Whether administered orally or subcutaneously, sumatriptan has a plasma half-life of about 2 hours (Fowler *et al.*, 1991).

Oral sumatriptan. Sumatriptan 100 mg orally, given when migraine headache was es-tablished, relieved the headache in 2 hours in 51 per cent of patients compared with 19 per cent of those given placebo in a double-blind crossover study (Goadsby *et al.*, 1991). The Oral Sumatriptan Dose-Defining Study Group (1991) reported that 50 per cent of patients were relieved 2 hours after 100 mg sumatrip-tan and 75 per cent after 4 hours (59 per cent of whom had taken a second tablet 2 hours after the first), compared with 19 per cent and 30 per cent, respectively, of those given placebo. Studies with lower doses (25 and 50 mg) have demonstrated clear efficacy against placebo for both doses (Cutler *et al.*, 1995; Pfaffenrath *et al.*, 1997; Sargent *et al.*, 1995). A meta-analysis of published and abstracted clinical studies with sumatriptan 50 mg has shown a 2-hour headache response (severe or moderate headache becomes nil or mild) of 56 per cent (95 per cent confidence in-terval 51–62 per cent) with a therapeutic gain (active response minus placebo) of 33 per cent (95 per cent CI 26–40 per cent) (Tfelt-Hansen, personal communica-tion). Similarly, the headache response at 2 hours for 100 mg in the same meta-analysis was 58 per cent (95 per cent CI 56–60 per cent). The differences between the doses is not remarkable, although given the choice patients tend to drift from 25 mg to 50 or 100 mg over time (Salonen, 1997).

Intranasal sumatriptan. In order to provide an alternative formulation for patients requiring quick delivery of sumatriptan, and particularly in those in whom nausea is a significant problem, a nasal form of sumatriptan was developed (Finnish Su-matriptan Group and the Cardiovascular Clinical Research Group, 1991). It has been studied across a range of doses (2.5 to 20 mg) (Becker, 1995) with doses of 10 and 20 mg being focused on in later development (Hernandez-Gallego, 1995). At 2 hours after dosing, 55 per cent of patients taking 20 mg intranasal sumatrip-tan compared with 25 per cent on placebo had a headache response, while at the same time 24 per cent were headache-free on 20 mg and 4 per cent were headache-free on placebo (Hernandez-Gallego, 1995). In a direct comparison with oral su-matriptan (100 mg) the 2-hour headache response rates were comparable at 70 per cent for 100 mg orally and 67 per cent for 20 mg intranasally (Massiou, 1996). The main difference was the more rapid onset of action of intranasal sumatriptan with a response rate of 18 per cent at 15 minutes compared to 6 per cent for oral sumatriptan. It should be noted that the high response rates when compared to other sumatriptan studies may reflect the fact that this comparison had no placebo arm. In a comparison with intranasal dihydroergotamine (DHE) the 2-hour re-sponse rate was 40 per cent for DHE and 51 per cent for sumatriptan in a direct comparison while the rate of headache recurrence was less on the DHE spray (Massiou, 1996).

Rectal sumatriptan. For similar reasons as the intranasal formulation, a rectal for-mulation of sumatriptan has been developed for patients who have marked nausea or vomiting, or both. The half life at 1.8 hours is similar to other forms of suma-triptan with a T_{max} of 1.5 hours (Hussey et al., 1995). This formulation has been studied in doses from 6 to 100 mg with the dose–response curve at a plateau be-yond 25 mg (Gobel, 1995). The rectal formulation is well tolerated but again head-ache recurrence is unaffected by formulation (Henriksson, 1995).

Subcutaneous sumatriptan. In a randomized double-blind trial involving 639 patients, the subcutaneous administration of sumatriptan 6 mg proved to be highly effec-tive, with 72 per cent of patients being relieved within 1 hour compared with 25 per cent given placebo (Ferrari, 1991). In a large single-blind trial, conducted in the USA (Cady et al., 1991), 734 patients were treated with sumatriptan 6 mg sub-cutaneously and 370 with placebo, with relief after 1 hour being 70 per cent and 22 per cent, respectively. Headache was abolished completely in 49 per cent of the sumatriptan group and 9 per cent of the placebo group. There was no demon-strable benefit from giving a second injection of sumatriptan. Side-effects were slight; some reaction at the injection site (about 60 per cent) and dizziness, tingling and sensations of warmth (each about 12 per cent). Subsequent clinical experience has confirmed that subcutaneous sumatriptan is both extremely effective and gen-erally well tolerated (Cady et al., 1993; Sheftell et al., 1994; Visser et al., 1996d).

Comparative studies of sumatriptan with other acute attack medications
Sumatriptan was also found to be superior to ergotamine, given in the form of two Cafergot tablets, each containing 1 mg of ergotamine tartrate (The Multinational Oral Sumatriptan and Cafergot Study Group, 1991). Similarly, sumatriptan was superior to the combination of aspirin/metaclopramide, but not in all attacks treated in a three-attack study (The Oral Sumatriptan and Aspirin plus Metoclopramide Comparative Study Group, 1992). When compared to lysine acetylsalicylate and metoclopramide oral sumatriptan 100 mg was no better in terms of efficacy at 2 hours (Tfelt-Hansen et al., 1995).

The side-effects of sumatriptan are usually mild and transient, comprising sensa-tions of heaviness in the head, tightness in the chest, heat or tingling. Of 4859 patients monitored, 3 per cent experienced pressure, tightness or pain in the chest without ECG (EKG) evidence of ischaemia (Brown et al., 1991). Since then, Willett et al. (1992) reported that a patient with a history of intermittent chest pain unrelated to exertion, being treated with methyscrgide for cluster headache, experienced severe chest pain within minutes of receiving an injection of sumatriptan 6 mg subcuta-neously. The pain was accompanied by ST elevation in the ECG, which returned to normal within 22 minutes without subsequent elevation of cardiac muscle enzymes. The issue of the coronary safety of sumatriptan and related compounds has been the subject of considerable discussion. There is little doubt that as a class the *triptans* constrict human coronary arteries (Macintyre et al., 1992; Macintyre et al., 1993). However, given the selective over-representation of 5-HT$_{1B}$ receptors in the cranial over the coronary circulation this dose not represent a major clinical problem in most patients (Visser et al., 1996b). Based on these considerations it is contraindi-cated to administer sumatriptan to any patient suspected of having coronary artery disease or Prinzmetal angina, or any patient with uncontrolled hypertension, although its constrictor action is relatively selective for cranial vessels.

Naratriptan. Naratriptan, like sumatriptan, is a $5\text{-HT}_{1B/1D}$ agonist. Its basic pharmacological profile is the same as that of sumatriptan with the exception of increased lipophilicity and it is active in models used to select antimigraine activity (Connor *et al.*, 1997; Goadsby and Knight, 1997b). Naratriptan has better bioavailability than sumatriptan at 63–74 per cent, for males and females, respectively (Fuseau *et al.*, 1997). It has a longer $T_{1/2}$ but paradoxically, and without current explanation, a longer T_{max} at 2.5–3 hours (Kempsford *et al.*, 1997). Unlike sumatriptan its main route of elimination is by metabolism in the liver through P450 enzyme systems (Kempsford, 1997), meaning that there is no interaction with MAO inhibitors.

Naratriptan was characterized through a 100-fold dose range from 0.1 to 10 mg and deliberately developed to target clinical shortcomings associated with sumatriptan, in particular to improve tolerability and reduce headache recurrence. The headache response based on a meta-analysis of the phase II/III clinical trial programme for naratriptan was 48 per cent (95 per cent CI 45–51 per cent) at 2 hours with a therapeutic gain (active response minus placebo) of 21 per cent (95 per cent CI 18–24 per cent) and for the headache free endpoint, 23 per cent (95 per cent CI 20–26 per cent) with a corresponding therapeutic gain of 15 per cent (95 per cent CI 12–18 per cent) for the 2.5 mg (recommended clinical) dose (Goadsby, 1997b; Goadsby, 1988).

Formal data for consistency of the headache response within a patient demonstrates that 73 per cent of patients respond in two-thirds of attacks, compared with 75 per cent for sumatriptan and 22 per cent for placebo. These are, however, 4-hour data and no data for the 2-hour time-point are currently available. As an aside, 'consistency' as a term should probably be restricted to indicate within-patient consistency rather than the less meaningful concept of consistency on a population basis. Naratriptan has a slower onset of action than sumatriptan but has a lower rate of headache recurrence (Gobel *et al.*, 1997). It is important to note, given that headache recurrence has not been defined consistently across the *triptan* studies, that historical controls and comparisons are probably of little value and claims for a benefit in terms of headache recurrence are best based on head to head blinded studies, such as this one and those done for dihydroergotamine (Touchon *et al.*, 1996; Winner *et al.*, 1996). In common with sumatriptan (Korsgaard, 1995), naratriptan has no statistically significant benefit in the treatment of adolescents with acute migraine attacks (Rothner *et al.*, 1997). The International Headache Society criteria are somewhat less useful in adolescents and this, coupled with the shorter attacks, requires a re-evaluation of how studies are conducted in the younger population. Naratriptan at 2.5 mg is better tolerated than sumatriptan, with an adverse event rate across all the studies, corrected for placebo, of 0.1 per cent (95 per cent CI 4 to 4.2 per cent). It should be noted that the confidence interval crosses zero and that the incidence of adverse events at this dose in the controlled studies was very low.

Zolmitriptan. Zolmitriptan was the second of the 5-HT$_{1B/1D}$ class to be marketed after sumatriptan and was designed to more lipophilic (Hill *et al.*, 1995) and to be a potent partial agonist (Martin *et al.*, 1997). Both aims were achieved and its activity in preclinical models is well established as it has been a useful laboratory tool for addressing some issues in the field surrounding the potential central sites of action of this class of compounds (Goadsby and Edvinsson, 1994; Goadsby and Hoskin, 1996; Goadsby and Knight, 1997a). It has a $T_{1/2}$ of 3 hours (Seaber *et al.*, 1996) and a T_{max} of 1 hour (Thomsen *et al.*, 1996) with an oral bioavailability of 40 per cent (Palmer and Spencer, 1997). It is also metabolized through the P450 system but has an active metabolite (*N*-desmethyl-zolmitriptan) that is degraded by MAO-A. This does not create a clinically significant effect on initial dosing but does limit the total dose to 5 mg per day. There is an increase in the C_{max} of zolmitriptan with propranolol administration (160 mg/day) (Palmer and Spencer, 1997) but again this does not limit use of the 5 mg dose. Based on a meta-analysis of the phase II/III placebo-controlled studies zolmitriptan has, at 2 hours, a headache response of 64 per cent (95 per cent CI 59–69 per cent) with a therapeutic gain of 34 per cent (27–41 per cent) for 2.5 mg and a headache response of 66 per cent (95 per cent CI 62–70 per cent) with a corresponding therapeutic gain of 37 per cent (30–44 per cent) for the 5 mg dose (Goadsby, 1998). For comparison the headache-free endpoint at two hours was 25 per cent (95 per cent CI 21–29 per cent) with a therapeutic gain of 19 per cent (14–24 per cent) and 34 per cent (95 per cent CI 30–38 per cent) with a therapeutic gain of 28 per cent (23-33 per cent), for the 2.5 mg and 5 mg doses, respectively.

Given the corresponding adverse event rates, the therapeutic penalty rates are 17 per cent (95 per cent CI 11–23 per cent) and 29 per cent (95 per cent CI 23–35 per cent), for 2.5 mg and 5 mg, respectively. On this basis the recommended starting dose of 2.5 mg provides the best balance of benefit and side-effects, but there is a group of patients who may benefit from the 5 mg dose. A meta-analysis of the placebo-controlled data suggests that it may also have the benefit of a lesser rate of recurrent headache (Goadsby, 1997a) but this requires formal study, while any hopes of an answer to the question of its comparison with sumatriptan were dashed in a study with a high placebo response that rendered no useful outcome (Diener, Third European Headache Federation Meeting, Sardinia, 1996). It certainly has an early onset of action and in practice many patients find it a useful treatment.

Rizatriptan. Rizatriptan is a potent 5-HT$_{1B/1D}$ agonist (Beer *et al.*, 1995) that is active both in peripheral (Williamson *et al.*, 1997a, 1997b) and central (Cumberbatch *et al.*, 1997) models predictive of antimigraine efficacy. It is more lipophilic than sumatriptan (Rance *et al.*, 1997) and has a $T_{1/2}$ of 2–3 hours and a T_{max} of 1 hour. The oral bioavailability is 40 per cent and it is largely MAO metabolized. The compound has been studied across a range of doses up to 40 mg (Visser, Lines and Reines, 1996) with the optimium clinical doses being 5 and 10 mg (Gijsman *et al.*, 1997; Visser *et al.*, 1996a). Quoted response rates for the 10 mg dose are superior to sumatriptan 100 mg (Visser *et al.*, 1996) while the placebo-corrected aggregate responses for 5 and 10 mg were 28 and 38%, respectively, in placebo-controlled studies. Given that the compound was further encapsulated for blinding in these studies, these outcomes are likely to underestimate the dry effect (Gijsman *et al.*, 1997). The compound is well tolerated generally and a more detailed analysis of its place in clinical practice will be possible when it is available for use.

Eletriptan. Eletriptan is a potent partial $5\text{-HT}_{1B/1D}$ agonist (Gupta *et al.*, 1996a) which is active in preclinical models that predict antimigraine efficacy (Gupta *et al.*, 1996a). It is in late phase III development so that its clinical profile is not yet completely delineated. It is certainly an effective antimigraine agent and a high dose (80 mg) was more effective in a phase II study than sumatriptan 100 mg (Jackson, 1996). Further studies are awaited with interest.

Comparison of the triptans

The age of the *triptans* is upon clinicians. In addition to those mentioned above, almotriptan (Cabarrocas, 1997) and VML-251 (SB 209 509 or frovatriptan; Ryan and Keywood, 1997) are also in development, but there is much less data upon which to base any assessment. Each of the additions to treatment thus far have brought a particular utility while supplying some interesting questions. The sumatriptan nasal spray is a helpful adjunct that finds particular use with a more rapid onset of action than oral sumatriptan and the benefit for some patients of not having to resort to an injection. If one is thinking of the sumatriptan injection the spray should at least be considered and, if headache recurrence is an additional issue, the combined clinical problem should make one think of the dihydroergotamine spray where it is available. Naratriptan is an ideal drug in patients sensitive to side-effects or in whom headache recurrence on sumatriptan is an important issue. It would *not* be a wise choice if speed of onset were an important consideration or if they had already failed to respond to sumatriptan. Zolmitriptan is a very useful addition to the therapeutic options, combining high efficacy rates, which are probably at least equal to sumatriptan, although this has not been properly tested, with rapid onset of action and good tolerability. While we would not get a patient who is safely and successfully using sumatriptan to change to zolmitriptan, if efficacy or speed are issues and the patient wants to examine other options, it would be the obvious first step which may obviate the need for a nasal spray or injection. When rizatriptan and then eletriptan become available similar issues and discussions will arise, although when all is said and done what the patient says when they return will dictate the course of treatment, just as it should.

Non-specific treatments of acute migraine attacks

Non-steroidal anti-inflammatory drugs (NSAIDs)

Aspirin. Aspirin reduces prostaglandin synthesis but it is not known whether this is related to its action in relieving headache. Aspirin can be an effective agent in migraine, providing that it can be adequately absorbed. Volans (1974) showed that the absorption of aspirin was impaired in 19 out of 42 migraine patients during headache, which has led to the use of metoclopramide 10 mg being given intramuscularly to facilitate the absorption of ergotamine tartrate and aspirin in the management of the acute attack of migraine. An intravenous form of aspirin (D,L-lysine-acetylsalicylate), each vial containing about 500 mg, has been used in Japan and Europe (Fukuda and Izumikawa, 1988) and the oral form is particularly effective when combined with metaclopramide (Chabriat *et al.*, 1994; Tfelt-Hansen *et al.*, 1995) as had been advocated by Wilkinson (1983).

Fenemates. Flufenamic acid in doses of 250 mg every 2 hours, up to a maximum of 1000 mg, gave symptomatic relief in 195 of 200 migraine headaches (Vardi *et al.*, 1976), although upper abdominal discomfort was experienced by eight of 26 patients and another two patients had severe nausea and vomiting, one with mel aena.

Tolfenamic acid in doses of 200 mg was found to be as effective as ergotamine tartrate 1 mg in relieving migraine (Hakkarainen *et al.*, 1979). Both drugs were more effective than aspirin, which in turn was superior to placebo. It has also been reported to be useful in reducing patient overuse of ergotamine (Ala-Hurula *et al.*, 1981) and may be more useful when given in combination with caffeine (Hakkarainen *et al.*, 1982).

Indomethacin. Indomethacin, when given in large dosage (150–200 mg daily), is said to be beneficial in preventing migraine (Sicuteri *et al.*, 1964) but produces a high incidence of gastrointestinal side-effects. We did not find it helpful in more modest doses of 25 mg three times daily (Anthony and Lance, 1968). Indomethacin finds a place in the management of paroxysmal hemicranias (see Chapter 11), 'ice-pick' head pains and exertional vascular headache (see Chapter 12). The continued usage of indomethacin may sometimes induce daily headache.

Naproxen. Nestvold (1986) summarized the results of four controlled trials, including his own, of naproxen in the management of acute migraine. The dosage of naproxen in his own trial was 750 mg initially with another 250–500 mg taken later if necessary. While the results were significantly better than placebo medication, total relief from headache was rare.

Diclofenac. Diclofenac was shown to relieve migraine more readily than placebo with 27 per cent of attacks being aborted by the active drug (Massiou *et al.*, 1991). In another active-controlled study the response rate to 75 mg of diclofenac intramuscularly was 88 per cent (Karachalios *et al.*, 1992).

Other NSAIDs. Ketorolac 60 mg intramuscularly was found to be as effective as mecperidine (pethidine) 75 mg and Promezathine 25 mg intramuscularly in relieving migraine by Davis and colleagues (1995). Ibuprofen and other NSAIDs have also been used for the treatment of migraine headache.

Other agents

Lignocaine (lidocaine). Lignocaine 100 mg intravenously has been reported to relieve migraine and cluster headache for approximately 20 minutes (Maciewicz *et al.*, 1988) and our custom is to continue a lignocaine infusion at 2 mg/minute for as long as necessary to control pain which may be 2–3 days. This can be combined with DHE 0.5 mg intravenously given 8 hourly into the drip. One report (Reutens *et al.*, 1991) failed to confirm the effective use of lignocaine when given in a lower dose of 1 mg/kg intravenously. Patients should be under observation with regular blood pressure recordings during lignocaine infusion.

Phenothiazines. Chlorpromazine 12.5 mg intravenously repeated at 20 minute intervals to a total of 37.5 mg was compared with DHE 1 mg intravenously (repeated in 30 minutes if necessary) and lignocaine 50 mg intravenously (repeated at 20 minute intervals to a maximum of 150 mg if needed) in the management of acute migraine headache (Bell *et al.*, 1990). Chlorpromazine-treated patients fared significantly better than those on the two other medications with 15 of the 24 having persistent relief when contacted 12–24 hours later. Lane (1989) reported the use of chlorpromazine at 0.1 mg/kg intravenously as adjuvant therapy in 24 patients, six of whom responded to one injection, with nine requiring two doses and nine needing three doses at 15 minute intervals. Prochlorperazine 10 mg intravenously is also an effective agent for the treatment of acute migraine headache (Jones *et al.*, 1989). Of 42 patients, 80 per cent had complete or partial relief of headache compared with 45 per cent given placebo.

Metoclopramide 10 mg intramuscularly or a 20 mg suppository relieved nausea more effectively than placebo in a double-blind trial but did not by itself improve migraine headache (Tfelt-Hansen *et al.*, 1980). Dystonic reactions may occur after many phenothiazines, and benztropine mesylate (1.0–2.0 mg intravenously) should be on hand to counter this problem if it arises.

Isometheptene mucate. The sympathomimetic amine, isometheptene, in a preparation combined with analgesics (Midrid) relieved migraine headache more effectively than ergotamine in a double-blind crossover trial (Yuill *et al.*, 1972). Isometheptene has also been shown to be more effective than placebo in treating acute attacks of migraine, producing a response in 42 per cent of patients compared to 29 per cent on placebo (Diamond and Medina, 1975).

5-HT$_3$ antagonists. Thus far, no 5-HT$_3$ antagonist has proved to be both safe and clearly effective in the management of migraine either as an acute or prophylactic medication. Granisetron is a potent anti-emetic in cancer chemotherapy and a selective 5-HT$_3$ receptor antagonist (Joss and Dott, 1993). In an initial early study of seven attacks in six patients results were promising (Couturier *et al.*, 1991) and in a placebo-controlled study of 28 patients the effects were less impressive when compared to control (Rowat *et al.*, 1991). Similarly, MDL-72222 has been studied in a small group and showed some promise (Loisy *et al.*, 1985).

The place of opioids in the management of acute attacks

The use of narcotics, particularly pethidine (meperidine), for the relief of migraine in general practice is common in the USA as in many countries (Ziegler, 1997). The case for injection of opioids rests on the presence of opioid receptors in the brain's endogenous pain control pathways and the fact that some patients claim that their migraine headaches respond rapidly to the injection of a narcotic agent but not to the other measures described above. When their use is confined to infrequent attacks of migraine accompanied by obvious signs of distress in a stable personality, pethidine appears to be a safe, cheap and often effective remedy. The case against the use of narcotics rests on the short duration of their action and their tendency to induce tolerance, dependence or addiction if used often.

There have been a number of comparative trials to show that other treatments such as dihydroergotamine and metoclopramide were as effective or more effective than pethidine (Klapper and Stanton, 1993; Scherl and Wilson, 1995) but the fact remains that some patients do respond to opioids and no other therapies without showing any indication of addiction. Pethidine may be the treatment of choice during pregnancy when the use of ergotamine or similar preparations is to be avoided.

It is difficult to formulate a set of rules to govern if, when and how often a narcotic should be administered to a particular patient. If patients are manipulative, seeking injections of narcotics more and more frequently or visiting different doctors to obtain narcotics, they are best referred to a drug and alcohol advisory clinic. On the other hand, if a patient is known to be emotionally stable and to suffer genuine migraine that responds solely to narcotics, it is only humane to administer them appropriately. One cardinal rule is that the patient should have a single prescribing practitioner or medical practice. If attention is required out of hours by a 24 hour medical clinic or emergency service and narcotics are used in treatment, the primary prescriber should be notified so that a check is maintained on the frequency of administration.

Agents used for prophylactic (interval) therapy

If migrainous headaches are recurring twice a month or more, and not responding to ergotamine, sumatriptan or other agents mentioned above, there is a good case for the daily administration of medication with a view to reducing the frequency or severity of attacks. The International Headache Society Committee on Clinical Trials in Migraine (1991) has laid down guide lines for the design of controlled trials to determine the effectiveness of a particular medication. It should be borne in mind that a drug which may prove to be more effective than a placebo in a double-blind trial may still be fairly useless clinically, leaving the patient with a slightly reduced frequency of devastating headaches. The results of clinical trials may also be confounded by a lack of patient compliance (Steiner et al., 1994).

Beta-noradrenergic antagonists
Beta-blocking agents have been used in the prophylaxis of migraine for 20 years and remain the first line of defence in non-asthmatic patients. Those without intrinsic

sympathomimetic (agonist) activity have proven effective but whether they act by beta-blockade or another mechanism remains an open question. They comprise the non-selective beta-blockers propranolol, nadolol and timolol as well as the selective beta$_1$-blockers atenolol and metoprolol (Tfelt-Hansen, 1989). Beta-blockers are best avoided in those patients with a prolonged aura or severe focal neurological symptoms because there have been reports of migrainous stroke in such instances (Bardwell and Trott, 1987).

Propranolol. Since propranolol was first reported to be efficacious in preventing migraine attacks (Weber and Reinmuth, 1971), there have been many confirmatory trials cited by Pascual, Polo and Berciano (1989), who studied the effect of dosage on response. Of 53 patients treated with low doses of 1 mg/kg body weight, commonly 20 mg three times daily, 39 experienced 50 per cent or greater improvement in frequency and intensity of attacks. Ziegler *et al.* (1993) found that propranolol reduced the frequency but not the severity of headache and that the results did not correlate with plasma levels. Postural hypotension, asthenia, muscle cramps and vivid dreams have been encountered as side-effects in reported series of treatment with propranolol and other beta-blockers.

Timolol. Timolol 10 mg twice daily proved to be as effective as propranolol 80 mg twice daily, and better than placebo in a three-way double-blind crossover trial involving 96 patients (Tfelt-Hansen, 1986; Tfelt-Hansen *et al.*, 1984). Headache frequency per month was reduced from a baseline of about six to about five on placebo and about 3.5 on the active drugs, so significant disability still remained. The authors suggested starting patients on one-quarter of the above dosage and increasing slowly.

Nadolol. Nadolol has a plasma half-life of 20–24 hours and is therefore administered only once daily. Sudilovsky *et al.* (1987) studied 140 patients with classical and common migraine, comparing the effect of nadolol 80–160 mg once daily with propranolol 80 mg twice daily. Of the 98 patients who completed the trial all those on active medication had a decrease of blood pressure and heart rate. Headache days per month were reduced to half or less from baseline in approximately 30 per cent of patients on propranolol and the lower dose of nadolol, and about 60 per cent after 2 months on the higher dose of nadolol. Side-effects were experienced by 4 per cent of patients on nadolol and 9 per cent of patients on propranolol.

Metoprolol. A double-blind parallel study of 71 patients taking the selective beta-blocker metoprolol 200 mg (slow-release formation) or placebo once daily was reported by Andersson *et al.* (1983). The number of migraine days per month was reduced from about eight to about 5.5 on the active drug but remained at the baseline level in those on placebo medication. Side-effects, including insomnia and nightmares, were experienced equally by both groups. A clinical trial limited to patients with classical migraine (migraine with aura) was conducted by Kangasniemi *et al.* (1987), using the same dose and form of metoprolol in a crossover study against placebo. The monthly frequency of attacks was significantly reduced (1.8 versus 2.5) as was the average duration of attacks (6 hours versus 8 hours).

Atenolol. A double-blind crossover study against placebo demonstrated the efficacy of atenolol 100 mg once daily (Forssman *et al.*, 1983). The monthly frequency of headache diminished to about five on the active drug compared with about seven on placebo. Attacks were reduced to less than half the previous frequency in seven of the 20 patients. As with all beta-blockers the results were statistically significant but by no means dramatic.

Drugs acting on 5HT mechanisms

Pizotifen and cyproheptadine. Pizotifen (pizotyline) is a benzocycloheptathiophene derivative which is structurally similar to cyproheptadine and the tricyclic antidepressants. It has an elimination half-life of about 23 hours and can therefore be given as a single nocturnal dosage. Pizotifen and cyproheptadine are 5-HT_2 and histamine-1 antagonists. They probably have a similar efficacy in the prevention of migraine and share the same side-effects of drowsiness, increased appetite and weight gain. Pizotifen has proven effective in controlled trials (Speight and Avery, 1972), although less potent than methysergide. An early open study of our own (Curran and Lance, 1964) followed 100 patients taking 12–24 mg daily for a period of 6 months, and found that 15 became headache-free and 31 were substantially improved. This success rate of 46 per cent compared with 64 per cent for 150 patients treated with methysergide 2–6mg daily for 6 months and 20 per cent of 50 patients given placebo medication for 1 month. Placebo-controlled studies have confirmed the utility of pizotifen (Arthur and Hornabrook, 1971; Capildeo and Rose, 1982; Lawrence *et al.*, 1977). A comparative trial, incorporating a placebo group, demonstrated that pizotifen 0.5 mg three times daily and naproxen sodium 550 mg twice daily were of equal value in prophylaxis (Bellevance and Meloche, 1990) and that both were more effective than placebo. The number of headache days was reduced to about half by naproxen and to about two-thirds on pizotifen. A study comparing flunarizine 10 mg nocte and pizotifen 2–3 mg daily did not show any significant difference in reduction in headache frequency, with both compounds being effective (Louis and Spierings, 1982).

Methysergide. Methysergide (l-methyl-D-lysergic acid butanolamide) is an ergot derivative with an elimination half-life of about 3 hours. It breaks down to methylergometrine (methylergonovine), which is probably responsible for its sustained beneficial effect in the prophylaxis of migraine. Methysergide is a 5-HT_2 antagonist but also has agonist properties on 5-HT receptors. It has been proven effective in the prevention of migraine in two double-blind trials (Lance *et al.*, 1963; Pedersen and Moller, 1966).

Graham (1967) reported that retroperitoneal fibrosis, pleural fibrosis or cardiac valvular fibrosis had developed in about 100 patients of the half-million who were estimated to have been treated with methysergide at that time. In 35 years of using methysergide extensively, we have known seven patients with retroperitoneal fibrosis, three with pleural fibrosis and one patient who developed a cardiac murmur while under observation. It must be borne in mind that other agents may cause fibrotic syndromes and that in some cases no cause may be apparent. Lewis *et al.* (1975) reported a retrospective study of seven patients with retroperitoneal fibrosis from the London Hospital. None had ever taken methysergide but four of the seven had taken excessive amounts of analgesics. Those cases that are associated with methysergide usually resolve completely once treatment is ceased.

The fibrotic complications of methysergide may well be the result of its 5-HT-like action. Graham (1967) commented on the similarity of the appearance at operation of valvular fibrosis in methysergide-treated patients to that seen in carcinoid syndrome and in this context the recent report of valvular fibrosis with fenfluramine-phentermine treatment is of interest (Connolly *et al.*, 1997). The administration of 5-HT to rats either decreases or increases granuloma formation, depending upon the function of the adrenal gland (Bianchine and Eade, 1967). Excessive fibrosis appears only if adrenal insufficiency is induced. This raises the question of whether there might be adrenal insufficiency in patients who develop fibrotic syndromes in response to 5-HT or methysergide. It is possible that any drug which relies upon a 5-HT-simulating action for the treatment of migraine has the potential for producing excessive fibrosis in susceptible subjects. It is recommended that patients cease medication with methysergide for 1 month every 6 months to minimize the possibility of fibrotic complications.

Amitriptyline. Amitriptyline blocks the re-uptake of 5-HT and noradrenaline at central synapses. Apart from its use as an antidepressant, it has been employed in the management of tension headache (see Chapter 10) and other pain syndromes such as post-herpetic neuralgia (see Chapter 17). It is effective in the prevention of migraine (Couch *et al.*, 1976; Gomersall and Stuart, 1973; Ziegler *et al.*, 1993) independent of its antidepressant effect.

Individual responses to amitriptyline vary greatly. Some patients are unable to tolerate as little as 10 mg given as a nocturnal dose because of intolerable drowsiness the next day, whereas others experience no side-effects while taking 150 mg in divided doses or a single nocturnal dose. Plasma levels on a given dosage vary widely (as much as 10-fold) but a steady state is reached 7–14 days after a fixed dosage is achieved (Ziegler *et al.*, 1977). Apart from drowsiness and a 'drugged feeling', gain in weight and dryness of the mouth may be troublesome side-effects. The addition of amitriptyline to propranolol does not improve the results in migraine headache but the combination is superior to either preparation alone in the management of headaches combining the features of migraine and tension headache (Mathew *et al.*, 1982).

Monoamine oxidase inhibitors. Since platelet 5-HT levels are lowered in migraine, the use of a drug which maintains or increases 5-HT levels is a logical form of treatment. Anthony and Lance (1969) treated 25 patients who had failed to respond to other forms of interval medication with phenelzine, 45 mg daily, for periods up to 2 years. The frequency of headache was reduced to less than half in 20 of the 25 patients. Although mean platelet 5-HT increased by about 50 per cent, there was

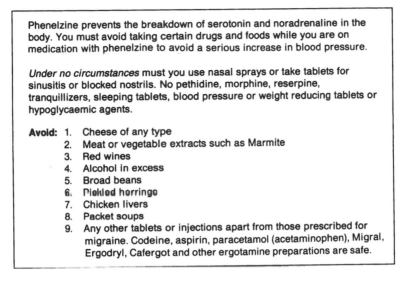

Phenelzine prevents the breakdown of serotonin and noradrenaline in the body. You must avoid taking certain drugs and foods while you are on medication with phenelzine to avoid a serious increase in blood pressure.

Under no circumstances must you use nasal sprays or take tablets for sinusitis or blocked nostrils. No pethidine, morphine, reserpine, tranquillizers, sleeping tablets, blood pressure or weight reducing tablets or hypoglycaemic agents.

Avoid: 1. Cheese of any type
2. Meat or vegetable extracts such as Marmite
3. Red wines
4. Alcohol in excess
5. Broad beans
6. Pickled herrings
7. Chicken livers
8. Packet soups
9. Any other tablets or injections apart from those prescribed for migraine. Codeine, aspirin, paracetamol (acetaminophen), Migral, Ergodryl, Cafergot and other ergotamine preparations are safe.

Figure 9.2 List of foods and drugs to be avoided while taking monoamine oxidase inhibitors

no correlation between the 5-HT level and the response of each individual patient. We have continued to use this form of treatment in patients resistant to other therapy. Patients are issued with a notice specifying the foods and drugs to be avoided while on MAO (A) inhibitors (Figure 9.2). Diamond (1995) has prescribed sumatriptan for acute attacks in patients maintained on phenelzine without encountering untoward reactions, but caution is advisable. Naratriptan and, at 5 mg or less a day, zolmitriptan, are safe to use with MAO (A) inhibitors, while rizatriptan should probably be avoided. Phenelzine has been used in conjunction with the beta-blocker atenolol with advantage in that the side-effect of postural hypotension is less frequent (Merikangas and Merikangas, 1995). The MAO-B inhibitor selegiline, which prevents the breakdown of dopamine and phenylethylamine, is not helpful in the management of migraine (Kuritzky *et al.*, 1992).

Specific serotonin uptake inhibitors (SSRIs)

This newer group of antidepressants is not as effective in treatment of migraine as the tricyclics. The combination of the two is to be avoided because cases of the 'serotonin syndrome' have been reported, with agitation, myoclonus and other movement disorders (Mathew *et al.*, 1996). Fluoxetine is a high profile antidepressant that specifically blocks 5-HT reuptake. A small controlled trial against placebo, using doses varying from 20 mg every second day to 40 mg daily, showed a significant improvement in the fluoxetine group (Adley *et al.*, 1992). A larger trial involving 58 migraine patients given 20 mg daily (Saper *et al.*, 1994) did not demonstrate any improvement compared with placebo, although another group with chronic daily headache showed some response. Side-effects of fluoxetine included sleep disturbance, tremor and abdominal pain.

Other medications

Calcium channel blocking agents

Despite initial enthusiastic reports concerning the benefit of calcium channel blockers in migraine, the subject remains controversial. The Migraine Nimodipine European Study Group (1989) was unable to demonstrate any significant effect of nimodipine 40 mg three times daily over placebo in migraine without aura or migraine with aura, although made the reservation that a larger sample in the latter trial may possibly have yielded a positive result. Solomon (1989) summarized the results of three small controlled studies, which found verapamil more effective than placebo and reported that a dosage of 320 mg per day was more effective than 240 mg per day. Constipation and swollen ankles are the main side-effects. Flunarizine is a calcium channel blocker with dopamine antagonist properties and a very long half-life. Double-blind studies have demonstrated its efficacy at a dose of 10 mg per day (Leone et al., 1991). Side-effects include fatigue, depression and the development of Parkinsonian symptoms after prolonged use. A trial of cyclandelate did not show any advantage over placebo (Diener et al., 1996).

Non-steroidal anti-inflammatory drugs (NSAIDs)

Aspirin has been used for the prevention as well as the treatment of migraine attacks. Of a group of physicians taking low-dose aspirin (325 mg every 2 days), 6.0 per cent reported suffering from migraine at some time after randomization compared with 7.4 per cent of those in the placebo group (Buring et al., 1990). This reduction of 20 per cent was modest but significant. Masel et al. (1980) conducted a controlled crossover trial of aspirin 325 mg twice daily, combined with dipyridamole, 25 mg three times daily, finding that the frequency and severity of migraine attacks were significantly reduced compared with the placebo period.

Much attention has been devoted to naproxen as a prophylactic agent. A crossover double-blind trial established that naproxen 275 mg, two tablets given morning and night, gave significantly better results than placebo, with freedom from severe headaches being achieved by 59 per cent of patients on naproxen compared with 19 per cent on placebo (Welch, 1986). Naproxen 550 mg twice daily was also found to be useful in the management of menstrual migraine but a significant difference from the placebo response occurred only after 3 months of treatment (Sances et al., 1990).

Feverfew

The herbal remedy feverfew, which inhibits the release of 5-HT from platelets among other activities, has been in vogue in the United Kingdom as a remedy for migraine. A double-blind study against placebo has confirmed that the daily consumption of one capsule of dried leaves was effective in reducing the number and severity of attacks (Murphy et al., 1988).

Histamine antagonists

In a carefully controlled double-blind trial, we were unable to demonstrate any worthwhile effects of the histamine-1 blocking agent, chlorpheniramine, or the histamine-2 blocking agent, cimetidine, in preventing migraine (Anthony et al., 1978).

Anticonvulsants

The suggested link between migraine and epilepsy has led to paroxysmal outbursts of advocacy of anticonvulsant agents in the management of migraine. Carbamazepine was mooted as being a useful prophylactic agent but a comparative trial in our own clinic was unable to substantiate this (Anthony and Lance, 1972). Clonazepam 1–2 mg daily proved no better than placebo in preventing migraine (Stensrud and Sjaastad, 1979).

Sodium valproate has been advocated as a means of suppressing migraine headache Sorensen (1988) and a controlled trial (Hering and Keritsky, 1992), demonstrated that the attack frequency and severity were reduced to half while patients were taking 400 mg twice daily over a 2-month period. The effectiveness of valproate (divalproex) has been subsequently confirmed in two large controlled studies (Jensen *et al.*, 1994; Mathew *et al.*, 1995). In practice it is an effective compound that is particularly useful in patients with frequent headache (Mathew and Ali, 1991). Silberstein (1996) has summarized clinical experience with valproate. Side-effects include gastrointestinal disturbances, weight gain and either hyperexcitability or drowsiness. About 3 per cent of women complain of their hair falling out but it grows back and we have never encountered an unbecoming baldness. Hepatic toxicity has occurred in children on polypharmacy but does not present a problem in adults on monotherapy (Silberstein and Wilmore, 1996).

Valproate has also been referred to as overcoming the vexing problem of visual disturbance persisting for weeks or months after a migrainous aura (Rothrock, 1997). Unfortunately, we have not had this happen in the few patients with this distressing condition that we have treated, although we have had significant amelioration of other persistent aura symptoms.

An open trial of gabapentin (Mathew and Lucker, 1996) in doses of 900–1800 mg per day has given promising results and awaits controlled evaluation.

Magnesium

There have been conflicting reports about the efficacy of oral magnesium. Peikert, Willimzig and Kohne-Volland (1996) found that 600 mg of trimagnesium citrate reduced attack frequency by 42 per cent compared with 16 per cent on placebo after 2 months. On the other hand, Pfaffenrath *et al.* (1996) could not demonstrate any benefit from a slightly smaller dose given over 3 months. As might be expected, diarrhoea was the main side-effect.

Riboflavin

On the ground that mitochondrial phosphorylation is reduced in migraineurs, riboflavin 400 mg daily has been tested for efficacy. Schoenen, Jacquy and Lennaerts (1998) showed that headache frequency and severity was reduced to half in the riboflavin group.

Clonidine

Clonidine is an α_2-adrenoceptor agonist, which was proposed as a prophylactic agent for migraine. Initial optimistic reports were followed by a series of negative trials. Of 11 published reports one gave positive results (Kallanranta *et al.*, 1977), four gave negative results, three were equivocal and three provided insufficient data to form an opinion. It remains doubtful whether clonidine has any place in the management of migraine, although this may be because of its dose-limiting side-effects rather than incorrect mechanism of action.

The practical management of migraine

Pre-emptive treatment

If premonitory symptoms give 6–12 hours warning of a migraine attack, the administration of domperidone 30–40 mg at the onset of symptoms is said to prevent the development of migraine headache in about 60 per cent of cases (Waelkens, 1981; Waelkens, 1984). Those patients who experience mood changes or a craving for sweet foods predictably on the evening before they awaken with migraine headache may prevent the development of headache by taking a nocturnal dose of ergotamine tartrate.

Treatment of the acute attack

Some patients respond rapidly to aspirin or a similar analgesic agent that is administered at the first sign of an attack, particularly if 10 mg metoclopromide is given by mouth or by the intramuscular route at the same time to promote gastric absorption and reduce nausea. The intravenous use of aspirin is worth further exploration. NSAIDs, such as naproxen 500 mg can be given orally or by suppository as an alternative to aspirin (Nestvold, 1986). Ketorolac 60 mg intramuscularly can be effective in minimizing an attack (Davis et al., 1995). The patient should then rest and, preferably, sleep. Unfortunately, severe migraine headaches are usually resistant to these measures.

Sumatriptan is now the most efficacious medication that is widely available to terminate an acute attack of migraine. One tablet of 50 mg may be taken at the onset of pain, or even if the headache is well established. Some patients will require 100 mg while others may have a response to 25 mg. A second or third tablet can be taken within a 24-hour period if a headache recurs once the effect of sumatriptan wears off.

For those patients who do not respond to the oral form, the alternative *triptans* are effective and certainly rizatriptan (5 or 10 mg) or zolmitriptan (2.5 or 5 mg) are useful options. Generally naratriptan 2.5 mg is not useful in patients who do not respond to sumatriptan but may be particularly useful in patients who, while responding to any of the *triptans*, experience marked side-effects or frequent headache recurrence. If oral medications fail or drug absorption is a particular problem, such as in patients who vomit early, the sumatriptan nasal spray (20 mg) can be helpful and, where available, the suppository form may also be useful. An auto-injector administering 6 mg subcutaneously can be used if patients do not respond to oral medications, or cannot tolerate or fail to administer the intranasal route. The injection can be repeated within 24 hours if required. Some patients respond to sumatriptan on some occasions but not others (Visser et al., 1996a) so that it is worth trying this medication for at least three attacks to ascertain its value for each individual. If the headache is not relieved by sumatriptan, there is no advantage in repeating an oral dose on that occasion.

The major indication for the use of the *triptans* is for those patients who are incapacitated by their migraine headache in spite of the use of ergotamine and analgesics or who do not tolerate those medicines. Certainly, there are many patients for whom a triptan is cost-effective and many patients prefer these medications over ergotamine and analgesics. There is still a place for regular prophylactic medication (tricyclic antidepressants, beta-blockers, pizotifen, methysergide, valproate) to treat those patients who are subject to very frequent attacks. At the moment it is advised not to use *triptans* in patients partly controlled by methysergide but there is no evidence of major interaction with propranolol, flunarizine, pizotifen, valproate or oral dihydroergotamine (which acts mainly on venous capacitance vessels). It is recommended that sumatriptan not be administered until 24 hours after the last dose of ergotamine tartrate because the vasoconstrictive effects of each drug may be additive. On the other hand, ergotamine can be administered 6 hours after sumatriptan because of the latter's short half life and timing can be similarly adjusted for the half-lives of the other triptans. In this setting it can be useful for preventing the recurrence of headache once the effect of sumatriptan wears off.

The most remarkable effect of sumatriptan in our experience is the ability of the injectable form to abolish migraine headaches of a severity that has previously required narcotic agents to provide relief. This has proven a boon to the harassed general practitioner or staff of an accident and emergency unit who are frequently confronted with the dilemma of whether or not it is justifiable to administer narcotics to a particular person. Sumatriptan has also proven useful in the control of migraine headaches during withdrawal from excessive use of ergotamine and analgesics (Diener *et al.*, 1991).

Ergotamine tartrate is cheaper but less effective than sumatriptan and should be given in optimal dosage at the first indication of an attack developing. If the patient is not nauseated, ergotamine 1–2 mg may be given by mouth, alone or in combination with caffeine (Cafergot) or caffeine plus an anti-emetic agent in a variety of preparations. The trade names of these preparations differ from country to country (Table 9.1) and it is advisable to check whether the pill or suppository prescribed contains 1 or 2 mg of ergotamine tartrate, since repetition of the higher dose often causes nausea. Because gastric absorption is often impaired in migraine, the gastric route may be bypassed with a pressure-pack inhaler or a suppository. Most inhalers deliver 0.36–0.45 mg of ergotamine tartrate and the inhalation may be repeated once or twice at intervals of 5 minutes. The most commonly available suppository is Cafergot, which contains 2 mg of ergotamine tartrate and may cause nausea and aching in the legs. This can be avoided by instructing the patient to place the suppositories in a refrigerator to harden, then slicing them in half. One half suppository can be inserted at the onset of an attack and the other half later on if the headache does not abate. It is said that no more than 10 mg of ergotamine should be taken in 1 week, but individual tolerance varies and vascular side-effects are uncommon.

Patients who use ergotamine frequently may run into the problem of daily re-bound headaches and feel generally unwell, in which case the drug is best ceased completely – at least for a period – to allow the previous intermittent pattern of headache to re-establish itself.

Dihydroergotamine (DHE) 1 mg intramuscularly can be given as the attack begins or repeated 8-hourly if headache continues. Similarly, DHE can now be used in-tranasally and is particularly useful in patients who experience headache recurrence. DHE acts on venous capacitance vessels rather than arteries and is usually free of vasoconstrictive side-effects. There is also evidence that it has a central action on pain pathways.

Metoclopramide 10 mg intravenously or intramuscularly, or prochlorperazine 12.5 mg intramuscularly may be given for the relief of nausea and vomiting; pro-chlorperazine 10 mg intravenously has also been reported to abort headache. Chlor-promazine 12.5 mg intravenously has proven useful in the treatment of headaches as described earlier in this chapter.

We have found intravenous lignocaine, given slowly as a bolus of 100 mg, fol-lowed by an intravenous infusion of 2 mg/minute, useful in terminating continuing migraine headache ('status migrainosus'). This can be combined with the intrave-nous injection of DHE 0.5 mg 8-hourly. There should be less need for these measures with the advent of sumatriptan because the injection of sumatriptan 6 mg subcuta-neously is usually sufficient to stop such headaches (Jauslin et al., 1991).

Corticosteroids have been used in combination with other agents for the treatment of intractable migraine headache (Gallagher, 1985).

The use of narcotic agents is to be avoided as habituation can become a problem. One must be aware of 'smiling migraineurs' who state that they have an intolerable headache requiring an injection of narcotics while appearing to be in the best of health. In the case of those patients who have not responded to other measures and who show objective signs of distress, narcotics should not be withheld. Morphine is usually less effective than meperidine (pethidine) in migrainous patients. Pentazocine may cause hallucinations.

Prophylactic therapy for frequent migraine attacks

If migraine headaches can be prevented from developing by the use of sumatriptan, ergotamine or NSAIDs, there is no need for the patient to take prophylactic medica-tion (interval therapy; Figure 9.3). If these agents are not completely effective and if the frequency of attacks warrants it (say two or more each month) it is worthwhile for the patient to take daily medication in an attempt to suppress headaches or reduce their frequency and severity. Many patients with frequent headache over-use analgesics and, in particular, overuse of compound analgesics can make patients refractory to the effects of prophylactic medications. It is imperative that a careful drug history be obtained and that the patient's use of both prescription and non-prescription compounds be assessed so that they may be advised to reduce or elim-inate the intake so as to provide a window of opportunity for prophylactic medicines.

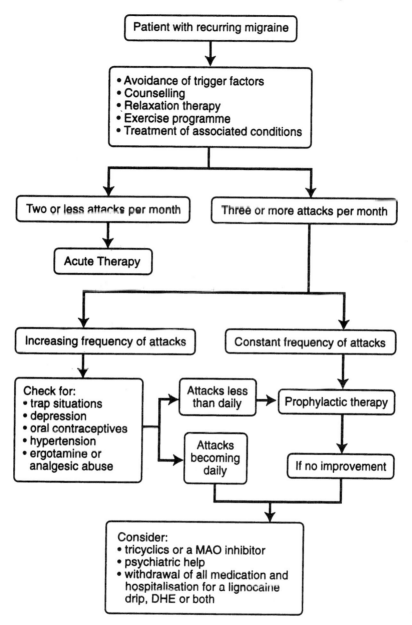

Figure 9.3 Treatment of migraine

Providing the patient is not overweight pizotifen or cyproheptadine is worth trying first. Tablets of pizotifen containing 0.5 mg are available and the dose can be increased slowly from one to six tablets at night if necessary, keeping at a level that does not cause morning drowsiness. Alternatively, cyproheptadine 4 mg one to two tablets at night can be prescribed. Increase in appetite with resulting weight gain is a common side-effect of both drugs. If the patient has not improved after 1 month on the optimum dose, our own policy is to change to a beta-blocker, such as propranolol (Inderal), after checking that the patient is not asthmatic. Some patients respond to as little as 10 mg twice daily of propranolol, but others require full beta-blocking doses. For those patients who do not respond to beta-blockers, naproxen 250–500 mg twice daily can be given a trial. Valproate is an extremely useful preventative agent and often controls patients who have not responded to first-line agents, but the dose must often be pushed to 1000–1500 mg and maintained for 6–8 weeks.

When migraine is mixed with tension headache or is recurring often, tricylic antidepressants are useful even for those patients who are not depressed. Amitriptyline is probably the most effective but should be given at night or about 12 hours prior to when the patient wishes to wake up and the dose increased slowly because many patients complain of morning drowsiness. The patient can start with a tablet of 10 mg, or half of a 25 mg tablet, at night and increase to 75 mg or even 150 mg each night if the medication is well tolerated. Its use may be limited by dryness of the mouth and tremor as well as sedation. In this case dothiepin or imipramine can be employed instead. Valproate can also be very useful in this setting of very frequent headache.

Methysergide is a highly effective antimigrainous agent, but treatment must be started cautiously to minimize the incidence of side-effects. Patients are well advised to cut a pill in half as a small test dose, because about 40 per cent of patients experience side-effects such as epigastric discomfort, muscle cramps, vasoconstrictive phenomena or mood changes if the full dosage schedule of 1–2 mg three times a day is taken immediately.

Methysergide suppresses migraine completely in about 25 per cent of patients and reduces the frequency of headaches by half or more in another 40 per cent. If the patient's symptoms are substantially relieved, methysergide therapy is usually continued for 4 months and then reduced slowly and substituted by another prophylactic agent for a period of 1 month before being recommenced. The reason for this precaution is the rare complication of retroperitoneal or pleural fibrosis.

Some patients choose to continue methysergide therapy because attempts at withdrawal lead to a severe and debilitating recrudescence of migraine. In such cases the patient should be aware of the possibility of fibrotic side-effects, and should report for a physical examination and a blood urea or creatinine estimation every 3 months; patients must notify their medical adviser immediately should any symptoms appear. With these precautions, methysergide is a safe and useful form of migraine prophylaxis for many patients. It is uncertain whether methysergide benefits migraine by maintaining tonic constriction of large arteries or by acting on the central nervous system.

Some patients experience side-effects, chiefly abdominal discomfort and muscle cramps, when treatment is first started but these usually pass off after some days or weeks. Less common side-effects include insomnia, depression, hair loss, a sensation of swelling in the face or throat, increase in the venules over nose and cheeks and gain in weight (Curran et al., 1967). About 10 per cent of patients are unable to tolerate methysergide because of persistent unpleasant symptoms or the appearance of peripheral vasoconstriction with pallor of the extremities, intermittent claudication or, very rarely, angina pectoris.

Peripheral vascular disease, coronary artery disease, hypertension, a history of thrombophlebitis or peptic ulcer, and pregnancy, are all contraindications to the use of methysergide. The reason for avoiding methysergide in the first four conditions is fairly clear, since arterial vasoconstriction is a recognized side-effect. The administration of methysergide was found to double basal gastric secretion of hydrochloric acid in patients with peptic ulcer, and hence its use is best avoided in this condition. There is no evidence to suggest that methysergide is harmful to mother or fetus, but it has been our own practice to suspend its use if pregnancy is planned or occurs unexpectedly.

Some 80 per cent of patients with migraine who have proved to be resistant to other forms of therapy respond to phenelzine 15 mg three times a day. A list of foods and drugs to be avoided while taking monoamine oxidase inhibitors should be issued to each patient (Figure 9.2). Particular mention should be made of oral or inhaled nasal decongestant or bronchodilator agents which commonly contain monoamines.

Migrainous auras (migrainous equivalents)

Since auras are associated with a low cerebral blood flow they are best treated with a vasodilator. A capsule of nifedipine 10 mg can be bitten and several drops swallowed as soon as the visual disturbance or other neurological symptoms begin. Inhalation of an isoprenaline spray or a tablet of glycerol trinitrate 0.6 mg may also hasten the resolution of the aura.

Menstrual migraine and pregnancy

Hormonal methods of treating menstrual migraine are aimed at overcoming the sudden fall in plasma oestradiol that takes place before menstruation. The subcutaneous implantation of pellets of oestradiol, starting with 100 mg, inhibits ovulation and maintains oestradiol levels, while regular monthly periods can be induced by cyclical oral progestogens. Using this method, Magos, Zilkha and Studd (1983) rendered 20 out of 24 patients virtually headache-free over a follow-up period of 5 years.

The application of a gel containing 1.5 mg oestradiol to the skin 48 hours before the expected onset of menstruation prevented 18 of 26 menstrual headaches compared with only one of seven in the patients using a placebo gel (De Lignières et al., 1986).

Tamoxifen has complex effects on ovarian function, competing at oestrogen and anti-oestrogen binding sites, as well as having calcium channel blocking properties. O'Dea and Davis (1990) reported a pilot open trial in which five of eight patients improved markedly and two moderately when treated with tamoxifen citrate 10–20 mg daily preceding and during menstruation. Continuous therapy with bromocriptine 2.5 mg three times daily reduced the frequency of premenstrual migraine in 18 of 24 women followed for a year (Herzog, 1997).

Table 9.4 Proprietary names of some drugs commonly used in the treatment of migraine

Generic term	Proprietary names								
	USA and Canada (c)	UK	France	Italy	Germany	Scandinavia	Brazil	Japan	Australia
Sumatriptan	Imitrex	Imigran	Imigrane Montase	Imigran	Imigran	Imigran	Imigran	Imigran	Imigran
Ergotamine alone	Ergostat Ergomar	Lingraine Medihaler			Medihaler	Medihaler			Ergodryl (mono)
& Caffeine	Cafergot	Cafergot	Gynergene-Cafeine	Cafergot	Cafergot Celatil	Cafergot Ergokoffin	Cafergot	Cafergot	Cafergot
& Caffeine & Anti-emetic	Wigraine Megral (c)	Migril	Migwell						Migral Ergodryl
Dihydroergotamine	DHE 45	Dihydergot	Oxeterone Nocertone	Diidergot	Dihydergot	Dihydergot	Dihydergot	Dihydergot	Dihydergot
5-HT$_2$ blockers: Pizotifen, Pizotyline	Sandomigran (c)	Sanomigran	Sanmigran	Sandomigran	Sandomigran	Sandomigran	Sandomigran		Sandomigran
Cyproheptadine	Periactin	Periactin	Periactine	Periactin	Periactinol	Periactin	Periactin	Periactin	Periactin
Methysergide	Sansert	Deseril	Deseril	Deserril	Deseril	Deseril	Deserila		Deseril

Beta-blockers: β₁, β₂ Propranolol	Inderal	Inderal	Avlocardyl	Inderal	Dociton Beta-Tablinen	Inderal	Inderal	Inderal	Inderal
Timolol	Blocadren	Blocadren	Timacor		Temserin	Timicar	Blocadren	Timoptol	Blocadren
Nadolol	Corgard	Corgard	Corgard	Corgard			Corgard	Nadic	
β₁ Metoprolol	Lopresor	Lopresor Betaloc	Lopresor Seloken	Soloken	Beloc	Soloken	Soloken	Lopresor	Lopresor Betaloc
Atenolol	Tenormin	Tenormin	Tenormin	Tenormin Atenol	Tenormin		Atenol	Tenormin	Tenormin
Ca channel blockers: Verapamil	Isoptin Calan	Cordilox	Isoptine		Isoptin		Dilacoron	Vasolan	Isoptin
Flunarizine	Sibelium (c)		Sibelium		Sibelium		Sibelium	Flunar	Sibelium
Antidepressants: Amitriptyline	Elavil	Tryptizol	Elavil Laroxyl		Saroten	Saroten	Tryptanol	Tryptanol	Tryptanol Laroxyl
Phenelzine	Nardil	Nardil							Nardil
Anticonvulsants: Valproic acid Valproate	Depakote Depakene (c)	Epilim	Depakine		Ergenyl		Depakene Valpakine Valprin	Depakene	Epilim

Our own practice is to use interval medication as described earlier for a few days before and during the menstrual period before attempting hormonal therapy.

Migraine headaches cease in the second and third trimesters of pregnancy in two-thirds of women. There is no evidence that any of the agents used in the treatment of migraine are harmful to the fetus but our own practice is to discontinue medication during pregnancy. Ergotamine has only a weak oxytocic effect but is best avoided lest any natural complication of pregnancy be attributed to its use.

Migraine in childhood

Episodic headaches in children and adolescents are often thought erroneously to be of the tension variety even though they are associated with nausea, photophobia or other migrainous characteristics. Tensions at school and at home may certainly contribute to the frequency of migraine in childhood and the excitement of going to a birthday party often triggers an attack. Good, Taylor and Mortimer (1991) found that migrainous children wearing rose-tinted glasses at school reduced their monthly headache frequency from 6.2 to 1.6 per month over a period of 4 months whereas wearing density-matched blue glasses had no effect. Improvement was attributed to the red tint reducing exposure to short-wavelength flicker from fluorescent lights. Attention must be paid to any psychological factors as well as to physical relaxation (Duckro and Cantwell-Simmons, 1989).

The child's posture should be checked. If the height of chair and desk are mismatched so that children have to crane their heads awkwardly to write or see the blackboard at school, aching of the neck muscles may lead on to a migraine attack. Diet and regular mealtimes may play a more important part in childhood than in adult life but the child should not be denied pharmacotherapy.

While some children find that their headaches are eased by an analgesic and disappear with sleep, many do not. In these less fortunate children, ergotamine tartrate can be given at the onset, orally or by inhalation. A medihaler of ergotamine is easy for children to use and carries no stigma, if not actually a status symbol. Nasal sprays of dihydroergotamine or sumatriptan may well prove to be useful for the same reasons. When migraine recurs frequently in children, interval therapy can be used as in adults, usually starting with pizotifen or cyproheptadine (if the child is not overweight) or propranolol (if there is no tendency to asthma). Once migraine is brought under control in children it goes into remission in about 60 per cent of cases, although it may recur in later years in about 20 per cent of individuals.

Conclusions

The variety of medications employed in the treatment of migraine is an indication that none is entirely effective. Nevertheless, most patients can be relieved by a combination of behavioural management and drug therapy. The advent of the selective 5-HT$_{1B/1D}$ agonists is the start of a new era promising more specific and efficacious management of acute attacks. For those patients who do not respond satisfactorily to sumatriptan, the newer *triptans*, ergotamine derivatives or analgesics, and whose frequency of attacks exceeds two a month, a thorough trial of prophylactic therapy is indicated with the aim of reducing the intensity and frequency of attacks, or eliminating them completely.

References

Adley, C., Straumanis, J. and Chasson, A. (1992). Fluoxetine prophylaxis of migraine. *Headache* **32**,101–104

Aellig, W. H. and Berde, B. (1969). Ergot compounds and vascular resistance. *Br. J. Pharmacol.* **36**, 561–570

Ala-Hurula, V., Myllylä, V. V., Hokkanen, E. and Tokola, O. (1981). Tolfenamic acid and ergotamine abuse. *Headache* **21**, 240–242

Andersen, A. R., Tfelt-Hansen, P. and Lassen, N. A. (1987). The effect of ergotamine and dihydroergotamine on cerebral blood flow in man. *Stroke* **18**, 120–123

Anderson, J. A. D., Basker, M. A. and Dalton, R. (1975). Migraine and hypnotherapy. *Int. J. Exp. Hypnosis* **23**, 48–58

Andersson, P. G., Hansen, J. H., Hansen, P. E. *et al.* (1983). Prophylactic treatment of classical and non-classical migraine with metoprolol – a comparison with placebo. *Cephalalgia* **3**, 207–212

Anthony, M. and Lance, J. W. (1968). Indomethacin in migraine. *Med. J. Aust.* **1**, 56–77

Anthony, M. and Lance, J. W. (1969). Monoamine oxidase inhibition in the treatment of migraine. *Arch. Neurol.* **21**, 263–268

Anthony, M. and Lance, J. W. (1972). A comparative trial of pindolol, clonidine and carbamazepine in the interval therapy of migraine. *Med. J. Aust.* **1**, 1343–1346

Anthony, M., Lord, G. D. A. and Lance, J. W. (1978). Controlled trials of cimetidine in migraine and cluster headache. *Headache* **18**, 261–264

Arthur, G. P. and Hornabrook, R. W. (1971). The treatment of migraine with BC-105 (Pizotifen), a double-blind trial. *N.Z. Med. J.* **73**, 5–9

Baischer, W. (1995). Acupuncture in migraine. Long term outcome and predicting factors. *Headache* **35**, 472–474

Bardwell, A. and Trott, J. A. (1987). Stroke in migraine as a consequence of propranolol. *Headache* **27**, 381–383

Becker, W. J. (1995). A placebo-controlled, dose-defining study of sumatriptan nasal spray in the acute treatment of migraine. *Cephalalgia* **15** (Suppl. 14), 239

Beer, M., Middlemiss, D., Stanton, J. *et al.* (1995). *In vitro* pharmacological profile of the novel 5-HT$_{1D}$ receptor agonist MK-462. *Cephalalgia* **15** (Suppl. 14), 203

Bell, R., Montoya, D., Shuaib, A. and Lee, M. A. (1990). A comparative trial of three agents in the treatment of acute migraine headache. *Ann. Emerg. Med.* **19**, 1079–1082

Bellevance, A. J and Meloche, J. P. (1990). A comparative study of naproxen sodium, protyline and placebo in migraine prophylaxis. *Headache* **30**, 710–715

Benedict, C. R. and Robertson, D. (1979). Angina pectoris and sudden death in the absence of atherosclerosis following ergotamine therapy for migraine. *Am. J. Med.* **67**, 177–178

Benson, H., Klemchuk, H. P. and Graham, J. R. (1974). The usefulness of the relaxation response in the therapy of headache. *Headache* **14**, 49–52

Berde, B. and Schild, H. O. (1978). Ergot alkaloids and related compounds. In *Handbook of Experimental Pharmacology*, Vol. 49, Eds G. V. R. Born, O. Eichler, A. Farah, H. Herken and A. D. Welch. Berlin, Springer-Verlag

Bianchine, J. R. and Eade, N. R. (1967). The effect of 5-hydroxytryptamine on the cotton pellet local inflammatory response in the rat. *J. Exp. Med.* **125**, 501–510

Blanchard, E. B., Appelbaum, K. A., Radnitz, C. L. *et al.* (1990). A controlled evaluation of thermal biofeedback and thermal biofeedback combined with cognitive therapy in the treatment of vascular headache. *J. Consulting in Clin. Psychol.* **58**, 216–224

Brown, E. G., Endersby, C. A., Smith, R. N. and Talbot, J. C. C. (1991). The safety and tolerability of sumatriptan: an overview. *Eur. Neurol.* **31**, 339–344

Buring, J. E., Peto, R. and Hennekens, C. H. (1990). Low-dose aspirin for migraine prophylaxis. *J. Am. Med. Assoc.* **264**, 1711–1713

Cabarrocas, X. (1997). First efficacy data on subcutaneous almotriptan, a novel 5-HT$_{1B/D}$ agonist. *Cephalalgia* **17**, 420

Cady, R. K., Dexter, J., Sargent, J. D. *et al.* (1993). Efficacy of subcutaneous sumatriptan in repeated episodes of migraine. *Neurology* **43**, 1363–1368

Cady, R. K., Wendt, J. K., Kirchner, J. R., Sargent, J. D., Rothrock, J. F. and Skaggs, H. (1991). Treatment of acute migraine with subcutaneous sumatriptan. *J. Am. Med. Assoc.* **265**, 2831–2835

Callaham, M. and Raskin, N. (1986). A controlled study of dihydroergotamine in the treatment of acute migraine headache. *Headache* **26**, 168–171

Capildeo, R. and Rose, F. C. (1982). Single-dose pizotifen, 1.5 mg nocte: a new approach in the prophylaxis of migraine. *Headache* **22**, 272–275

Chabriat, H., Joire, J. E., Danchot, J., Grippon, P. and Bousser, M. G. (1994). Combined oral lysine acetylsalicylate and metoclopramide in the acute treatment of migraine: a multicentre double-blind placebo-controlled study. *Cephalalgia* **14**, 297–300

Connolly, H. M., Crary, J. L., McGoon, M. D. *et al.* (1997). Valvular heart disease associated with fenfluramine-phentermine. *N. Eng. J. Med.* **337**, 581–588

Connor, H. E., Feniuk, W., Beattie, D. T. *et al.* (1997). Naratriptan: biological profile in animal models relevant to migraine. *Cephalalgia* **17**, 145–152

Connor, H. E., Stubbs, C. M., Feniuk, W. and Humphrey, P. P. A. (1992). Effect of sumatriptan, a selective 5-HT1-like receptor agonist, on pial vessel diameter in anaesthetised cats. *J. Cereb. Blood Flow Metabol.* **12**, 514–519

Couch, J. R., Ziegler, D. K. and Hassanein, R. (1976). Amitriptyline in the prophylaxis of migraine. Effectiveness and relationship of antimigraine and antidepressant drugs. *Neurology* **26**, 121–127

Couturier, E. G. M., Hering, R., Foster, C. A., Steiner, T. J. and Rose, F. C. (1991). First clinical study of selective 5-HT$_3$, antagonist, granisetron (BRL, 43694), in the acute treatment of migraine headache. *Headache* **31**, 296–297

Cumberbatch, M. J., Hill, R. G. and Hargreaves, R. J. (1997). Rizatriptan has central antinociceptive effects against durally evoked responses. *Eur. J. Pharmacol.* **328**, 37–40

Curran, D. A., Hinterberger, H. and Lance, J. W. (1967). Methysergide. *Res. Clin. Stud. Headache* **1**, 74–122

Curran, D. A. and Lance, J. W. (1964). Clinical trial of methysergide and other preparations in the management of migraine. *J. Neurol. Neurosurg. Psychiat.* **27**, 463–469

Cutler, N., Mushet, G. R., Davis, R., Clements, B. and Whitcher, L. (1985). Oral sumatriptan for the long-term treatment of migraine: clinical findings. *Neurology* **45** (Suppl. 7), S5–S9

Cyriax, J. (1962). *Textbook of Orthopaedic Medicine*, Vol. 1. London, Cassell

Davis, C. P., Torre, P. T., Williams, C. *et al.* (1995). Ketorolac versus meperidine plus promethazine treatment of migraine headaches: evaluation by patients. *Am. J. Emerg. Med.* **13**, 146–150

De Lignières, B., Mauvais-Javis, P., Mas, J. M. L., Toubout, P. J. and Bousser, M. G. (1986). Prevention of menstrual migraine by percutaneous oestradiol. *Br. Med. J.* **293**, 1540

Diamond, S. (1995). The use of sumatriptan in patients on monoamine oxidase inhibitors. *Neurology* **45**, 1039–1040

Diamond, S. and Medina, J. L. (1975). Isometheptene – a non-ergot drug in the treatment of migraine. *Headache* **16**, 212–213

Diener, H. C., Foh, M., Iaccarino, C. *et al.* (1996). Cyclandelate in the prophylaxis of migraine: a randomised parallel, double-blind study in comparison with placebo and propranolol. *Cephalalgia* **16**, 441–447

Diener, H. C., Haab, J., Peters, C., Ried, S., Dichgans, J. and Pilgrim, A. (1991). Subcutaneous sumatriptan in the treatment of headache during withdrawal from drug-induced headache. *Headache* **31**, 205–209

Duckro, P. N. and Cantwell-Simmons, E. (1989). A review of studies evaluating biofeedback and relaxation training in the management of paediatric headache. *Headache* **29**, 428–433

Edvinsson, L., Jansen, I. and Olesen, J. (1991). Analysis of the vasoconstrictor effects of sumatriptan on human cranial arteries. *Cephalalgia* **11**, 210–211

Feniuk, W., Humphrey, P. P. A., Perren, M. J., Connor, H. E. and Whalley, E. T. (1991). Rationale for the use of 5-HT1-like agonists in the treatment of migraine. *J. Neurol.* **238**, S57–S61

Ferrari, M. D. (1991). Treatment of migraine attacks with sumatriptan. *N. Eng. J. Med.* **325**, 316–321

Ferrari, M. D., Caekebeke, J. F. V., Haan, J. *et al.* (1991). Effect of sumatriptan on cerebral blood flow during and outside migraine attacks: a Tc-99m HMPAO SPECT and transcranial Doppler study. *Cephalalgia* **11** (Suppl. 11), 205

Finnish Sumatriptan Group and the Cardiovascular Clinical Research Group (1991). A placebo-controlled study of intranasal sumatriptan for the acute treatment of migraine. *Eur. Neurol.* **31**, 332–338

Forssman, B., Lindbald, C. J. and Zbornikova, V. (1983). Atenolol for migraine prophylaxis. *Headache* **23**, 188–190.

Fowler, P. A., Lacey, L. F., Thomas, M., Keene, O. N., Tanner, R. J. N. and Baber, N. S. (1991). The clinical pharmacology, pharmacokinetics and metabolism of sumatriptan. *Eur. Neurol.* **31**, 291–294

Friberg, L., Olesen, J., Iversen, H. K. and Sperling, B. (1991). Migraine pain associated with middle cerebral artery dilatation – reversal by sumatriptan. *Lancet* **338**, 13–17

Fukuda, Y. and Inumikawa, K. (1988). Intravenous aspirin for intractable headache and facial pain. *Headache* **28**, 47–50

Fuseau, E., Baille, P. and Kempsford, R. D. (1997). A study to determine the absolute oral bioavailability of naratriptan. *Cephalalgia* **17**, 417

Gallagher, M. (1996). Acute treatment of migraine with dihydroergotamine nasal spray. Dihydroergotamine Working Group. *Arch. Neurol.* **53**, 1285–1291

Gallagher, R. M. (1985). Emergency treatment of intractable migraine. *Headache* **25**, 164

Gijsman, H., Kramer, M. S., Sargent, J. *et al.* (1997). Double-blind, placebo-controlled, dose-finding study of rizatriptan (MK-462) in the acute treatment of migraine. *Cephalalgia* **17**, 647–651

Goadsby, P. J. (1997a). 311C90, a novel 5-HT$_{1B/D}$ agonist – the assessment of efficacy and tolerability in the acute treatment of migraine. *Neurology* **48**(3), A86

Goadsby, P. J. (1997b). Place of naratriptan in clinical practice. *Cephalalgia* **17**, 472–473

Goadsby, P. J. (1998). A Triptan too far. *J. Neurol. Neurosurg. Psych.* **64**, 143–147.

Goadsby, P. J. and Edvinsson, L. (1993). The trigeminovascular system and migraine: studies characterising cerebrovascular and neuropeptide changes seen in man and cat. *Ann. Neurol.* **33**, 48–56

Goadsby, P. J. and Edvinsson, L. (1994). Peripheral and central trigeminovascular activation in cat is blocked by the serotonin (5HT)-1D receptor agonist 311C90. *Headache* **34**, 394–399

Goadsby, P. J. and Gundlach, A. L. (1991). Localization of [^{3}H]-dihydroergotamine binding sites in the cat central nervous system: relevance to migraine. *Ann. Neurol.* **29**, 91–94

Goadsby, P. J. and Hoskin K. L. (1996). Inhibition of trigeminal neurons by intravenous administration of the serotonin (5HT)-1-D receptor agonist zolmitriptan (311C90): are brain stem sites a therapeutic target in migraine? *Pain* **67**, 355–359

Goadsby, P. J. and Knight, Y. E. (1997a). Direct evidence for central sites of action of zolmitriptan (311C90): an autoradiographic study in cat. *Cephalalgia* **17**, 153–158

Goadsby, P. J. and Knight, Y. E. (1997b). Naratriptan inhibits trigeminal neurons after intravenous administration through an action at the serotonin (5HT$_{1B/1D}$) receptors. *Br. J. Pharmacol.* **122**, 918–922

Goadsby, P. J. and Olesen, J. (1996). Migraine: diagnosis and treatment in the 1990's. *Br. Med. J.* **312**, 1279–1282

Goadsby, P. J., Zagami, A. S., Donnan, G. A. *et al.* (1991). A double-blind placebo controlled crossover study of sumatriptan in the treatment of acute migraine attacks. *Lancet* **ii**, 782–783

Gobel, H. (1995). A placebo-controlled, dose-defining study of sumatriptan suppositories in the acute treatment of migraine. *Cephalalgia* **15** (Suppl. 14), 232

Gobel, H., Boswell, D., Winter, P. and Crisp, A. (1997). A comparison of the efficacy, safety and tolerability of naratriptan and sumatriptan. *Cephalalgia* **17**, 426

Gomersall, J. D. and Stuart, A. (1973). Amitriptyline in migraine prophylaxis. Changes in pattern of attacks during a controlled clinical trial. *J. Neurol. Neurosurg. Psychiat.* **36**, 684–690

Good, P. A., Taylor, R. H. and Mortimer, M. J. (1991). The use of tinted glasses in childhood migraine. *Headache* **31**, 533–536

Graham, J. R. (1967). Cardiac and pulmonary fibrosis during methysergide therapy for headache. *Am. J. Med. Sci.* **254**, 23–24

Gupta, P., Brown, D., Butler, P. *et al.* (1996a). Preclinical *in vivo* pharmacology of eletriptan (UK-116,044): a potent and selective partial agonist at the $5HT_{1D}$-like receptor. *Cephalalgia* **16**, 386

Gupta, P., Scatchard, J., Shepperson, N., Wallis, R. and Wythes, M. J. (1996b). *In vitro* pharmacology of eletriptan (UK-116,044), a potent partial agonist at the '$5HT_{1D}$ -like' receptor in the dog saphenous vein. *Cephalalgia* **16**, 386

Hakkarainen, H., Parantainen, P., Gothoni, G. and Vapaatalo, H. (1982). Tolfenamic acid and caffeine: a useful combination in migraine. *Cephalalgia* **2**, 173–177

Hakkarainen, H., Vapaatolo, H., Gothoni, G. and Parantainen, J. (1979). Tolfenamic acid is as effective as ergotamine during migraine attacks. *Lancet* **2**, 326–328

Hartig, P. R., Hoyer, D., Humphrey, P. P. A. and Martin, G. R. (1996). Alignment of receptor nomenclature with the human genome: classification of 5HT-1B and 5-HT-1D receptor subtypes. *Trends Pharmacol. Sci.* **17**, 103–105

Henkes, H., May, A., Kuhne, D., Berg-Dammer, E. and Diener, H.-C. (1996). Sumatriptan: vasoactive effect on human dural vessels, demonstrated by subselective angiography. *Cephalalgia* **16**, 224–230

Henriksson, A. (1995). The efficacy and tolerability of 12.5 mg and 25 mg sumatriptan suppositories in the acute treatment of migraine. *Cephalalgia* **15** (Suppl. 14), 235

Hering, R. and Keritsky, A. (1992). Sodium valproate in the prophylactic treatment of migraine: a double blind study versus placebo. *Cephalalgia* **12**, 81–84

Hernandez-Gallego, J. (1985). The efficacy and tolerability of sumatriptan 10 mg and 20 mg nasal sprays in the acute treatment of migraine. *Cephalalgia* **15** (Suppl. 14), 240

Herzog, A. G. (1997). Continuous bromocriptine therapy in menstrual migraine. *Neurology* **48**, 101–102

Hill, A. P., Hyde, R. M., Robertson, A. D., Woollard, P. M., Glen, R. C. and Martin, G. R. (1995). Oral delivery of 5-HT1D receptor agonists: towards the discovery of 311C90, a novel antimigraine agent. *Headache* **34**, 308

Hokkanen, E., Myllyla, V. V. and Ala-Hurula, V. (1982). Clinical aspects of the pharmacokinetics of ergotamine. In *Advances in Migraine, Research and Therapy*, Ed. F. Clifford Rose. pp. 181–185. New York, Raven Press

Holroyd, K. A. and Penzien, D. B. (1990). Pharmacological versus non-pharmacological prophylaxis of recurrent migraine headache: a meta-analytic review of clinical trials. *Pain* **42**, 1–13

Hoskin, K. L., Kaube, H. and Goadsby, P. J. (1996). Central activation of the trigeminovascular pathway in the cat is inhibited by dihydroergotamine: a c-*Fos* and electrophysiology study. *Brain* **119**, 249–256

Hoyer, D., Clarke, D. E., Fozard, J. R. *et al.* (1994). International Union of Pharmacology classification of receptors for 5-hydroxytryptamine (serotonin). *Pharmacol. Rev.* **46**, 157–203

Humphrey, P. P. A., Feniuk, W., Marriott, A. S., Tanner, R. J. N, Jackson, M. R. and Tucker, M. L. (1991). Preclinical studies on the anti-migraine drug, sumatriptan. *Eur. Neurol.* **31**, 282–290

Hussey, E. K., Aubert, B., Richard, I., Kunk, R. L. and Fowler, P. (1995). The clinical pharmacology of sumatriptan suppositories. *Cephalalgia* **15** (Suppl. 14), 233

International Headache Society Committee on Clinical Trials in Migraine (1991). Guidelines for controlled trials of drugs in migraine. *Cephalalgia* **11**, 1–12

Jackson, N. C. (1996). A comparison of oral eletriptan (UK-116,044) (20-80 mg) and oral sumatriptan (100 mg) in the acute treatment of migraine. *Cephalalgia* **16**, 368–369

Jauslin, P., Goadsby, P. J. and Lance, J. W. (1991). The hospital management of severe migrainous headache. *Headache* **31**, 658–660

Jensen, R., Brinck, T. and Olesen, J. (1994). Sodium valproate has a prophylactic effect in migraine without aura: a triple blind, placebo-controlled crossover study. *Neurology* **44**, 647–651

Jones, J., Sklar, D., Dougherty, J. and White, W. (1989). Randomized double-blind trial of intravenous prochlorperazine for the treatment of acute headache. *J. Am. Med. Assoc.* **261**, 1174–1176

Joss, R. A. and Dott, C. S. (1993). Clinical studies with granisetron, a new 5-HT_3 receptor antagonist for the treatment of cancer chemotherapy-induced emesis. The Granisetron Study Group. *Eur. J. Cancer* **29A** (Suppl. 1), S22–S29

Jost, W. H., Raulf, F. and Müller-Lobeck, H. (1991). Anorectal ergotism. Induced by migraine therapy. *Acta Neurol. Scand.* **84**, 73–74

Kallanranta, T., Hakkarainen, H., Hokkanen, E. and Tuovinen, T. (1977). Clonidine in migraine prophylaxis. *Headache* **17**, 169–172

Kangasniemi, P., Andersen, A. R., Andersson, P. G. *et al.* (1987). Classic migraine: effective prophylaxis with metoprolol. *Cephalalgia* **7**, 231–238

Karachalios, G. N., Fotiadou, A., Chrisikos, N., Karabetsos, A. and Kehagioglou, K. (1992). Treatment of acute migraine attack with diclofenac sodium: a double-blind study. *Headache* **32**, 98–100

Kempsford, R. (1997). Clinical pharmacology and pharmacokinetics of naratriptan. *Cephalalgia* **17**, 473

Kempsford, R. D., Baille, P. and Fuseau, E. (1997). Oral naratriptan tablets (2.5 mg–10 mg) exhibit dose-proportional pharmacokinetics. *Cephalalgia* **17**, 408

Klapper, J. A. and Stanton, J. (1993). Current emergency treatment of severe headaches. *Headache* **33**, 560–562

Korsgaard, A. G. (1995). The tolerability, safety and efficacy of oral sumatriptan 50 mg and 100 mg for the acute treatment of migraine in adolescents. *Cephalalgia* **16**, 98

Kuritzky, A., Zoldan, Y. and Melamed, E. (1992). Selegeline, a MAO B inhibitor, is not effective in the prophylaxis of migraine without aura – an open study. *Headache* **32**, 416

Lance, J. W., Fine, R. D. and Curran, D. A. (1963). An evaluation of methysergide in the prevention of migraine and other vascular headache. *Med. J. Aust.* **1**, 814–818

Lane, P. L., McLellan, B. A. and Baggoley, C. J. (1989). Comparative efficacy of chlorpromazine and meperidine with dimenhydrinate in migraine headache. *Ann. Emerg. Med.* **18**, 360–365

Lataste, X., Taylor, P. and Notter, M. (1989). DHE nasal spray in the acute management of migraine attacks. *Cephalalgia* **9** (Suppl. 10), 342–343

Lawrence, E. R., Hossain, M. and Littlestone, W. (1977). Sanomigran for migraine prophylaxis; controlled multicenter trial in general practice. *Headache* **17**, 109–112

Leone, M., Grazzi, L., Mantia, L. L. and Bussone, G. (1991). Flunarizine in migraine: a mini review. *Headache* **31**, 388–391

Lewis, C. T., Molland, E. A., Marshall, V. R., Tresidder, G. C. and Blandy, J. P. (1975). Analgesic abuse, ureteric obstruction and retroperitoneal fibrosis. *Br. J. Med.* **2**, 76–78

Little, P. J., Jennings, G. L., Skews, H. and Bobik, A. (1982). Bioavailablility of dihydroergotamine in man. *Br. J. Pharmacol.* **13**, 785–790

Loh, L., Nathan, P. W., Schott, G. D. and Zilkha, K. J. (1984). Acupuncture versus medical treatment for migraine and muscle tension headache. *J. Neurol. Neurosurg. Psychiat.* **47**, 333–337

Loisy, C., Beorchia, S., Centonze, V., Fozard, J. R., Schechter, P. J. and Tell, G. P. (1985). Effects on migraine headache of MDL 72,222, an antagonist at neuronal 5-HT receptors. Double-blind, placebo-controlled study. *Cephalalgia* **5**, 79–82

Louis, P. and Spierings, E. L. H. (1982). Comparison of flunarizine (Sibelium®) and pizotifen (Sandomigran®) in migraine treatment: A double-blind study. *Cephalalgia* **2**, 197–203

Maciewicz, R., Borsook, S. and Strassman, A. (1988). Intravenous lidocaine relieves acute vascular headache. *Headache* **28**, 309

Macintyre, P. D., Bhargava, B., Hogg, K. J., Gemmill, J. D. and Hillis, W. S. (1992). The effect of i.v. sumatriptan, a selective 5-HT$_1$-receptor agonist on central haemodynamics and the coronary circulation. *Br. J. Clin. Pharmacol.* **1992**, 541–546

Macintyre, P. D., Bhargava, B., Hogg, K. J., Gemmill, J. D. and Hillis, W. S. (1993). Effect of subcutaneous sumatriptan, a selective 5-HT$_1$-receptor agonist, on the systemic, pulmonary, and coronary circulation. *Circulation* **87**, 401–405

Magee, R. (1991). Saint Anthony's fire revisited. Vascular problems associated with migraine medication. *Med. J. Aust.* **154**, 145–149

Magos, A. L., Zilkha, K. J. and Studd, J. W. W. (1983). Treatment of menstrual migraine by oestradiol implants. *J. Neurol. Neurosurg. Psychiat.* **46**, 1044–1046

Malaquin, F., Urbun, T., Ostinelli, J., Ghedita, H. and Lacronique, J. (1989). Pleural and retroperitoneal fibrosis from dihydroergotamine. *N. Eng. J. Med.* **321**, 1760

Martin, G. R., Robertson, A. D., MacLennan, S. J. *et al.* (1997). Receptor specificity and trigemino-vascular inhibitory actions of a novel 5-HT$_{1B/1D}$ receptor partial agonist, 311C90 (zolmitriptan). *Br. J. Pharmacol.* **121**, 157–164

Masel, B. E., Chesson, A. L., Peters, B. H., Levin, H. S. and Alperin, J. B. (1980). Platelet antagonists in migraine prophylaxis. A clinical trial using aspirin and dipyridamole. *Headache* **20**, 13–18

Massiou, H. (1996a). A comparison of sumatriptan nasal spray 20 mg and oral sumatriptan 100 mg in the acute treatment of migraine. *Third European Headache Federation Meeting*, Sardinia

Massiou, H. (1996b). A comparison of sumatriptan nasal spray and intranasal dihydroergotamine (DHE) in the acute treatment of migraine. *Functional Neurol.* **11**(2/3), 151

Massiou, H., Serrurier, D., Lasserre, O. and Bousser, M. G. (1991). Effectiveness of oral diclofanac in the acute treatment of common migraine attacks: a double-blind study versus placebo. *Cephalalgia* **11**, 59–63

Mathew, N. T. and Ali, S. (1991). Valproate in the treatment of persistent chronic daily headache. An open label study. *Headache* **31**, 71–74

Mathew, N. T. and Lucker, C. (1996). Gabapentin in migraine prophylaxis: a preliminary open label study. *Neurology* **46**, A169

Mathew, N. T., Saper, J. R., Silberstein, S. D. *et al.* (1995). Migraine prophylaxis with divalproex. *Arch. Neurol.* **52**, 281–286

Mathew, N. T., Stubits, E. and Nigam, M. (1982). Transformation of migraine into daily headache: analysis of factors. *Headache* **22**, 66–68

Mathew, N. T., Tiejen, G. E. and Lucker, C. (1996). Serotonin syndrome complicating migraine pharmacotherapy. *Cephalalgia* **16**, 323–327

McQueen, J., Loblay, R. J., Swain, A. R., Anthony, M. and Lance, J. W. (1989). A controlled trial of dietary modification in migraine. In *New Advances in Headache Research*, Ed. F. Clifford Rose. pp. 235–242. London, Smith-Gordon

Merikangas, K. R. and Merikangas, J. R. (1995). Combination monamine oxidase inhibitor and β-blocker treatment of migraine. *Biol. Psychiat.* **37**, 1–8

Migraine Nimodipine European Study Group (MINES) (1989). European multicenter trial of nimodipine in the prophylaxis of common migraine (migraine without aura). *Headache* **29**, 633–638, 639–642

Mitchell, K. R. and Mitchell, D. M. (1971). Migraine: an exploratory treatment application of programmed behaviour therapy techniques. *J. Psychosom. Res.* **15**, 137–157

Mitchell, K. R. and White, R. G. (1976). The control of migraine headache by behavioural self-management: controlled case study. *Headache* **16**, 178–184

Muller-Schweinitzer, E. and Fanchamps, A. (1982). Effects on arterial receptors of ergot derivatives used in migraine. In *Advances in Neurology*, Vol. 33, Ed. M. Critchley. pp. 343–355. New York, Raven Press

Multinational Oral Sumatriptan and Cafergot Study Group (1991). A randomized, double-blind comparison of sumatriptan and Cafergot in the acute treatment of migraine. *Eur. Neurol.* **31**, 314–322

Murphy, J. J., Heptinstall, S. and Mitchell, J. R. A. (1988). Randomized double-blind placebo-controlled trial of feverfew in migraine prevention. *Lancet* **2**, 189–192

Nestvold, K. (1986). Naproxen and naproxen sodium in acute migraine attacks. *Cephalalgia* **6** (Suppl. 4), 81–84

O'Dea, J. P. K. and Davis, E. H. (1990). Tamoxifen in the treatment of menstrual migraine. *Neurology* **40**, 1470–1471

Oral Sumatriptan and Aspirin plus Metoclopramide Comparative Study Group (1992). A study to compare oral sumatriptan with oral aspirin plus metoclopramide in the acute treatment of migraine. *Eur. Neurol.* **32**, 177–184

Oral Sumatriptan Dose-Defining Study Group (1991). Sumatriptan – an oral dose-defining study. *Eur. Neurol.* **31**, 300–305

Palmer, K. J. and Spencer, C. M. (1997). Zolmitriptan. *CNS Drugs* **7**, 468–478

Parker, G. B., Pryor, D. S. and Tupling, H. (1980). Who does migraine improve during a clinical trial? Further results from a trial of cervical manipulation for migraine. *Aust. N.Z. J. Med.* **10**, 192–198

Parker, G. B., Tupling, H. and Pryor, D. S. (1978). A Controlled trial of cervical manipulation for migraine. *Aust. N.Z. J. Med.* **8**, 589–593

Pascual, K., Polo, J. M. and Cerciano, J. (1989). The dose of propranolol for migraine prophylaxis. Efficacy of low doses. *Cephalalgia* **9**, 287–291

Pedersen, E. and Möller, C. E. (1966). Methysergide in migraine prophylaxis. *Clin. Pharmacol. Therap.* **7**, 520–526

Peikert, A., Wilimzig, C. and Kohne-Volland, R. (1996). Prophylaxis of migraine with oral magnesium: results from a prospective, multi-center, placebo-controlled and double-blind randomized study. *Cephalalgia* **16**, 257–263

Peroutka, S. J. (1990). The pharmacology of current anti-migraine drugs. *Headache* **30**, 5–11

Pfaffenrath, V., Cunin, G., Sjonell, G., Prendergast, S., Hassani, H. and Bertin, L. (1998) Efficacy and safety of sumatriptan tablets (25 mg, 50 mg, 100 mg) in the acute treatment of migraine: defining the optimum doses of oral sumatriptan. *Headache*, **38**, 184–190

Pfaffenrath, V., Wessely, P., Mener, C. *et al.* (1996). Magnesium in the prophylaxis of migraine – a double-blind placebo-controlled study. *Cephalalgia* **16**, 436–440

Phebus, L. A., Johnson, K. W., Audia, J. E. *et al.* (1996). Characterization of LY334370, a potent and selective 5-HT$_{1F}$ receptor agonist, in the neurogenic dural inflammation model of migraine pain. *Proc. Soc. Neurosci. (USA)* **22**, 1331

Rance, D., Clear, N., Dallman, L., Llewellyn, E., Nuttall, J. and Verrier, H. (1997). Physicochemical comparison of eletriptan and other 5-HT$_{1D}$-like agonists as a predictor of oral absorption potential. *Headache* **37**, 328

Raskin, N. H. (1986). Repetitive intravenous dihydroergotamine as therapy for intractable migraine. *Neurology* **36**, 995–997

Reutens, D. C., Fatovich, D. M., Stewart-Wynne, E. G. and Prentice, D. A. (1991). Is intravenous lignocaine clinically effective in acute migraine? *Cephalalgia* **11**, 245–247

Rothner, A., Edwards, K., Kerr, L., DeBussey, S. and Asgharnejad, M. (1997). Efficacy and safety of naratriptan tablets in adolescent migraine. *J. Neurol. Sci.* **150**, S106

Rothrock, J. F. (1997). Successful treatment of persistent migraine aura with divalproex sodiem. *Neurology* **48**, 261–262

Rowat, B. M. T., Merrill, C. F., Dais, A. and South, V. (1991). Double-blind comparison of granisetron and placebo for the treatment of acute migraine in the emergency department. *Cephalalgia* **11**, 207–213

Ryan, R. and Keywood, C. (1997). A preliminary study of VML251 (SB209509) a novel 5-HT$_{1B/1D}$ agonist for the treatment of acute migraine. *Cephalalgia* **17**, 418

Salonen, R. (1997). Patient preference among 25 mg, 50 mg, and 100 mg oral sumatriptan. *J. Neurol. Sci.* **150** (Suppl.), S36

Sances, G., Martignoni, E., Floroni, L., Blandini, F. M., Facchinetti, F. and Nappi, G. (1990). Naproxen sodium in menstrual migraine prophylaxis; a double-blind placebo controlled study. *Headache* **30**, 705–709

Saper, J. R., Silberstein, S. D., Lake, A. E. and Winters, M. E. (1994). Double-blind trial of fluoxetine: chronic daily headache and migraine. *Headache* **34**, 497–502

Sargent, J., Kirchner, J. R., Davis, R. and Kirkhart, B. (1995). Oral sumatriptan is effective and well tolerated for the acute treatment of migraine: results of a multicenter study. *Neurology* **45** (Suppl 7), S10–S14

Scherl, E. R. and Wilson, J. F. (1995). Comparison of dihydroergotamine with metoclopramide versus meperidine with promethazine in the treatment of acute migraine. *Headache* **35**, 256–259

Schoenen, J., Jacquy, J. and Lenaerts, M. (1998). Effectiveness of high-dose riboflavin in migraine prophylaxis – A randomized controlled trial. *Neurology* **50**, 466–470

Seaber, E., On, N., Phillips, S., Churchus, R., Posner, J. and Rolan, P. (1996). The tolerability and pharmacokinetics of the novel antimigraine compound 311C90 in healthy male volunteers. *Br. J. Clin. Pharmacol.* **41**(2), 141–147

Selby, G. and Lance, J. W. (1960). Observations on 500 cases of migraine and allied vascular headache. *J. Neurol. Neurosurg. Psychiat.* **23**, 23–32

Sheftell, F. D., Weeks, R. E., Rapoport, A M., Siegel, S., Baskin, S. and Arrowsmith, F. (1994). Subcutaneous sumatriptan in a clinical setting: The first 100 consecutive patients with acute migraine in a tertiary care center. *Headache* **34**, 67–72

Sicuteri, F., Michelacci, S. and Anselmi, B. (1964). Indiviuazione della poprietà vasoattive ed antiemicraniche dell'indomethacin, nuovo antiflogistico di derivazione indolica. *Settim. Med.* **52**, 335–345

Silberstein, S. D. (1996). Divalproex sodium in headache: literature review and clinical guidelines. *Headache* **36**, 547–553

Silberstein, S. D. and Wilmore, J. (1996). Divalproex sodium: migraine treatment and monitoring. *Headache* **36**, 239–242

Sleight, A. J., Cervenka, A. and Peroutka, S. J. (1990). *In vivo* effects of sumatriptan (GR 43175) on extracellular levels of 5-HT in the guinea pig. *Neuropharmacology* **29**, 511–513

Solomon, G. D. (1989). Verapamil in migraine prophylaxis – a five-year review. *Headache* **29**, 425–427

Sorensen, K. V. (1988). Valproate: a new drug in migraine prophylaxis. *Acta Neurol. Scand.* **78**, 346–348

Speight, T. M. and Avery, G. S. (1972). Pizotifen (BC-105): a review of its pharmacological properties and its therapeutic efficacy in vascular headaches. *Am. J. Med. Sci.* **240**, 327–331

Steiner, T. J., Catarci, T., Hering, R., Whitmarsh, T. and Couturier, E. G. M. (1994). If migraine prophylaxis does not work, think about compliance. *Cephalalgia* **14**, 463–464

Stensrud, P. and Sjaastad, O. (1979). Clonazepam (Rivotril) in migraine prophylaxis. *Headache* **19**, 333–334

Sudilovsky, A., Elkind, A. H., Ryan, R. E., Stern, M. A. and Meyer, J. H. (1987). Comparative efficacy of nadolol and propranolol in the management of migraine. *Headache* **27**, 421–426

Tfelt-Hansen, P. (1986). Efficacy of beta-blockers in migraine. A critical review. *Cephalalgia* **6** (Suppl. 5), 15–24

Tfelt-Hansen, P. (1989). Therapy of migraine. *Curr. Opin. Neurol. Neurosurg.* **2**, 212–216

Tfelt-Hansen, P., Henry, P., Mulder, L. J., Scheldewaert, R. G., Schoenen, J. and Chazot, G. (1995). The effectiveness of combined oral lysine acetylsalicylate and metoclopramide compared to oral sumatriptan for migraine. *Lancet* **346**, 923–926

Tfelt-Hansen, P., Ibraheem, J. J. and Psalzow, L. (1982). Clinical pharmacology of ergotamine studied with a high performance liquid chromatographic method. In *Advances in Migraine, Research and Therapy*, Ed. F. Clifford Rose. pp. 173–179. New York, Raven Press

Tfelt-Hansen, P., Olesen, J., Aebelholt-Krabbe, A., Melgaard, B. and Veilis, G. (1980). A double-blind study of metaclopramide in the treatment of migraine attacks. *J. Neurol. Neurosurg. Psychiat.* **43**, 369–371

Tfelt-Hansen, P., Standnes, B., Kanagasneimi, P., Hakkareinen, H. and Olesen, J. (1984). Timolol versus propranolol versus placebo in common migraine prophylaxis: a double-blind multicenter trial. *Acta Neurol. Scand.* **69**, 1–8

Thomsen, L. L., Dixon, R., Lassen, L. H. *et al.* (1996). 311C90 (Zolmitriptan), a novel centrally and peripheral acting oral 5-hydroxytryptamine-1D agonist: a comparison of its absorption during a migraine attack and in a migraine-free period. *Cephalalgia* **16**(4), 270–275

Touchon, J., Bertin, L., Pilgrim, A. J., Ashford, E. and Bes, A. (1996). A comparison of subcutaneous sumatriptan and dihydroergotamine nasal spray in the acute treatment of migraine. *Neurology* **47**, 361–365

Vardi, Y., Rabey, I. M., Streifer, M., Schwartz, A., Lindner, H. R. and Zor, U. (1976). Migraine attacks. Alleviation by an inhibitor of prostaglandin synthesis and action. *Neurology* **26**, 447–450

Visser, W. H., de Vriend, R. H., Jaspers, N. H. and Ferrari, M. D. (1996a). Sumatriptan-nonresponders: a survey in 366 migraine patients. *Headache* **36**, 471–475

Visser, W. H., Jaspers, N. M., de Vriend, R. H. and Ferrari, M. D. (1996b). Chest symptoms after sumatriptan: a two-year clinical practice review in 735 consecutive migraine patients. *Cephalalgia* **16**, 554–559

Visser, W. H., Lines, C. R. and Reines, S. A. (1996). Dose-finding studies of rizatriptan (MK-462) in the acute treatment of migraine. *Cephalalgia* **16**, 359–360

Visser, W. H., Terwindt, G. M., Reines, S. A., Jang, K., Lines, C. R. and Ferrari, M. D. (1996c). Rizatriptan vs. sumatriptan in the acute treatment of migraine. *Arch. Neurol.* **53**, 1132–1137

Visser, W. H., Vriend, R. H. Md., Jaspers, N. M. W. H. and Ferrari, M. D. (1996d). Sumatriptan in clinical practice. *Neurology* **47**, 46–51

Volans, G. N. (1974). Absorption of effervescent aspirin during migraine. *Br. Med. J.* **2**, 265–269

Waelkens, J. (1981). Domperidone in the prevention of complete classical migraine. *Br. Med. J.* **284**, 944

Waelkens, J. (1984). Dopamine blockade with domperidone: bridge between prophylactic and abortive treatment of migraine? A dose-finding study. *Cephalalgia* **4**, 85–90

Warner, G. and Lance, J. W. (1975). Relaxation therapy in migraine and tension headache. *Med. J. Aust.* **1**, 298–301

Weber, R. B. and Reinmuth, O. M. (1971). The treatment of migraine with propranolol. *Neurology* **21**, 404–405

Welch, K. M. A. (1986). Naproxen sodium in the treatment of migraine. *Cephalalgia* **6** (Suppl. 4), 85–92

White, J. C. and Sweet, W. H. (1955). *Pain: Its Mechanisms and Neurosurgical Control*. Springfield, Springfield Publishing Co

Wilkinson, M. (1983). Treatment of the acute migraine attack – current status. *Cephalalgia* **3**, 61–67

Willett, F., Curzen, N., Adams, J. and Armitage, M. (1992). Coronary vasospasm induced by subcutaneous sumatriptan. *Br. Med. J.* **304**, 1415

Williamson, D. J., Hargreaves, R. J., Hill, R. G. and Shepheard, S. L. (1997a). Intravital microscope studies on the effects of neurokinin agonists and calcitonin gene-related peptide on dural blood vessel diameter in the anaesthetized rat. *Cephalalgia* **17**, 518–524

Williamson, D. J., Hargreaves, R. J., Hill, R. G. and Shepheard, S. L. (1997b). Sumatriptan inhibits neurogenic vasodilation of dural blood vessels in the anaesthetized rat – intravital microscope studies. *Cephalalgia* **17**, 525–531

Winner, P., Ricalde, O., Force, B. L., Saper, J. and Margul, B. (1996). A double-blind study of subcutaneous dihydroergotamine vs subcutaneous sumatriptan in the treatment of acute migraine. *Arch. Neurol.* **53**, 180–184

Wolff, H. G. (1963). *Headache and Other Head Pain.* New York, Oxford University Press

Yuill, G. M., Swinburn, W. R. and Liversedge, L. A. (1972). A double-blind crossover trial of isomethepplene muoate compound and ergotamine in migraine. *Br. J. Clin. Pract.* **26**, 76–79

Ziegler, D., Ford, R., Kriegler, J. *et al.* (1994). Dihydroergotamine nasal spray for the acute treatment of migraine. *Neurology* **44**, 447–453

Ziegler, D. K. (1997). Opioids in headache treatment. Is there a role? In *Neurologic Clinics of North America*, Vol. 15, Ed. N. T. Mathew. pp. 199–207. Philadelphia, W. B. Saunders

Ziegler, D. K., Hurwitz, A., Preskorn, S., Hassanein, R. and Seim, J. (1993). Propranolol and amitriptyline in prophylaxis of migraine. Pharmacokinetic and therapeutic effects. *Arch. Neurol.* **50**, 825–830

Ziegler, V. E., Clayton, P. J. and Biggs, J. T. (1977). A comparative study of amitriptyline and nortriptyline with plasma levels. *Arch. Gen. Psychiat.* **34**, 707–712

Chapter 10

Tension-type headache

Definition

Tension headache may be defined as a constant tight or pressing sensation, usually bilateral, which may initially be episodic and related to stress but can recur almost daily in its chronic form without regard to any obvious psychological factors. Such a definition amounts to saying that tension headache is a chronic headache without migrainous features (such as vomiting, blurring of vision and focal neurological symptoms) and thus bypasses the question of whether tension headache and migraine form a continuum, with vomiting and neurological disturbance only appearing when headaches are acute and severe.

Ziegler and Hassanein (1982) analysed the symptoms of 1200 patients attending a headache clinic and were unable to isolate any particular combination of characteristics that clearly defined migraine and tension headache as separate entities. They concluded that the most reliable features for the diagnosis of migraine were the episodicity and relative brevity of attacks. Patients who suffer from both tension headache and migraine usually distinguish the two forms of headache on the grounds of severity and associated symptoms much in the same way as a clinician taking a case history but this does not throw light on whether the two conditions share the same pathophysiology.

Drummond and Lance (1984) analysed the case histories of 600 patients presenting with the complaint of headache to a neurology clinic, comparing their clinical diagnosis with that made by a computer which correlated the symptoms and other features of the headache. The clinical and computer diagnosis had no trouble in agreeing on the diagnosis of cluster headache and migraine with aura but found difficulty in finding a dividing line between migraine and tension-type headache. For example, of episodic headaches recurring up to once per week, 55 per cent were unilateral and most were accompanied by the usual migrainous symptoms of nausea and photophobia. Of those headaches recurring daily, 20 per cent were unilateral, nausea was still a feature in about 25 per cent and photophobia in about 50 per cent (Figure 10.1). The explanation for this may have been the inclusion of patients whose frequency of migraine has increased until it became daily, described as 'transformed migraine' by Mathew, Reuveni and Perez (1987). We agree with Mathew (1993) and Silberstein, Lipton and Sliwinski (1996) that this is a common cause of chronic daily headache.

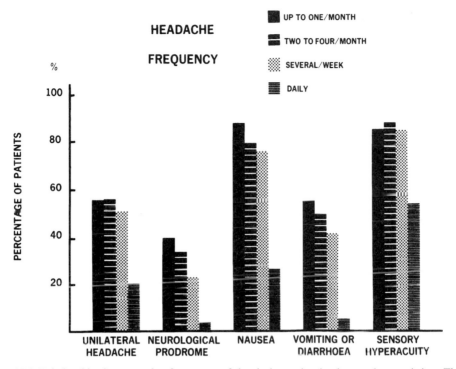

Figure 10.1 Relationship between the frequency of headache and migrainous characteristics. The percentage of patients with each symptom diminishes as headache frequency increases. (From Drummond and Lance, 1984, by permission of the editor of *Journal of Neurology, Neurosurgery and Psychiatry*)

Until the pathophysiology of headache is fully understood, tension-type headache can be recognized as an entity separate from migraine by the criteria put forward by the Headache Classification Committee of the International Headache Society (1988). The Committee divided tension-type headaches into episodic and chronic varieties, with a subclassification for those patients with and without evidence of excessive contraction of the jaw and scalp muscles. The episodic type of tension headache is characterized by a frequency of less than 15 headache days each month. Both episodic and chronic types must have at least two of the following features:

1. A pressing or tight (non-pulsatile) quality.
2. Mild or moderate intensity, which inhibits but does not prevent daily activities.
3. Bilateral distribution.
4. Not aggravated by routine physical activity.

Chronic daily headache

The term 'chronic tension-type headache' is applied to those patients with 15 or more such headaches each month. Some progress to have headaches every day but not all chronic daily headaches are of the tension type. The following varieties may be distinguished.

1. Chronic daily headache: Tension-type headache with the characteristics described above, often becoming daily as the result of excessive consumption of analgesics or the onset of a depressive state.
2. Transformed migraine: Patients whose frequency of typical migraine headache increases until it recurs daily, still retaining some migrainous features such as unilaterality or nausea (Mathew, Reuveni and Perez, 1987; Jauslin, Goadsby and Lance, 1991).
3. New daily persistent headache: Patients, previously headache-free, who develop a headache (often at a particular time on a particular day) that persists daily thereafter without any obvious psychological or physical factors to account for it. An occult viral infection has been considered as a possible cause.
4. Hemicrania continua: A constant unilateral headache of uncertain cause responsive to indomethacin (Sjasastad and Spierings, 1984).

Clinical features of tension-type headache

Prevalence, age and sex distribution

Most people have probably been aware of a dull headache at some time of their lives after exposure to glare, flickering light, eye-strain, noise or a succession of harassing incidents. Of the 740 normal subjects interviewed, Rasmussen et al. (1991) found a lifetime prevalence of tension-type headache in 578 (78%), fulfilling the IHS criteria for episodic tension-type in 488, and most of those criteria in 66. The remaining 24 patients had chronic tension-type headache. The latter group are more heavily represented in medical practice as most people with occasional mild headaches usually treat themselves with analgesics or simply put up with their discomfort.

Tension-type headache may start in childhood, affecting some 10 per cent (Rasmussen, 1993) or 15 per cent (Lance, Curran and Anthony, 1965) by the age of 10 years (see Figure 7.1). The condition may be intractable and continue throughout life. Many patients have suffered from headaches almost every day for 10, 20 or 30 years. As in the case of migraine, more patients with chronic tension-type headache are women.

Family history

Some 18 per cent of patients with tension headache give a family history of migraine (Lance and Anthony, 1966), which is much the same as for the general population. However, a family background of some form of headache is found in the history of 40 per cent of tension headache patients (Friedman, von Storch and Merritt, 1964).

Past health

There is no evidence that allergic disorders or childhood vomiting attacks are more common in patients complaining of tension headache than in the general community, but psychosomatic disorders such as irritable bowel syndrome may be associated (Martin, Rome and Swenson, 1967).

Site of headache

Headache was bilateral in 80 per cent of the patients with chronic daily headache in the series analysed by Drummond and Lance (1984), and in almost 90 per cent in the population-based analysis of tension-type headache by Rasmussen *et al.* (1991).

Quality of headache

The pain is usually dull and persistent in tension headache, and undulates in intensity during the day. It is often described as a feeling of heaviness, pressure, weight on the head or tightness rather than pain and may extend like a band around the head. Some patients experience sudden jabs of pain on one side or at the back of the head ('ice-pick pains') superimposed on a general background of discomfort. About one-quarter of tension headache patients, whose headaches become severe and assume a pulsating quality at times, form a group intermediate between muscle-contraction headache and migraine, which was called 'tension-vascular headache' by Lance and Curran (1964). About 10 per cent of patients with tension headache are also subject to frank migraine.

The intensity of headache experienced and the reaction of the patient to pain was found to vary with the mood of the patient in a study by Hunter and Phillips (1981), the symptoms being more severe when the patient was depressed.

Time and mode of onset

In episodic cases, the headache develops during or after recognizable stress. In more severe cases, the headache comes on in anticipation of some unpleasant situation, such as a distasteful interview. Contemplation of the day's tasks may be enough to start a headache while travelling to work. In Lewis Carroll's *Through the Looking Glass*, Tweedledum remarked before the projected battle with Tweedledee: 'I'm very brave generally, only today I happen to have a headache!'.

In the chronic form, the patient either awakens with the headache or notices it shortly after getting up, and it remains throughout the day, without regard to the emotional content of the day's activities. Some 10 per cent of patients, not necessarily those who are depressed, may be woken up by headache between 1 and 4 a.m. in the manner of a migrainous patient.

Frequency and duration

Of 466 patients attending our neurological clinic for the treatment of tension headache, the headache recurred less than 10 times each month in 49 patients, from 10 to

30 times each month in 64 patients and was present every day in the remaining 354 patients (Lance and Curran, 1964). This contrasts with the population-based study of Rasmussen *et al.* (1991) which found that only 3 per cent of 740 people questioned suffered from chronic tension-type headache (defined as more than 180 headache days each year). It is apparent that patients attending clinics are those who are most severely affected and that figures from clinics do not necessarily reflect the pattern of tension headache as seen by the general practitioner. The spectrum of tension headache extends from headache of half an hour's duration recurring every few months to a perpetual, unremitting ache present 'all day and every day'.

Associated phenomena

Tension headache is not accompanied by any of the focal neurological symptoms that add a distinctive character to most attacks of migraine. There is often a constant mild photophobia, not severe enough to make the patient retreat to a darkened room but often sufficient to encourage the wearing of sunglasses on all but the gloomiest day. Other symptoms are those of an anxiety state. Slight nausea may be present in the early mornings, or when the headache is severe, but vomiting is rare. Giddiness or lightheadedness usually indicates a tendency to overbreathe in times of anxiety. Abdominal distension, excessive belching and passing of flatus are commonly the result of unnoticed air swallowing. The patient often speaks of difficulty in concentrating and a lack of interest in work or hobbies. There may be more flagrant depressive symptoms which are attributed to the presence of headache. Pain under the left breast, pain in the back or coccygeal region, and indigestion are other psychosomatic symptoms commonly associated with tension headache. The patient may awaken with a bruised sensation inside the mouth lateral to the posterior upper molar tooth as the result of extreme mandibular movements during sleep (Every, 1960).

Underlying precipitating, aggravating and relieving factors

It is deceptively easy to think of all patients with tension headache as having an inadequate personality. This is certainly true of some patients who are ill-equipped by nature or education to cope with life's ramifications, but there are others who have considerable achievements to their credit. It may be that the meticulous energetic personality which has made a person prey to tension headache has also made him or her a leader in business or industry. Men with exclusively sedentary occupations have a higher prevalence of tension-type headache (Rasmussen, 1993).

Approximately one-third of patients with tension headache have symptoms of depression (Lance and Curran. 1964). Most are conscious of the fact that they are never really relaxed and are rarely elated. Many patients with tension headaches are 'born two drinks down on life'.

There may be obvious trigger factors for tension headache but in many patients the headache is not limited to times of emotional overload. The headache is usually made worse by any superimposed anxiety, stress, noise or glare. Coping with minor hassles in day to day living appears to be a more potent factor in perpetuating headache than major life events (De Benedittis and Lorenzetti, 1992). The pressure of working against time was found to be an important precipitating cause in women and exposure to fumes in men, while fatigue was a factor in both sexes in the study by Rasmussen (1992). A headache which is relieved by intake of alcohol is almost invariably of the tension variety, whereas most vascular headaches become more severe. Tension-type headache is often relieved by analgesics but commonly recurs after some hours. This may lead to repeated self-medication with subsequent risk of habituation and toxicity.

Physical examination

Formal neurological examination is usually normal, but signs of muscular over contraction are found in many patients. Some patients look the part, with deep wrinkles on face and forehead where time has etched their personality traits. The temporal and masseter muscles may stand out and twitch, and the hands may clench their chair firmly or the fingers move restlessly during the interview. Other patients may have a bland appearance which gives no indication of the tendency to headache. A simple test of the ability to relax is to lift the patient's arm up in one's hands and to tell the patient that he or she must imagine it is resting on an armchair. The aim is to let the limb go completely loose so that when the examiner's hands are removed the arm will flop lifelessly downwards to the patient's side. In fact, the vast majority of tension headache patients assure the examiner that the arm is completely relaxed and are surprised to find that it still rests on the imaginary armchair once the supporting hands are taken away.

Similar to the 'armchair sign' is the 'invisible pillow'. A patient who is instructed to let the head loll back in the examiner's hands will frequently maintain the head rigidly in position above the couch and can only put it down by a conscious voluntary extension movement of the neck. It should be possible to relax the legs so that they can be bent freely at the knees or rolled from side to side. Many patients with tension headache are quite unable to do this.

The patient can be asked to let the jaw hang down so that it can be moved rapidly up and down through a small range by the examiner. Most tension headache patients hold the jaw so rigidly that the whole head moves with the mandible. Auscultation over the temporal muscles will confirm the presence of inappropriate contraction.

The constant driving from above of spinal mechanisms may induce such hyper-activity of stretch reflexes that the examiner may feel a sensation akin to the rigidity of Parkinson's disease on manipulating a joint through its range of movement. If the patient also has an exaggerated physiological tremor as part of an anxiety state, then the similarity to Parkinson's disease may be heightened by the superimposition of a cog-wheel effect on the increased muscle tone. Indeed, the mechanism is probably a functional or reversible overactivity of descending motor pathways, which are thrown permanently into action in Parkinson's disease by anatomical and biochemical changes.

The elicitation of these physical signs of nervous tension is important not only for diagnosis but also to demonstrate to the patient that muscular hyperactivity is present and to prepare the way for relaxation exercises as a part of treatment.

Yawning, sighing, gasping or rapid respiration may be noticed while the history is being taken. These signs of overbreathing warrant management in their own right (see Appendix A).

Neck movements should be tested, the completeness of dentition and the balance of biting movements checked, and the temporomandibular joints palpated, looking for abnormalities that could initiate reflex muscle contraction and thus contribute to tension headache. Posture should be observed as craning the neck forward can be responsible for nuchal and occipital pain.

Pathophysiology

Psychological factors

Martin, Rome and Swenson (1967) studied 25 patients in detail and found that 22 described tension situations, usually involving dependence, sexuality and control of anger. These problems were exemplified by difficulty in leaving home, submission to a domineering spouse, broken marriages, impotence, frigidity and a poor work record, as well as specific emotional problems. The comment 'he's a pain in the neck' was often applied to a family member without realization of its literal application. Eight of the 25 patients had sexual problems, such as premature ejaculation, dyspareunia and aversion to sexual intercourse. Nine patients were depressed. No fewer than 22 of the 25 patients had various psychosomatic disorders such as duodenal ulcer, vasomotor rhinitis, obesity and irritable bowel syndrome. Nowdays one could add chronic fatigue syndrome to this list. Minnesota Multiphasic Personality Inventory (MMPI) tests showed no significant qualitative differences from the general population but the intensity of reaction was more, with the emphasis on hypochondriasis, depression and hysteria. Similar findings were obtained by Kudrow and Sutkus (1979) who were able to distinguish patients with tension headache from those with migraine, but not from those with post-traumatic and conversion headaches, on the grounds of MMPI scores. Another study (Gainotti, Cianchetti and Taramelli, 1972) compared 104 patients suffering from tension headache with 79 migraine patients. Symptoms of anxiety and depression were present in 95 per cent of the tension headache group compared with 54 per cent of the migraine patients.

The evidence from psychological tests clearly points to anxiety, depression and hypochondriasis being common factors in tension-type headache, as well as suppressed anger (Hatch et al., 1991) and feelings of inadequacy (Passchier et al., 1991). Rasmussen (1992) found a higher index of neuroticism than in migrainous patients. Patients with chronic headache resemble those with chronic pain from other sources in that they deny general life problems. As the headaches become more frequent and severe, the patients are more inclined to view their illness as somatic rather than psychological in origin (Demjen and Bakal, 1981).

External forces are obviously important. One of us can recall a day's consulting in which three women said that their headaches began when they were married and stopped when they separated!

Muscle contraction

It is probable that some forms of headache do arise from afferent fibres in muscle. Many patients describe a sensation of tension or pressure in the frontalis muscle after excessive frowning, which passes away when the forehead is relaxed. Others become aware of a similar sensation in the masseter or temporalis muscles after clenching the jaw, which is eased by ceasing muscle contraction. Jensen and Rasmussen (1996) reported that 87 per cent of patients with chronic tension-type headache and 66 per cent with the episodic form had increased pericranial muscle tenderness and/or EMG activity, both indications of excessive muscle contraction.

When 58 patients prone to tension-type headache clenched their jaws for 30 minutes, 69 per cent developed a headache, compared with 17 per cent of control subjects (Jensen and Olesen, 1996). Muscle tenderness increased in those patients who developed headache but their tolerance to painful pressure and heat remained unchanged, whereas pain and thermal pain thresholds actually increased in those subjects who remained headache-free. This suggests that excessive muscle contraction plays some part in the genesis of tension-type headache in those subjects with defective mobilization of their endogenous pain control system. A logical extension of this thought is that EMG biofeedback would be most effective in reducing pain in those patients who do have consistent overcontraction of muscles. However, Schoenen et al. (1991b) could not find any such correlation. They recorded the EMG of frontal, temporal and trapezius muscles in 32 patients with chronic tension-type headaches and 20 healthy volunteers and found that muscle activity was, on average, significantly higher in the patients but did not correlate with headache severity, anxiety or response to biofeedback.

Every (1960) has drawn attention to nocturnal fang-sharpening movements of the jaw that occur during sleep as a manifestation of repressed aggression. The latter syndrome may be recognized by the association of chronic headache with pain in the temporomandibular joints and jaw muscles and a raw tender spot on the buccal mucosa opposite the posterior part of the upper gum, which results from excessive lateral movement of the mandible during sleep. This disorder responds to psychological management and nocturnal medication with tricyclics rather than measures directed solely to malocclusion.

Vascular factors

There is no evidence for sustained vasoconstriction causing tension headache. On the contrary, sensitivity to painful vascular dilatation appears to be intermediate between that of migraine patients and normal controls. Martin and Mathews (1978) reported that the inhalation of amyl nitrite increased the severity of tension headache on 43 per cent of occasions and did not alter the intensity on 48 per cent of occasions, whereas no patients reported any increase after the inhalation of a placebo substance. In another study, Krabbe and Olesen (1980) found that the intravenous infusion of histamine produced a pulsating headache in 14 of 25 migraine patients, five out of 10 tension headache patients and none of 13 normal controls. In spite of this apparent susceptibility to vascular pain in tension headache patients, no significant change in cortical or extracranial blood flow has been demonstrated in tension headache by the xenon-133 inhalation method (Sakai and Meyer, 1978). Acetazolamide increases cerebral blood flow and provokes headache in migrainous but not in tension-type headache patients (Shirai *et al*, 1996).

It is not uncommon for typical episodic migrainous headache to become progressively more frequent until it is recurring daily in the same site, often unilateral, and sometimes still accompanied by nausea and photophobia. While this may be attributed to nervous tension, depression or the abuse of ergotamine or analgesics, it is not always the case. This syndrome of 'transformed' or 'evolutive' migraine was described by Mathew, Reuveni and Perez (1987) and presents a difficult problem in management (Jauslin, Goadsby and Lance, 1991).

Humoral factors

The platelet content of 5-hydroxytryptamine (5-HT) was reported to be low in patients with tension-type headache by Rolf, Wiele and Brune (1981), Anthony and Lance (1989), and Shimomura and Takahashi (1990), but to be normal by Shukla *et al*. (1987) and Ferrari *et al*. (1990). A possible explanation for this discrepancy is that platelet 5-HT concentration is diminished in patients with analgesic-induced headache (Srikiatkhachorn and Anthony, 1996). The low values obtained in tension-type headache are thus liable to be influenced by the consumption of analgesics. It is possible that low platelet 5-HT could reflect a 5-HT deficiency in pain control pathways.

Tension headache patients were found to have a low platelet content and high plasma levels of methionine-enkephalin by Ferrari *et al*. (1990), which may have implications for pain control mechanisms.

Central factors

Pressure-pain threshold
There has been some dispute in the past about the susceptibility of tension headache patients to painful stimuli. Drummond (1987) found that muscle tenderness was increased at the site of headache but that the pain threshold to finger pressure was the same as in normal controls. Schoenen *et al*. (1991a) confirmed that the pain threshold in pericranial sites (forehead, temple and occipital region) was diminished in chronic tension-type headache and also found greater sensitivity to pressure over the Achilles tendon. The pain threshold has also been reported to be diminished in chronic tension-type headache by Langemark *et al*. (1989) and Jensen and Rasmussen (1996), suggesting that central pain mechanisms might be impaired.

Langemark *et al*. (1993) used measurements of the flexor withdrawal reflex in response to sural nerve stimulation as another index of pain control. The median threshold for this protective reflex was significantly lower in 36 patients with chronic tension-type headache than in 26 matched control subjects. Curiously, the reflex could not be obtained in four headache patients and three controls who were excluded from the analysis. Sicuteri (1981) compared chronic tension headache to the syndrome of abstinence from narcotics, and postulated a defect in pain control pathways, possibly involving opioid receptors and serotonergic transmission. How-ever, the intensity of headache remains unaltered by the intravenous injection of naloxone 4 mg (Langemark, 1989).

Inhibition of jaw clenching

If one bites firmly on a hard object jaw closure is mercifully inhibited to protect the teeth. A similar reflex inhibition can be elicited by electrical stimulation of trigeminal innervated territory, the usual site being lateral to the lips, while the jaws are clenched. Two silent periods in the EMG of the temporalis muscle may be detected in this way and these have been designated as exteroceptive suppressions 1 and 2 (ES1 and ES2). Schoenen *et al.* (1987) compared these silent periods in 25 chronic tension headache patients, 20 suffering from migraine without aura and 22 control subjects. The latency of ES1 was similar in all groups. The latency of ES2 was also similar in all groups, but the duration was significantly shorter in the tension head-ache patients. This could not be confirmed by Zwart and Sand (1995) or Bendtsen *et al.* (1996), which raises questions on the duration of ES2 being a measure of dimin-ished central pain control.

An infectious origin for new daily persistent headache?

Some patients fulfilling the criteria for chronic tension-type headache state that their headaches started one day without obvious cause and have recurred daily since. Diaz-Mitoma, Vanast and Tyrell (1987) investigated 32 patients with this syndrome of 'new daily persistent headaches' and compared the results of virus studies with those in 32 control subjects. Of the 32 patients, 25 complained of severe fatigue, 12 had a history of infectious mononucleosis and 20 were found to be excreting Epstein–Barr (E–B) virus in the oropharynx (compared with four of the controls). When an early antigen titre of greater than 1 : 32 was also considered, 27 (84 per cent) of the patients had evidence of active E–B infection as opposed to eight (25 per cent) of the control group. While it is possible that patients with chronic daily headache are more susceptible to infection by the E–B virus, it would seem most likely that infection was responsible for headache. The E–B virus is a member of the human herpes virus group and the propensity of herpes zoster to induce persistent neuralgic pain is well known.

Santoni and Santoni-Williams (1993) investigated headaches that had persisted daily for about 2 weeks and found evidence of systemic infections in 108 patients, chiefly involving an adenovirus, salmonella and urinary *E. coli* but some with E–B virus, toxoplasmosis and herpes zoster. Whether lingering infection can be respon-sible for daily headaches lasting for months or years remains to be determined. Further studies along these lines in chronic daily headache and in atypical facial pain may throw light on these puzzling syndromes.

Conclusion

In some patients with tension-type headache, psychological factors appear para-mount, often associated with excessive contraction of neck, forehead and jaw muscles. There also appears to be a central deficit of pain control with lowering of the pain threshold in some cases. What part amine depletion or subclinical infection plays in the genesis of chronic daily headache is still uncertain.

Treatment

Many patients suffering from chronic muscle-contraction headache suspect that they have a cerebral tumour or other serious intracranial disorder. The first step in treatment is to give patients a good hearing and careful examination to give them confidence that their complaint is being taken seriously and that the doctor is not jumping to a facile conclusion in order to prescribe an antidepressant and move on to the next patient.

The second step in treatment is to check whether the scalp and facial muscles are indeed contracting for much of the time without reason. This can be achieved partly by questions at the end of history-taking. Do your friends comment that you always look serious or worried? Do you find yourself clenching your jaw, grinding your teeth, making a tight fist with your hands? The answers to these questions can be quite surprising. Some patients have had to seek dental attention because their teeth are tender or chipped from unremitting pressure of their jaws. The authors have had patients who had broken their dentures repeatedly by the same mechanism. Some state that they notice their fingers flexed firmly or jaw clenched even on awakening from sleep.

The presence of the unnecessary muscular contraction can be shown to the patient at the end of physical examination. Most are unable to relax the jaw muscles so that the jaw cannot be moved freely by the physician. They are unable to let the head loll back when the shoulders are supported because the neck muscles remain rigid. They cannot permit their elevated arm to fall limply to the couch when requested by the examiner.

Correction of various physical factors may be necessary to help patients reach their goal of muscular relaxation. Correction of a refractive error or orthoptic treatment for a latent ocular imbalance may remove the factors of eye-strain which set up a pattern of wasteful muscle activity. Dental treatment may be important to open a closed bite, restore a chewing surface or improve dentures so that the bite is evenly distributed. Cervical traction or manipulation may be useful if neck pain from degenerated intervertebral discs is triggering the tension headache. Observation by patients of their posture in sitting at a desk or driving a car can be important in correcting a tendency to overcontract muscles unnecessarily.

The management of the patient with tension headache must by necessity be psychological, physiological (aimed at relaxation of the facial and scalp muscles) and usually pharmacological as well.

Psychological management

It may be argued that all patients with muscle-contraction headache should be referred to a psychiatrist in the first instance. This is certainly the authors' policy with any patient who shows signs of serious mental disturbance, but it is neither practical for every tense patient to be seen by a psychiatrist, nor would it be desirable because many patients are resentful of the implication of mental illness.

Most can be managed by the doctor of first contact providing he or she has the time and interest to take a history and counsel the patient. Some patients will not admit to any problem or source of anxiety, and may simply have a longstanding habit of muscle contraction in response to the ordinary pressures of everyday life. Others may have easily identifiable worries and anxieties concerned with their work or home life, which may respond to sympathetic discussion. Some tension headaches clear up as soon as the patient goes on vacation. One woman told me that her symptoms mysteriously eased as soon as her husband went away on a business trip only to return as soon as he did. The man or woman with marital or relationship problems or the victims of verbal or physical abuse lives with a constant provocation to headache which may be hard to remove by any amount of psychological counselling. Careful thought about the patient and his or her reactions to stress, combined with advice about personal problems and adjustment of work pattern and lifestyle, may help to ease the patient's anxiety. The use of social agencies to provide support for those who are slowly losing the struggle for existence on their own is also part of the doctor's role in helping the patient to overcome the symptom of headache. Referral of an individual or couple for expert sexual counselling can often be very useful because, even in these enlightened and liberated times, there are many whose lives are lived in ignorance or blighted by feelings of inadequacy, shame or guilt, which are often eased by confiding in their medical adviser.

Martin and Rome (1967) consider that anxiety is often a secondary response to anger in patients with muscle-contraction headaches and relates to multiple conflicts that are usually evident. They emphasize that a careful, unhurried history and an appreciation of the factors causing stress are essential for psychological management, which may require only a 'single corrective emotional experience', or may involve long-term psychotherapy or group therapy.

The authors' view is to combine simple counselling at the first interview with an explanation of how the patient's emotional conflicts are translated into headache by muscular activity. This is then followed by some form of relaxation therapy, considered as physiological management.

Hyperventilation is a common accompaniment of tension headache (and migraine). Most patients can overcome this with explanation and advice (see Appendix A).

Hypnosis

Melis *et al.* (1991) treated 26 patients with chronic tension headache by 1-hour sessions each week for 1 month. Trances were induced by eye fixation, and suggestions were then made to transfer pain from the head to some other part of the body where it would be more easily tolerated. Headaches were reduced in frequency, duration and intensity when compared with a waiting-list group. No mention is made of pain being experienced in other areas to which it has been supposedly transferred.

Physiological management: relaxation and biofeedback

Relaxation exercises, usually modified from those described by Jacobsen (1938), have become generally accepted as the most direct means of overcoming the habitual overcontraction of muscles in tension headache. Warner and Lance (1975) combined relaxation therapy with some of the techniques of transcendental meditation in the treatment of 17 patients with chronic tension headache. Personal tuition was followed by the patient practising at home with the help of tape recordings of the instructor's voice. When the patients were followed up after 6 months, four were headache-free, seven were subject to one to four headaches each month (instead of 12–30) and only six were unimproved. Only three required analgesics or tranquillisers whereas 14 were habitual users before relaxation therapy.

Feedback techniques may guide the patient in controlling muscle activity and promoting relaxation. Feedback from the electromyogram (EMG) of the frontal or temporal muscles has been the most popular method. The amplified EMG signal is played back to the patient through a loudspeaker or earphones, either directly or transformed into a clicking, humming or buzzing noise, which varies in intensity in proportion to the integrated EMG activity. Controlled trials of EMG feedback have found that it is effective in reducing the frequency and severity of headache (Blanchard et al., 1980; Bruhn, Olesen and Melgaard, 1979; Jessup, Neufeld and Merskey, 1979). Arena et al. (1995) reported that EMG feedback from the upper trapezius muscles was more effective than using the frontal muscles or than relaxation therapy alone.

Feedback can be regarded as a technique to assist relaxation training in reducing the general level of anxiety and associated vascular changes, as well as any specific effect it has on muscular contraction.

There are probably many ways in which the patient can be made aware of nervous tension and ways of relieving it. Our own practice is to explain the relaxation process to the patients along the lines of Appendix B. Some patients are referred to physiotherapists or psychologists who take a particular interest in relaxation therapy. This approach may occasionally be sufficient to relieve tension headache without any need for tranquillisers or antidepressant agents.

Acupuncture

Acupuncture and physiotherapy (relaxation, massage, cryotherapy and transcutaneous nerve stimulation) were compared in the management of 62 female patients with chronic tension headache (Carlsson, Fahlrantz and Augustinsson, 1990). Headache was reduced in both groups, more in those undergoing physiotherapy, but even so, the headache score was reduced only from 3.7 (out of a maximum of 5) to 2.5.

Pharmacological management

Episodic tension headache often responds promptly to aspirin or paracetamol (acetaminophen). The occasional use of analgesics presents no real problem, except for epigastric pain from gastric irritation as a side-effect of aspirin in some patients.

When analgesic tablets are taken daily, they may lead to rebound headaches as the effect wears off, and therefore predispose to chronic daily headache. The object of regular interval (prophylactic) therapy is to rid the patient of headache if possible, or at least to reduce its intensity and frequency while reserving the use of analgesics for acute episodes. Pharmacotherapy should go hand in hand with psychological counselling and relaxation training.

The most widely used agent for the management of chronic tension headache is amitriptyline, shown to be effective in an open and a double-blind crossover trial (Lance and Curran, 1964). Improvement in this trial was not correlated with the presence or absence of pre-existing depression. Of the 98 patients treated, 58 improved substantially, only 18 of whom had symptoms of depression. Surprisingly, a later trial of amitriptyline in the treatment of chronic tension-type headache (Pfaffenrath et al., 1992) did not demonstrate any advantage over placebo. The most recent controlled trial reaffirmed the value of amitriptyline in reducing the frequency and duration of chronic tension-type headache but could not demonstrate any benefit from the use of the specific serotonin uptake inhibitor citalopram (Bendtsen, Jensen and Olesen, 1996).

Blood levels of amitriptyline vary 10-fold with the same dose per kg body weight, so the dose must be titrated carefully for each patient. Our own practice is to start with 10 mg or half of a 25 mg tablet at night and to ask patients to increase the nocturnal dose slowly to 75 mg each night if they can tolerate this without morning drowsiness. Patients who respond lose their headaches or notice substantial improvement from 2 to 14 days after starting treatment and are advised to continue for at least 6 months and then wean off the medication slowly over a period of 2–3 months. Amitriptyline may cause dryness of the mouth, tremor and weight gain. Its use should be avoided in patients with glaucoma or prostate hypertrophy because of its atropine-like side-effects, and in cardiac dysrhythmias and epilepsy. For those patients unable to tolerate amitriptyline, dothiepin or imipramine are worth a trial. Protriptyline 20 mg daily has been suggested as an option for the management of tension-type headache since it is less sedative and patients tend to lose rather than gain weight (Cohen, 1997).

Mathew and Ali (1991) reported that sodium valproate in doses of 1000–2000 mg daily given for 3 months reduced the index of chronic daily headache to half or less in 18 of 30 patients, with the mean number of headache-free days each month increasing from 5.5 to 17.7. These promising results could not be replicated by Vijayan and Spillane (1995) who treated 16 patients with chronic daily headache unresponsive to other forms of treatment. Only two of the group improved while eight of the 16 reported side-effects. The withdrawal of analgesics and ergotamine under supervision in hospital proved beneficial for 38 patients whose chronic daily headache was attributed to excessive intake of these drugs (Schnider et al., 1996). At a 5-year follow-up, 18 patients were virtually headache-free and the frequency of headache was reduced to eight or less each month in another 19 patients.

For patients resistant to these measures, pizotifen, cyproheptadine or beta-blockers may be used as for migraine but their effectiveness has not been substantiated by clinical trials. I have found phenelzine 15 mg, given two or three times daily, with the usual warnings about foods and drugs to be avoided while on monoamine oxidase inhibitors, useful in some cases. Benzodiazepines are also helpful but there is a high risk of habituation with continued use.

Chronic daily headache of the 'transformed migraine' variety was found to be associated with an elevated CSF pressure in 12 out of 85 patients investigated by Mathew, Ravishankar and Sanin (1996). Such patients improved clinically with the addition of acetazolamide or frusemide to their medication.

The local application of a traditional Asian remedy ('Tiger Balm') proved more effective than a placebo liniment and provided relief comparable with that obtained with paracetamol (acetaminophen) when submitted to a controlled trial by Schattner and Randerson (1996).

Psychogenic headache

The term 'psychogenic headache' is used to describe the association of headache with florid psychiatric disturbance such as acute depression, schizophrenia or hysteria. Headache may be incorporated into the delusional system of such patients. There is no way in which a mechanism can be postulated for such headaches incorporating peripheral pain pathways. The headache is a concept of disordered thought processes and appears or disappears with the mental state that engendered it.

Conclusion

Certain personality characteristics are more common in patients with tension-type headaches: anxiety, depression, suppressed anger and a feeling of inadequacy. Activity in frontal, temporal and nuchal muscles is often increased when the subject is at rest or under stress. Pericranial muscles are often unduly tender and their pain threshold is diminished; in some cases, the pain threshold to pressure or thermal stimuli may also be lowered in other parts of the body.

Tension headache patients are more susceptible to painful vascular dilatation than normal controls but less so than migraine patients. Migrainous headache may increase in frequency until it becomes a chronic daily headache. The platelet content of 5-HT is diminished in most patients taking excessive quantities of analgesics for chronic daily headaches. This may reflect low brain stem levels of 5-HT, which has a central inhibitory action in the pain control pathways, during headache. Some patients may develop persistent tension-type headache as the result of an infection by Epstein–Barr virus or other pathogens damaging central pain control pathways.

Tension-type headache appears to be a central disinhibitory phenomenon, probably with neurotransmitter changes underlying personality traits, defective pain control and sensitivity to both myofascial and vascular input.

Management includes psychological counselling, relaxation therapy, advice about hyperventilation when necessary, and the use of tricyclic antidepressants, of which amitriptyline is the most widely prescribed.

References

Anthony, M. and Lance, J. W. (1989). Plasma serotonin in patients with chronic tension headaches. *J. Neurol. Neurosurg. Psychiat.* **52**, 182–184

Arena, J. G., Bruno, G. M., Hannah, S. L. and Meador, K. Y. (1995). A comparison of frontal electromyographic feedback training, trapezius electromyographic feedback training and progressive muscle relaxation therapy in the treatment of tension headache. *Headache* **35**, 411–419

Bendtsen, L., Jensen, R., Brennum, J., Arendt-Nielsen, L. and Olesen, J. (1996). Exteroceptive suppression of temporal muscle activity is normal in chronic tension-type headache and not related to actual headache state. *Cephalalgia* **16**, 251–256

Bendtsen, L., Jensen, R. and Olesen, J. (1996). A non-selective (amitriptyline), but not a selective (citalopram), serotonin reuptake inhibitor is effective in the prophylactic treatment of chronic tension-type headache. *J. Neurol. Neurosurg. Psychiat.* **61**, 285–290

Blanchard, E. B., Andrasik, F., Ahles, T. A., Teders, S. J. and O'Keefe, D. (1980). Migraine and tension headache: a meta-analytic review. *Behav. Ther.* **11**, 613–631

Bruhn, P., Olesen, J. and Melgaard, B. (1979). Controlled trial of EMG feedback in muscle contraction headache. *Ann. Neurol.* **6**, 34–36

Carlsson, J., Fahlcrantz, A. and Augustinsson, L. E. (1990). Muscle tenderness in tension headache treated with acupuncture or physiotherapy. *Cephalalgia* **10**, 131–141

Cohen, G. L. (1997). Protriptyline, chronic tension-type headaches and weight loss in women. *Headache* **37**, 433–436

De Benedittis, G. and Lorenzetti, A. (1992). The role of stressful life events in the persistence of primary headache : major events vs. daily hassles. *Pain* **51**, 35–42

Demjem, S. and Bakal, D. (1981). Illness behaviour and chronic headache. *Pain* **10**, 221–229

Diaz-Mitoma, F., Vanast, W. J. and Tyrell, D. L. J. (1987). Increased frequency of Epstein–Barr virus excretion in patients with new daily persistent headaches. *Lancet* **i**, 411–415

Drummond, P. D. (1987). Scalp tenderness and sensitivity to pain in migraine and tension headache. *Headache* **27**, 45–50

Drummond. P. D. and Lance, J. W. (1984). Clinical diagnosis and computer analysis of headache symptoms. *J. Neurol. Neurosurg. Psychiat.* **47**, 128–133

Every, R. G. (1960) The significance of extreme mandibular movement. *Lancet* **ii**, 37

Ferrari, M. D., Fröhlich. M., Odink, J.-J., Tapparelli, C., Portielje, J. E. A. and Bruyn, G. W. (1987). Methionine-enkephalin and serotonin in migraine and tension headache. In *Current Problems in Neurology: 4. Advances in Headache Research*, Ed. F. Clifford Rose. pp. 227–234. London, John Libbey

Ferrari, M. D., Odink, J.-J., Fröhlich, M., Portielje, J. E. A. and Bruyn, G. W. (1990). Methionine-enkephalin in migraine and tension headache. Differences between classic migraine, common migraine and tension headache, and changes during attacks. *Headache* **30**, 160–164

Friedman, A., von Storch, T. J. C. and Merritt, H. H. (1964). Migraine and tension headaches. A clinical study of two thousand cases. *Neurology* **4**, 773–788

Gainotti, G., Cianchetti, C. and Taramelli, M. (1972). Anxiety level and psychodynamic mechanisms in medical headaches. *Res. Clin. Stud. Headache* **3**, 182–190

Hatch, J. P., Schoenfeld, L. S., Boutros, N. N., Seleshi, E., Moore, P. J. and Cyr-Provost, M. (1991). Anger and hostility in tension-type headache. *Headache* **31**, 302–304

Headache Classification Committee of the International Headache Society (1988). Classification and diagnosis criteria for headache disorders, cranial neuralgias and facial pain. *Cephalalgia* **8** (Suppl. 7), 29–34

Hunter, M. and Philips, C. (1981). The experience of headache – an assessment of the qualities of tension headache pain. *Pain* **10**, 209–219

Jacobsen, E. (1938). *Progressive Relaxation*. Illinois, University of Chicago Press

Jauslin, P., Goadsby, P. J. and Lance, J. W. (1991). The hospital management of severe migrainous headache. *Headache* **31**, 658–660

Jensen, R. and Hindberg, I. (1994). Plasma serotonin increase during episodes of tension-type headache. *Cephalalgia* **14**, 219–222

Jensen, R. and Olesen, J. (1996). Initiating mechanisms of experimentally induced tension-type headache. *Cephalalgia* **16**, 175–182

Jensen, R. and Rasmussen, B.K. (1996). Muscular disorders in tension-type headache. *Cephalalgia* **16**, 97–103

Jessup, B. A., Neufeld, R. W. J. and Merskey, H. (1979). Biofeedback therapy for headache and other pain: an evaluative review. *Pain* **7**, 225–270

Krabbe, A. A. and Olesen, J. (1980). Headache provocation by continuous intravenous infusion of histamine. Clinical results and receptor mechanisms. *Pain* **8**, 253–259

Kudrow, L. and Sutkus, B. J. (1979). MMPI pattern specificity in primary headache disorders. *Headache* **19**, 18–24

Lance, J. W. and Anthony, M. (1966). Some clinical aspects of migraine. *Arch. Neurol.* **15**, 356–361

Lance, J. W. and Curran. D. A. (1964). Treatment of chronic tension headache. *Lancet* i, 1236–1239

Lance, J. W., Curran, D. A. and Anthony, M. (1965). Investigations into the mechanism and treatment of chronic headache. *Med. J. Aust.* **2**, 909–914

Langemark, M. (1989). Naloxone in moderate dose does not aggravate chronic tension headache. *Pain* **39**, 85–93

Langemark, M., Bach, F. W., Jensen, T. S., Olesen, J. (1993). Decreased nociceptive flexion reflex threshold in chronic tension-type headache. *Arch. Neurol.* **50**, 1061–1064

Langemark, M., Jensen, K., Jensen, T. S. and Olesen, J. (1989). Pressure pain thresholds and thermal nociceptive thresholds in chronic tension-type headache. *Pain* **38**, 203–210

Martin, P. R. and Rome, H. P. (1967). Muscle-contraction headache: therapeutic aspects. *Res. Clin. Stud. Headache* **1**, 205–217

Martin, M. J., Rome, H. P. and Swenson, W. M. (1967). Muscle-contraction headache: a psychiatric review. *Res. Clin. Stud. Headache* **1**, 184–204

Martin, P. R. and Mathews, A. M. (1978). Tension headaches: psychophysiological investigation and treatment. *J. Pyschosom. Res.* **22**, 389–399

Mathew, N. T. (1993). Transformed migraine. *Cephalalgia* **13** (Suppl. 12), 78–83

Mathew, N. T. and Ali, S. (1991). Valproate in the treatment of persistent chronic daily headache. An open label study. *Headache* **31**, 71–74

Mathew, N.T., Ravishankar, K. and Sanin, L.C. (1996). Coexistence of migraine and idiopathic intracranial hypertension without papilloedema. *Neurology* **46**, 1226–1230

Mathew, N. T., Reuveni, U. and Perez, F. (1987). Transformed or evolutive migraine. *Headache* **27**, 102–106

Melis, P. M. L., Rooimans, W., Spierings, E. L. H. and Hoogduin, C. A. L. (1991). Treatment of chronic tension-type headache with hypnotherapy: a single-blind time controlled study. *Headache* **31**, 686–689

Passchier, J., Schouten, J., van der Donk, J. and van Romunde, L. K. J. (1991). The association of frequent headaches with personality and life events. *Headache* **31**, 116–121

Pfaffenrath, V., Diener, H.C., Isler, H., Meyer, C., Scholz, E., Taneri, Z., Wessely, P., Zaiser-Kaschel, H., Haase, W. and Fischer, W. (1994). Efficacy and tolerability of amitriptylinoxide in the treatment of chronic tension-type headache: a multi-centre controlled study. In *New Advances in Headache Research: 3*, Ed. F. Clifford Rose. pp. 265–274. London, Smith-Gordon

Rasmussen, B. K. (1992). Migraine and tension-type headache in a general population: psychosocial factors. *Int. J. Epidemiol.* **21**, 1138–1143

Rasmussen, B. K. (1993). Migraine and tension-type headache in a general population: precipitating factors, female hormones, sleep pattern and relation to lifestyle. *Pain* **53**, 65–72

Rasmussen, B. K., Jensen, R., Schroll, M. and Olesen, J. (1991). Epidemiology of headache in a general population – a prevalence study. *J. Clin. Epidemiol.* **44**, 1147–1157

Rolf, L.H., Wiele, G. and Brune, G.G. (1981). 5-Hydroxytryptamine in platelets of patients with muscle contraction headache. *Headache* **21**, 10–11

Sakai, F. and Meyer, J. S. (1978). Regional cerebral hemodynamics during migraine and cluster headache measured by the ^{133}Xe inhalation method. *Headache* **18**, 122–132

Santoni, J. R. and Santoni-Williams, C. J. (1993). Headache and painful lymphadenopathy in extracranial or systemic infection: etiology of new daily persistent headaches. *Int. Med.* **32**, 530–533

Schattner, P. and Randerson, D. (1996). Tiger Balm as a treatment of tension headache. *Aust. Family Physician* **25**, 216–222

Schnides, P., Aull, S., Baumgartner, C., Marterer, A., Wöber, C., Zeiler, K. and Wessely, P. (1996). Long-term outcome of patients with headache and drug abuse after inpatient withdrawal: five-year follow-up. *Cephalalgia* **16**, 481–485

Schoenen, J., Bottin, D., Hardy, F. and Gerard, P. (1991a). Cephalic and extracephalic pressure pain thresholds in chronic tension-type headache. *Pain* **47**, 145–149

Schoenen, J., Gerard, P., De Pasqua, V. and Juprelle, M. (1991b). EMG in pericranial muscles during postural variation and mental activity in healthy volunteers and patients with chronic tension-type headache. *Headache* **31**, 321–324

Schoenen, J., Jamart, B., Gerard, P., Lenarduzzi, P. and Delwaide, P. J. (1987). Exteroceptive suppression of temporalis muscle activity in chronic headaches. *Neurology* **37**, 1834–1836

Shimomura, T. and Takahashi, K. (1990). Alteration of platelet serotonin in patients with chronic tension-type headache during cold pressor test. *Headache* **30**, 581–583

Shirai, T., Meyer, J. S., Akiyama, H., Mortel, K. F. and Wills, P. M. (1996). Acetazolamide testing of cerebral vasodilator capacity provokes 'vascular' but not tension headaches. *Headache* **36**, 589–594

Shukla, R., Shanker, K., Nag, D., Verma, M. and Bhargava, K. P. (1987). Serotonin in tension headache. *J. Neurol. Neurosurg. Psychiat.* **50**, 1682–1684

Sicuteri, F. (1981). Opioid receptor impairment – underlying mechanism in 'pain diseases'. *Cephalalgia* **1**, 77–82

Silberstein, S. D., Lipton, R. B. and Sliwinski, M. (1996). Classification of daily and near-daily headaches: field trial of revised IHS criteria. *Neurology* **47**, 871–875

Sjaastad, O. and Spierings, E. L. H. (1984). Hemicrania continua: another headache absolutely responsive to indomethacin. *Cephalalgia* **4**, 65–70

Srikiatkhachorn, A. and Anthony, M. (1996). Platelet serotonin in patients with analgesic-induced headache. *Cephalalgia* **16**, 423–426

Vijayan, N. and Spillane, T. (1995) Valproic acid treatment of chronic daily headache. *Headache* **35**, 540–43

Warner, A. K. and Lance, J. W. (1975). Relaxation therapy in migraine and chronic tension headache. *Med. J. Aust.* **1**, 298–301

Zeigler, A. K. and Hassanein, R. S. (1982). Migraine muscle contraction headache dichotomy studied by statistical analysis of headache symptoms. In *Advances in Migraine Research and Therapy*, Ed. F. Clifford Rose. pp. 7–11. New York, Raven Press

Zwart, J.-A. and Sand, T. (1995). Exteroceptive suppression of temporalis muscle activity: a blind study of tension-type headache, migraine and cervicogenic headache. *Headache* **35**, 338–343

Chapter 11

Cluster headache and related conditions

Definition

Episodic cluster headache may be defined as a severe unilateral head or facial pain, which lasts from 15 minutes to 3 hours, associated commonly with ipsilateral conjunctival injection, lacrimation and blockage of the nostril, usually recurring once or more daily for a period of weeks or months. The term cluster headache derives from the tendency for the pain to appear in bouts, separated by intervals of complete freedom (Kunkle *et al.*, 1952). A chronic form, without remission, and other variations are now recognized (Headache Classification Committee of The International Headache Society, 1988) and are described later.

The headache

The nature of the attack and pattern of recurrence of cluster headache are so characteristic that it can readily be distinguished from migraine and trigeminal neuralgia. In spite of this many patients are referred to neurologists with the provisional diagnosis of one or other of these disorders, and the condition is often referred to in the British literature as 'migrainous neuralgia'. The subject has been reviewed in books by Kudrow (1980) and Sjaastad (1992).

Nomenclature

In 1840 Romberg first described as 'ciliary neuralgia' recurrent pain in the eye which was generally confined to one side and associated with photophobia (Romberg, 1840, translation 1853). 'The pupil is contracted. The pain not infrequently extends over the head and face. The eye generally weeps and becomes red. These symptoms occur in paroxysms of a uniform or irregular character, and isolated or combined with facial neuralgia and hemicrania.' Romberg considered that scrofula was the main cause of ciliary neuralgia but that it was also brought on by discharges, especially seminal emissions. The condition was first recorded in the English medical literature by Harris in 1925 as ciliary (migrainous) neuralgia and this description was later elaborated (Harris, 1936; Horton, MacLean and Craig, 1939).

The uncertainty about the nature and aetiology of this disorder is reflected by other names that have been used to describe similar syndromes over the past century, such as red migraine, erythroprosopalgia, erythromelalgia of the head, syndrome of hemicephalic vasodilation of sympathetic origin, autonomic faciocephalalgia, greater superficial petrosal neuralgia and histamine cephalalgia. Symonds (1956) used the noncommittal title of 'a particular variety of headache'. Sphenopalatine neurosis (Sluder, 1910) and vidian neuralgia (Vail, 1932) were described as affecting mostly female patients and appear more akin to lower half headache, now known as facial migraine, than to the syndrome under discussion. The extent to which the more peculiar syndromes were recognized we would now call paroxysmal hemicrania or even SUNCT (see below) is not clear and may never be certain.

Prevalence

Cluster headache is considerably less common than migraine but the ratio of one to the other varies from 1 : 6 to 1 : 50 in reports from different sources, depending on the interest and orientation of each clinic. Based on a screening of 6400 patient records in Olmsted County, Minnesota, Swanson et al (1994) found the incidence of cluster headache was approximately 9.8 per 100,000 per year or 1/25 that of migraine. Kudrow (1980) estimated that the prevalence of cluster headache in the USA was 0.4 per cent for men and 0.08 per cent for women. Ekbom, Ahlborg and Schele (1978) diagnosed cluster headache in 0.09 per cent of 18-year-olds called up for military service. D'Alessandro et al. (1986) studied the population of the Republic of San Marino (21,792 people) by reviewing medical records for the preceding 15 years and writing to every inhabitant. They found 15 cases (14 men, one woman), giving a prevalence of 69 cases per 100,000 population, i.e. 0.07 per cent.

Varieties of cluster headache

Episodic cluster headache

The episodic form recurs in periods lasting 7 days to 1 year, separated by pain-free periods lasting 14 days or more. Commonly, bouts last between 2 weeks and 3 months with remissions from 3 months to 3 years (Headache Classification Committee of The International Headache Society, 1988).

Chronic cluster headache

Some 10–20 per cent of patients experience recurrent cluster pains for more than 1 year with brief (shorter than 14 days) or no remissions. In some patients, the pain may be unremitting from the onset (primary chronic cluster) whereas it may develop from episodic cluster headache in others (secondary chronic cluster).

Clinical features

Sex distribution

Cluster headache is predominantly a male disease. Of 425 patients reported by Kudrow (1980), the male to female ratio was 5 : 1 and in a series of 400 patients described by Kunkel (1981) the ratio was 9 : 1. Most series report that about 85 per cent of patients were male.

Age of onset

The illness usually starts in the second to fourth decades of life but Kudrow (1980) described one child who developed typical symptoms at the age of 3 years and other cases have been reported to start at the age of 8 years (Ekbom, 1970; Lance and Anthony, 1971). Kudrow (1980) and Manzoni *et al.* (1983) found the peak age of onset to fall between the ages of 20 and 29 but the first bout may be delayed until the fifties and sixties.

Site of pain

The pain of cluster headache is unilateral, almost always affecting the same side of the head in each bout. In 32 of the 60 patients reported by Lance and Anthony (1971), the attacks were exclusively right-sided, in 23 left-sided and in five the side affected varied from bout to bout or on different days in the same bout. The pain is felt deeply in and around the eye by about 60 per cent of patients. It commonly radiates to the supraorbital region, temple, maxilla and upper gum on the same side of the face and may occasionally be limited to those areas, not involving the upper face (Ekbom, 1975). In some patients the ipsilateral nostril aches and burns, and a few complain of aching in the roof of the mouth. In other patients, the lower gum, jaw or chin are also involved. The pain may spread to the ear, the neck or 'the entire half of the head'. Presentation with pain in the gums or jaw may be interpreted as toothache (Brooke, 1978).

Quality of pain

The pain of cluster headache is peculiarly distressing and we have had many patients who have had other pain experiences, such as renal colic or childbirth, report that the pain of an attack of cluster headache is much worse. It may be throbbing or pulsating on occasions but the majority describe the pain as constant and severe. Common adjectives used to describe it are burning, boring, piercing, tearing and screwing. A dull background pain persists in the eye, temple or upper jaw between attacks or precedes a bout by some hours or days in some cases. About one-third of patients experience sudden jabs of pain in the affected areas at the time of headache.

Periodicity of bouts

About one-fifth of patients with the characteristic pain and accompaniments have a pattern of recurrence which resembles that of migraine without any long periods of freedom (chronic cluster headache). Four of the 60 patients described by Lance and Anthony (1971) were subject to attacks of pain from one to four times a week without ever having suffered a bout of regular daily episodes. The other eight of our chronic cluster headache patients had started in this manner but the frequency had increased until they were experiencing from one to five attacks daily. Most patients suffer one or two bouts each year. The periodicity of bouts in our series did not depend consistently upon the time of year. Of those who considered that their bouts had a seasonal incidence, five stated that they recurred in spring, six in summer, six in autumn and seven in winter.

Duration of bouts

The usual length of each bout is 4–8 weeks, but there is considerable variation from patient to patient.

Daily frequency of attacks during a bout

The usual number of attacks daily varies from one to three. Of our 60 patients, 52 stated that their attacks were liable to recur at a particular time of the day or night: 32 mentioned 'night-time', nine specifically from 10 p.m. to 2 a.m., and 13 from 2 a.m. to 6 a.m. Manzoni *et al.* (1983) found peaks at 1 a.m., 2 p.m. and 9 p.m.

Duration of attacks

Each particular episode usually starts suddenly, lasts for 10 minutes to 2 hours and may end abruptly or fade away more slowly. Occasional episodes may be sustained for 8 hours or more.

Associated features (Table 11.1)

Lacrimation and reddening of the eye on the affected side is common and is occasionally bilateral. Drooping of the ipsilateral eyelid and miosis are reported by about one-third of patients and have been observed in two-thirds of patients when examined during attacks (Ekbom, 1970; Kudrow, 1980). Ptosis and miosis may be apparent between attacks (see Figure 5.1) and can be demonstrated on the symptomatic side by pupillography in all patients between attacks (Drummond, 1988). Flushing of the periorbital area is not often observed clinically but an increase in skin temperature around the orbit, cheek and nose of about 0.25–1.5C can be measured by thermography during attacks (Drummond and Lance, 1984). The nostril is often blocked or running on one or both sides. A running nostril cannot be explained by lacrimation, because it is not always associated with a weeping eye. Autonomic symptoms sometimes start before pain.

Table 11.1 Associated features in 60 patients. (From Lance and Anthony, 1971)

Ocular			Vascular	
Lacrimation { unilateral		49	Flushing of face	12
Lacrimation { bilateral		3	Pallor of face	2
Conjunctival injection		27	Prominent, tender temporal artery	10
Partial Horner's syndrome		19	Prominent veins in forehead	2
Photophobia		12	Puffiness around eyes	6
Blurred vision		5	Lumps in mouth	2
			Cold hands and feet	1
Nasal			Polyuria	4
Blocked nostril { unilateral		28		
Blocked nostril { bilateral		4		
Running nostril { unilateral		9		
Running nostril { bilateral		1		
Epistaxis		1		
			Neurological	
Gastrointestinal			Hyperalgesia of scalp and face	10
Anorexia		2	Itching behind eye (preceding headache)	2
Nausea		26	Flashing lights in front of eyes	1
Vomiting { occasionally		9	Spots in front of eyes	1
Vomiting { regularly		9	Vertigo and mild ataxia	4
Diarrhoea		2	Mental confusion	1
			Unilateral carpal spasm	1

Gastrointestinal disturbances are less common than in migraine but about one-half of the patients feel nauseated and may vomit. Nausea may precede the onset of facial pain. Photophobia may be intense and patients may complain of phonophobia.

Hyperalgesia of the face and scalp is common and can be extreme in some cases, so that the patient cannot bear to touch the affected areas. Two of our patients had noticed an itching sensation behind the eye, one immediately preceding pain in the eye and the other for some weeks before a bout began. Others complained of a dull intermittent ache or jabs of pain behind the eye between severe paroxysms.

Focal neurological symptoms or signs, of the type which are common in migraine, are unusual in cluster headache. One of our patients mentioned occasional 'spots before the eyes' and another described 'little flashing lights in front of the eyes' during the headache. Four described a feeling of dizziness, giddiness or a 'rising feeling in the head' associated with impaired balance at the time of the attack. One patient had experienced a tonic seizure of the left arm on three occasions associated with a pain in the right eye and temple. The left hand assumed the position of carpal spasm for a period of minutes. Sutherland and Eadie (1972) reported a patient who was subject to scintillating scotomas before cluster headache, two patients with paraesthesiae on the side of the body opposite to the head pain, and one patient with twitching of the contralateral foot.

Precipitating factors

The only trigger factor that is consistently mentioned by patients is the taking of alcoholic drinks and this is only operative during a susceptible period, i.e. during a bout. Vasodilators, such as nitrates, will also precipitate an attack at this time. One of our patients who used carbon tetrachloride as a solvent in his daily work commented that inhalation of the fumes would induce an attack as readily as alcohol. Other factors mentioned by patients are stress, attacks of hay fever, heat, changes in weather, glare, missing a meal or sleeping late in the mornings.

Relieving factors

Some patients can find some ease from their pain by pressing on the superficial temporal arteries, by the application of heat or cold, or by pacing up and down with their hand clasped over one eye.

Past history and associated disorders

There is nothing very remarkable in the past health of patients with cluster headache other than an association with peptic ulcer and coronary disease. There is no convincing association with migraine or allergic disorders.

Peptic ulcer

Approximately 20 per cent of cluster headache patients have a history of peptic ulcer (Graham, 1972; Kudrow, 1980) compared with some 10 per cent of migraine patients.

Coronary artery disease

Graham (1972) and Manzoni et al. (1983) reported an increased prevalence of coronary artery disease in cluster headache patients. Kudrow (1980) found the prevalence to be double that of non-cluster controls but the numbers did not achieve statistical significance. Interestingly enough, angina may diminish in severity during bouts of cluster headache (Ekbom, 1970).

Trauma

Eight of our original 60 patients had experienced a head injury, and in four the site of injury could conceivably be relevant to the ensuing cluster headache. One patient had required extensive plastic surgery for facial and scalp lacerations following a car accident, and left-sided cluster headache started 21 months after injury. The second had gravel embedded in the right temple from a road accident at the age of 17 years, and cluster headaches involving the right temple and right side of the face began 7 years later. The third patient developed right frontotemporal cluster headache 30 years after a shotgun injury to the forehead, in which fragmented pellets were still embedded. The fourth patient experienced a blow to the forehead at the age of 22 years, following which he was subject to a dull right-sided headache for 3 years. Eight years after the injury, right-side cluster headaches developed, involving the right forehead and right side of the face.

We have seen subsequently patients with head injury that very often involves the ophthalmic division of the trigeminal nerve and particularly the supraorbital nerve prior to the onset of cluster headache. There are also clear reports, reviewed by Evers (1997), of the development of cluster headache after eye removal which may be considered a further form of trauma in this setting. Nevertheless, Kudrow (1980) has not found any correlation with head injury in his large series.

Family history

The prevalence of migraine in parents and siblings (22 per cent in our series) was not significantly greater than that of patients with tension headache (18 per cent), and much less than that of typical migraine patients (45 per cent) (Lance and Anthony, 1966). Ekbom (1970) found a family history of migraine in 16 per cent of patients with cluster headache compared with 65 per cent of migraine patients. It is unusual to find other examples of cluster headache in the family history. Kudrow (1980) reported that about 3 per cent of cluster headache patients have one relative affected by the disorder whereas a positive family history was found in 7 per cent by Russell, Andersson and Iselius (1996).

Segregation analysis suggested that cluster headache is transmitted by an auto-sominal dominant gene with a penetrance of 0.30–0.34 in males and 0.17–0.21 in females (Russell et al., 1995). There have been occasional reports of cluster headache in twins (Sjaastad, 1992). The distribution of HLA antigens in episodic cluster head-ache does not differ from that of a normal population but all five patients with chronic cluster headache examined by Cuypers and Altenkirch (1979) carried the HLA-A1 antigen, an observation that warrants a wider study of this subgroup.

The cluster headache personality

Graham (1972) drew attention to certain characteristics of the appearance of the longstanding cluster headache sufferer, which he described as 'leonine facies'. The patients tend to have a ruddy complexion and multi-furrowed thick skin. He con-sidered that they are usually a hard-drinking and hard-smoking lot, ambitious and hard-working, the prototype aggressive executive-type male. According to Graham this appearance conceals feelings of guilt, anger, inadequacy and dependency which shows itself in brief outbursts of hysterical behaviour during an attack of cluster headache.

Kudrow and Sutkus (1979) submitted 41 patients with cluster headaches to Min-nesota Multiphasic Personality Inventory (MMPI) testing in comparison with 217 patients suffering from other forms of headache. They could not find any difference between the characteristics of migraine and cluster headache patients but both of these groups gave significantly different results from patients with tension or post-traumatic headaches. An independent study, using the Freiburg Personality Inven-tory (Cuypers, Altenkirch and Bunge, 1981) came to much the same conclusion after comparing 40 cluster headache patients with 49 migraine patients. Cluster headache patients had a slightly increased score of nervousness and a slightly diminished score for traits of 'masculinity', which could simply reflect the impact of a painful relapsing disorder.

It may be concluded that cluster headache patients are not unduly neurotic, in spite of the strange behaviour of some at the height of their headaches.

Pathophysiology

The source of pain in cluster headache

Patients with cluster headache often state that they can relieve pain at one site, for example in the temple, by direct pressure over the site but that pain felt in or behind the eye persists or may become worse. The application of heat to the eye usually causes temporary relief of orbital pain. Pain does not arise in the eye itself because cluster headache may develop or persist after enucleation of the eye. Kunkle *et al.* (1952) injected normal saline intrathecally under pressure in two patients during cluster headache without relief of pain, which led them to conclude that the pain was not derived from dilatation of intracranial arteries. However, localization of pain to the eye is characteristic of other disorders involving the internal carotid artery and the frequency of involvement of the ocular sympathetic supply to produce a partial Horner's syndrome suggests that sympathetic fibres might be compromised in the pericarotid vascular plexus by dilatation, engorgement or oedema of the vessel wall (Kunkle and Anderson, 1961; Nieman and Hurwitz, 1961).

Localization of the lesion in the sympathetic pathway is aided by the sparing of sweating over the face (with the exception of the medial part of the forehead), which is mediated by fibres accompanying branches of the extracranial arteries. The site of entrapment must therefore lie distal to the bifurcation of the common carotid artery and is logically placed in the area surrounding the internal carotid artery or within the orbit. Ekbom and Greitz (1970) reported the angiographic appearance of localized narrowing of the lumen of the internal carotid artery, just beyond its entry into the skull, at the height of an attack of cluster headache. This was attributed to oedema or spasm of the vessel wall and persisted after pain had ceased. In contrast, the ophthalmic artery was dilated during the attack.

Ekbom (1975) assessed the relief of pain in cluster headache by various manoeuvres. Compression of the superficial temporal artery in 18 patients eased the pain in 8 patients, made it worse (commonly in the eye) in eight and had no effect in two. Common carotid compression in 20 patients reduced aching in the eye in 10 of them (and in the upper jaw in three) while the pain was more severe in five patients and unchanged in five. A rotatory head jolt accentuated the pain in only five of 17 patients and actually relieved the pain in seven. Ekbom concluded that the pain of cluster headache arises distally in the internal carotid circulation, in the region of the eye in most cases, but that branches of the external carotid artery were involved in some patients.

The pain and autonomic symptoms of cluster headache may be simulated by structural lesions in the vicinity of the cavernous sinus or in other cranial locations, including patients with an arteriovenous malformation in the occipital lobe (Mani and Deeter, 1982), a pituitary adenoma (Tfelt-Hansen, Paulson and Krabbe, 1982), orbito-sphenoidal aspergillosis (Heidegger *et al.*, 1997), upper cervical meningioma (Kuritzky, 1984), vertebral artery aneurysm (West and Todman, 1991) and dissection (Cremer, Halmagyi and Goadsby, 1995), and a pseudoaneurysm of the intracavernous carotid artery (Koenigsberg, Solomon and Kosmorsky, 1994). This phenomenon of symptomatic cluster headache must be of relevance to the pathophysiology of cluster headache in general, and the fact that both trigeminal and cervically innervated structures can be involved points to a central nervous system pathology rather than a primary disorder of the cavernous sinus. Indeed it has recently been demonstrated using PET that changes in cavernous sinus blood flow occur with pain experimentally induced by capsaicin injection into the forehead (May et al., 1998b) in a similar way to that seen in cluster headache (May et al., 1998a).

The trigeminal nerve is intact in patients with cluster headache and corneal responses to tactile stimulation are normal (Vijayan and Watson, 1985), but the corneal pain threshold was found by Sandrini et al. (1991) to be reduced ipsilaterally during attacks in 10 out of 15 patients. When 27 patients were examined carefully during cluster headache, 10 were found to have cutaneous hyperalgesia and 12 had deep hyperalgesia in the face, arm or whole body on the side of the pain (Procacci et al., 1989). These phenomena are presumably secondary to activation of the thalamus by trigeminothalamic pathways as has recently been demonstrated by PET scanning (May et al., 1998a).

Input from the upper cervical spine may also play a part in the pain of cluster headache given the overlap of sensory processing in the trigeminocervical complex (Goadsby and Hoskin, 1997; Goadsby, Hoskin and Knight, 1997). Some patients can precipitate attacks of cluster headache with neck movement. The injection of a local anaesthetic agent and long-acting corticosteroid into the ipsilateral greater occipital nerve can alter the pattern of recurrence of cluster headache (Anthony, 1987). A meningioma compressing the spinal cord at the level of the first and second cervical segments caused episodic pain with lacrimation and redness of the eye indistinguishable from cluster headache (Kuritzky, 1984). A syndrome resembling cluster headache was reported following whiplash injury to the neck in eight patients (Hunter and Mayfield, 1949). It is of interest that stimulation of the greater occipital nerve in rats produced ipsilateral conjunctival injection, lacrimation, ptosis or pupillary changes in one-third of the animals (Vincent et al., 1992).

Conclusion

It may be concluded that the spinal tract and nucleus of the trigeminal nerve, descending to the C_2 segment, becomes hyperactive unilaterally during cluster headache and that the main peripheral source of pain is the internal carotid artery and its proximal branches. Since afferents in upper cervical roots converge with trigeminal neurones in the second cervical segment of the spinal cord, they may also contribute to the level of excitation in central pain pathways. Based on the results of functional imaging studies with PET it is likely that the involvement of the carotid artery is due to its neurovascular connections and not a primary problem in the artery or the cavernous sinus.

Vascular changes

Reports on cerebral blood flow in cluster headache have not been consistent. Krabbe, Henriksen and Olesen (1984) did not observe any increase in mean cerebral blood flow in induced attacks but focal increases were noted in the central, basal and right parietotemporal region, which were attributed to non-specific activation by pain.

Studies include those of Hering *et al.* (1991) who found no change in intracranial or extracranial flow in 14 patients, two of whom were examined during an acute attack. In contrast, Meyer, Kawamura and Terayama (1991) described an increase in regional cerebral blood flow from a mean resting value of $73.1 \pm 5.2 \, \text{ml}/100 \, \text{g}$ brain per minute to a mean of 94.8 ± 12.4 during attacks in seven patients. Vasodilatation in response to CO_2 was impaired, particularly on the side of headache. Blood flow through grey matter was reduced by about one-third when 100 per cent oxygen was inhaled during the attack, compared with a 9 per cent reduction in normal controls. Dahl *et al.* (1990) found that regional cerebral blood flow did not increase in cluster attacks provoked by glyceryl trinitrate, 1 mg sublingually, but the velocity of blood flow in the middle cerebral arteries decreased, more so on the symptomatic side. A similar reduction in flow was noted in spontaneous attacks, suggesting that the artery became dilated during cluster headache. These findings are broadly consistent with our recent MRA experience but are not restricted to cluster headache (May *et al.*, 1998b). Gawel *et al.* (1990) reported that reactivity of the ipsilateral anterior cerebral artery to CO_2 was diminished during the cluster headache period.

Broch *et al.* (1970) measured internal carotid flow by the application of electromagnetic flow probes in one patient. No change in mean or pulsatile blood flow was recorded in either internal carotid artery during two typical episodes of cluster headache. In contrast, pulse-synchronous variations in ocular tension (the corneal indentation pulse recorded by dynamic tonometry) doubled on the affected side in the same patient and increased by about 30 per cent on the headache-free side. This is equivalent to a change in ocular volume from $4 \, \text{mm}^3$ to $8 \, \text{mm}^3$ on the headache side. Intraocular pressure increased within 1 minute of the onset of pain by 4–6 mmHg in the affected eye. The appearance of fluorescein in the retinal arteries was not delayed, indicating that the velocity of blood flow through internal carotid and ophthalmic arteries was unaltered during unilateral cluster headache. Similarly, we have seen no difference in fluorescein angiography in acute cluster headache when compared to a study performed outside of the attack (May *et al.*, 1998c).

Hørven and Sjaastad (1977) reported that corneal intraocular pressure and corneal temperatures all increased on the affected side during cluster headache, indicating intraocular vasodilatation. Drummond and Lance (1984) made thermographic observations on 11 patients with spontaneous attacks and 22 patients during attacks induced by nitroglycerin or alcohol. At the height of a spontaneous attack, the affected orbital region was 0.25–1.25°C warmer than the other side in seven patients but temperature remained symmetrical in four, while the ipsilateral cheek became 0.25–1.5°C warmer in 10 of the 11 patients. Similar changes were noted in induced attacks but pain felt behind the eye was not always correlated with increased heat loss from the area. Increase in cutaneous blood flow usually followed the onset of pain and was considered to be a secondary phenomenon, a vasodilator reflex mediated by the trigeminal nerve as the afferent limb and the greater superficial petrosal (GSP) nerve as the efferent limb (Goadsby and Lance, 1988).

The frequency of conjunctival injection and nasal blockage in cluster headache provides supporting evidence for dilatation of capillaries in the extracranial circulation. This may be associated with oedema, causing swelling of the periorbital region or buccal mucosa, described as 'little lumps in the mouth'. Skin biopsies taken from the temples of six patients with cluster headache showed an increased number of mast cells in comparison with those from three normal controls (Appenzeller, Becker and Ragaz, 1981). Dimitriadou *et al.* (1990) showed that mast cells surrounding temporal arteries removed from the symptomatic side of cluster headache patients were degranulated when compared with those obtained from normal control subjects. Mast cell changes may play a part in the mechanism of vasodilatation by releasing histamine.

Just as has been seen in migraine, certain vasoactive peptides are released in cluster headache. Calcitonin gene-related peptide (CGRP), a marker for trigeminal activation, and vasoactive intestinal polypeptide, a marker of cranial parasympathetic activation, are elevated in spontaneous (Goadsby and Edvinsson, 1994) and nitroglycerin-induced cluster attacks (Franciullacci *et al.*, 1995). This release confirms activation of the trigemino-parasympathetic reflex in humans during acute cluster headache. Given that it has been reported that parasympathetic activation may also lead to mast cell changes in animal models (Delepine *et al.*, 1996), it is likely that the degranulation observed in the temporal vessels is an epiphenomenon of either trigeminal or autonomic activation which is likely to be driven from the brain.

Conclusion

It may be concluded that cluster headache is associated with dilatation of proximal branches of the internal carotid artery, including the ophthalmic artery, without consistent changes in cerebral blood flow. Capillaries dilate in the ipsilateral conjunctiva, nasal mucosa and cutaneous circulation, particularly in the periorbital area.

The importance of vascular dilatation in the pathogenesis of cluster headache is indicated by the triggering of attacks during a bout by vasodilators such as alcohol, histamine (Horton, MacLean and Craig, 1939) and nitroglycerin (Ekbom, 1970), and the presence of dilatation in experimentally induced ophthalmic division pain in humans by local injection of capsaicin (May *et al.*, 1997b). Nevertheless the primary generator for cluster headache must lie within the brain.

Autonomic changes

During cluster headache heat loss increases from the eye and cheek on the affected side, the ipsilateral eye usually reddens or waters, while the nostril discharges fluid or blocks. These manifestations are usually associated, suggesting that they are produced by parasympathetic discharge through the greater superficial petrosal (GSP) nerve (Drummond, 1988; Drummond and Lance, 1985; Saunte, 1984), although Saunte (1984) has found that salivation is diminished during the attack. It is probable that sympathetic activity dominates parasympathetic action on the salivary glands but is unable to override its lacrimal and vascular functions.

Transient or permanent paralysis of the ocular sympathetic nerve supply, giving rise to a partial Horner's syndrome on the symptomatic side, is a common accompaniment of cluster headache. Kunkle and Anderson (1961) found miosis and sometimes ptosis in 14 out of 90 patients, persisting between attacks in seven. Nieman and

Hurwitz (1961) reported a permanent deficit in 10 of 50 patients. Careful investigation discloses a subtle sympathetic deficit in most patients. Fanciullaci *et al.* (1982) found that the pupil on the affected side dilated less after the instillation of tyramine drops in 26 patients examined between attacks and a further 19 patients between bouts. Since tyramine releases noradrenaline from nerve terminals, diminished pupillary dilatation indicates neuronal depletion resulting from a post-ganglionic sympathetic lesion. The demonstration of an excessive dilatation of the pupil in response to a dilute solution of a sympathomimetic agent, phenylephrine, shows that there is also denervation supersensitivity of receptors (Salvesen *et al.*, 1987). Drummond (1988) showed that the pupil on the symptomatic side dilated more slowly in darkness and constricted more rapidly in response to light than the opposite pupil between as well as during attacks, and that ptosis was also present on the side of cluster headache.

Salvesen, Sand and Sjaastad (1988) found that deficient pupillary dilatation in response to hydroxy-amphetamine (which, like tyramine, releases noradrenaline) and supersensitivity to phenylephrine were correlated with deficiency of sweating on the medial aspect of the forehead and overactivity of the sweat glands in this area in response to circulating pilocarpine. While denervation supersensitivity of the pupil may occur with central lesions its correlation with sweating changes limited to the medial part of the forehead clearly places the lesion in the postganglionic sympathetic neurone in the region of the carotid siphon (Lance and Drummond, 1987). The reasoning behind this is that facial sweating is mediated by post-ganglionic fibres, which are distributed to the periphery along branches of the external carotid artery, with the exception of the medial aspect of the forehead, where the sympathetic fibres derive from the internal carotid artery, leaving the siphon to accompany the first division of the trigeminal nerve and its frontal and supraorbital branches to the skin of the medial part of the forehead (Figure 11.1). Selective involvement of this area must implicate sympathetic fibres in the vicinity of the siphon.

Further evidence was obtained by Drummond and Lance (1992) who compared 11 cluster headache patients with another 24 patients who had a confirmed site of lesion in the cervical sympathetic pathway. Patients with a central or pre-ganglionic lesion had a normal mydriatic response to tyramine 2 per cent eye drops, which was diminished or absent in seven patients with a confirmed post-ganglionic lesion and in seven patients on the symptomatic side of cluster headache. Sweating and flushing in response to body heating was diminished on the medial aspect of the ipsilateral forehead in those patients but was excessive when lacrimation was evoked in the ipsilateral eye by the instillation of a soapy eye drop into the conjunctival sac. This can be explained by parasympathetic fibres in the vicinity of the internal carotid artery branching along the adjacent sympathetic fibres, which had degenerated as the result of a post-ganglionic lesion (Figure 11.1). Irritation of the eye that causes reflex lacrimation through the greater superficial petrosal nerve and its connections therefore causes excessive flushing and sweating in the medial aspect of the forehead comparable with that observed during some attacks of cluster headache. The only inconsistent feature in this investigation was that pulse amplitudes from the ipsilateral cheek, as well as from the medial forehead, were diminished after body heating in four out of six cluster headache patients studied, unlike the four patients

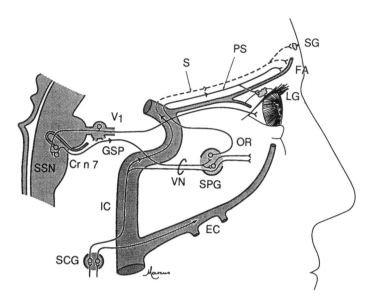

Figure 11.1 The mechanism of pathological sweating during cluster headache. (From Drummond and Lance, 1992, by permission of the publishers, Oxford University Press, Oxford)

Sympathetic fibres (S) arising from the superior cervical ganglion (SCG) are compromised in the wall of the internal carotid artery (IC), causing their peripheral distribution to the frontal arteries (FA) and sweat glands (SG) to degenerate.

Parasympathetic fibres, originating in the superior salivatory nucleus (SSN), traverse the facial nerve (Cr n 7) and the greater superficial petrosal nerve (GSP) to join the Vidian nerve (VN) and synapse in the sphenopalatine ganglion (SPG); post-ganglionic fibres then loop back as orbital rami (OR) to the cavernous sinus and internal carotid artery where they form a retro-orbital plexus with sympathetic and trigeminal fibres, before advancing to supply the lacrimal glands (LG) and cutaneous circulation of the forehead. Conjunctival irritation stimulates afferent fibres in the first division of the trigeminal nerve (V$_1$), which reflexly activates parasympathetic outflow to the lacrimal glands and forehead circulation. The dashed line represents the route taken by parasympathetic fibres that occupy the denervated sympathetic pathway and cause frontal sweating and flushing in response to the conjunctival stimulus.

with a confirmed postganglionic lesion from other causes, suggesting that the lesion in cluster headache might also affect the internal maxillary branch of the external carotid artery.

Russell and Storstein (1983) have plotted changes in cardiac rate and rhythm as an index of autonomic instability in cluster headache. Cardiac rate increases at the onset and slows during the attack. Of 27 patients monitored throughout an attack two developed conduction abnormalities, one experienced transient atrial fibrillation and another had an increased number of ventricular extrasystoles. Whether these changes indicate a disturbance of central autonomic innervation or are secondary to pain remains uncertain.

Conclusion

The most economical explanation of the partial Horner's syndrome in cluster headache is oedema of the wall of the internal carotid artery compromising post-ganglionic sympathetic neurones in the perivascular plexus. Narrowing of the lumen of this section of the internal carotid artery has been demonstrated angiographically in one patient with cluster headache by Ekbom and Greitz (1970) and has also been observed during an attack by Dr Fred Plum (personal communication). Gawel *et al.* (1990) demonstrated increased uptake of gallium in the region of the cavernous sinus in three out of six patients during the cluster period but such changes have also been reported in migraine patients and may therefore be non-specific (Sianard-Gainko *et al.*, 1994). No abnormality has been found in this area by magnetic resonance imaging during a bout of cluster headache but no examination has yet been recorded at the time of an acute attack (Sjaastad and Rinck, 1990).

Distension of the arterial wall could be caused by vasodilator peptides released from cells forming the internal carotid ganglion, lying on the ventrolateral surface of the human internal carotid artery as it enters the cranium, that are activated by the discharge along the GSP nerve which is responsible for lacrimation and for conjunctival, nasal and cutaneous vasodilatation (Suzuki and Hardebo, 1991). The fact that salivation is reduced during the attack suggests that secretion is inhibited by intact sympathetic fibres arising from the superior cervical ganglion. The effect of any generalized sympathetic arousal would not be expressed in those areas supplied from fibres in the pericarotid plexus. Section of the nervus intermedius, containing GSP fibres, does not always stop the recurrent pain of cluster headache. Indeed, even the autonomic symptoms may continue in some patients (Morgenlander and Wilkins, 1990; Rowed, 1990), possibly because the nerve is incompletely severed.

Humoral, metabolic and hormonal changes: where are the internal clocks?

There may be two biological clocks determining the pattern of cluster headache: one to switch on the bouts of episodic cluster and to switch them off after weeks or months; and the other to trigger the attacks within a bout, once or more in a 24-hour period. Alternatively, there may be one that switches the bout on with the daily periodicity being a function of normal circadian rhythms affecting susceptible central nervous system structures. Since many patients experience their attacks at a precise time of the day or night, and the timing of attacks varies if the patient moves from one time zone to another, it seems probable that the daily rhythm is set by the suprachiasmatic nucleus and hypothalamus. This notion is supported by the demonstration of increased metabolic activity in the ipsilateral hypothalamus by PET scanning (May *et al.*, 1998a). In view of this, hormonal changes have been studied as indicators of hypothalamic function. Boiardi *et al.* (1983) found basal growth hormone and prolactin levels to be normal in cluster headache patients and their response to insulin, levodopa and thyrotropin releasing hormone was the same as control subjects. The nocturnal maximal level of melatonin is lower during cluster periods and the cortisol level higher (Waldenlind *et al.*, 1987). Prolactin levels rise during headache and testosterone levels are lower in cluster periods than in remission, but not when compared with controls (Waldenlind and Gustafson, 1987). The thyrotropin response to TRH (thyrotropin releasing hormone) and the release of ACTH and cortisol during insulin-induced hypoglycaemia are reduced in cluster periods (Leone *et al.*, 1994), attributed by these authors to dysfunction of the hypothalamic paraventricular nuclei. Further studies using *m*-chlorophenylpiperazine (mCPP) have suggested that changes in cortisol levels in patients with cluster headache may be related to altered levels of central serotonergic activity in the central nervous system (Leone *et al.*, 1997). Hormonal changes and the complex chrono-biology of cluster headache were also summarized by Nappi and Martignoni (1988).

Studies of humoral agents have not provided any substantial clue to the mechanism of cluster headache. An acetylcholine-like substance was found in the CSF of four patients by Kunkle (1959). Platelet 5-HT increases during pain episodes (Medina, Diamond and Fareed, 1979) and decreases when cluster headache is successfully treated with lithium or other medication (Medina, Fareed and Diamond, 1980). Platelet noradrenaline and adrenaline are diminished in and between attacks (D'Andrea *et al.*, 1989). The mean blood level of histamine increases during cluster headache (Anthony and Lance, 1971; Medina, Diamond and Fareed, 1979) but treatment with H_1 and H_2 blocking agents has not proved to be helpful in management (Anthony, Lord and Lance, 1978; Russell, 1979). The part possibly played by endorphins and vasodilator peptides is considered by Ekbom, Hardebo and Waldenlind (1988) in their review of mechanisms.

Conclusion

Thus far, no changes have been reported in endocrine function or circulating humoral agents that could not be explained by the pain and disturbance of sleep pattern in bouts of cluster headache. The search for the biological clocks involved, or reliable markers of their activity, must continue. The most hopeful lead so far is the finding of increased metabolic activity in the ipsilateral hypothalamus (May *et al.*, 1998a).

General conclusions about the clinical features and pathophysiology of cluster headache

Cluster headache differs from migraine in many ways, as summarized in Table 11.2, which has been compiled from the data provided by Lance and Anthony (1966, 1971), Ekbom (1970) and Anthony and Lance (1971).

While the recurrence of migraine depends in some instances on an internal time-keeper that sets a frequency of monthly, weekly or sometimes even daily attacks, it is not subject to the rigid discipline that determines the pattern of cluster headache. The region of the ipsilateral hypothalamic grey matter that has been identified in recent PET studies to be active during acute attacks of cluster headache (May *et al.*, 1998a) is very likely to be the primary driving or permissive area for cluster headache.

Some patients become aware that an attack is about to start due to twinges of pain in the susceptible areas. Others detect a watering eye and stuffy nostril for half an hour or so before the pain begins. It is clear that the pain and the autonomic phenomena are independent variables, although one usually follows the other. They are compatible with paroxysmal discharge of central trigeminal, parasympathetic and sympathetic pathways with the ocular manifestations of sympathetic activity being blocked by a postganglionic lesion in the pericarotid plexus as a result of swelling of the internal carotid arterial wall. Dilatation of parts of the internal and external circulations are likely to be secondary to activity in vascular

Table 11.2 Differences between migraine and cluster headache

	Migraine	*Cluster headache*
Sex distribution (%)	Female 75	Male 85
Onset in childhood (%)	25	<1
Unilateral pain (%)	65	100
Recurrence in bouts (%)	0	80
Frequency of attacks	<1–12 per month	1–8 per day
Usual duration of pain	4–24 h	0.25–2 h
Associated features:		
Nausea, vomiting (%)	85	45
Blurring of vision (%)	Common	8
Lacrimation (%)	Uncommon	85
Blocked nostril (%)	Uncommon	50
Ptosis, miosis (%)	Uncommon	25
Hyperalgesia of face, scalp (%)	65	15
Teichopsia, photopsia (%)	40	<1
Polyuria (%)	30	7
Past health:		
Vomiting in childhood (%)	25	7
Family history:		
Migraine (%)	50	20
Biochemical changes:		
Fall in platelet serotonin (%)	80	0
Rise in plasma histamine (%)	0	90

Percentages refer to the number of patients with the symptom or sign in relation to the total studied.

projections from the brain stem as described in Chapter 5 and intensify pain by increasing input to the brain stem through trigeminal or upper cervical afferent fibres into the trigemino-cervical complex. As in the case of migraine, the pain can be eased by therapy directed at the dilated arteries or at central mechanisms. The fact that episodic pain may continue after surgical lesions of the trigeminal and GSP nerve clearly points to the primary defect being a central disturbance.

Treatment

The course of cluster headache does not appear to be influenced by psychological factors and does not respond to adjustment of lifestyle other than avoiding alcohol during a bout. Management is therefore directed towards suppressing bouts of episodic cluster headache, aborting any attacks that still occur, and reducing the frequency and severity of painful episodes in patients with chronic cluster headache, bearing in mind the lesions listed above that may mimic the disorder.

Episodic cluster headache

Suppression of bouts

Calcium channel blocking agents. Verapamil 80 mg four times daily is often effective in stopping a bout, with or without the addition of lithium. (See also under heading of Chronic cluster headache.)

Corticosteroids. The effectiveness of prednisone in stopping bouts of cluster headache was established in a double-blind trial by Jammes (1975). Kudrow (1980) reported that, of 77 episodic cluster patients unresponsive to methysergide, prednisone therapy relieved 76 per cent and partially improved 12 per cent. Kudrow uses prednisone 40 mg daily for 5 days, then 30 mg for 5 days, then reduces the dosage gradually over the next 11 days. Our custom has been to use higher doses than this, starting with 50–75 mg daily for 3 days, then reducing the daily dose at intervals of 3 days until the cluster headache starts to reappear. We have then stabilized the dose at a level just sufficient to prevent attacks.

Prednisone should be used with discretion, particularly if bouts are prolonged to the point when side-effects of treatment may appear. As in other disorders, the use of prednisone is contraindicated by a past history of tuberculosis or psychotic disturbance. The slight risk of delayed aseptic hip necrosis after courses of steroid therapy must be weighed against the immediate relief (in most cases) of a painful and debilitating disorder. The patient should however be warned of the possibility to forestall possible litigation if it occurs. As soon as the normal duration of a bout is reached, the treatment is gradually withdrawn. The mechanism of action is unknown.

Ergotamine tartrate and dihydroergotamine. Ergotamine tartrate is usually effective in the first one or two bouts of cluster headache, particularly if the headache is recurring at a predictable time. For example, many nocturnal attacks are prevented by taking ergotamine tartrate 1 mg, one or two tablets (or a combination tablet containing 2 mg), on retiring to bed. Alternatively, dihydroergotamine 1 mg may be administered by intramuscular injection once or twice daily at times appropriate for the prevention of the customary attacks. It must be stressed that the dose must be given at least half an hour before the predicted time of an attack to anticipate and abort the pain, and should not be delayed until the onset of pain.

Methysergide. Since bouts of cluster headache are usually shorter than 3 months in duration, it is safe to use methysergide in relatively high dosage for this brief period without concern about inducing fibrotic side-effects, which restrict its continuous long-term use in migraine. Assuming patients tolerate the medication well, the dose can be increased from 1 mg three times daily to two or three times this dose in order to suppress the attacks of pain. This regimen is effective in some 70 per cent of patients (Curran, Hinterberger and Lance, 1967).

Chlorpromazine. Chlorpromazine, in doses ranging from 75 to 700 mg daily, has been advocated for the suppression of bouts by Caviness and O'Brien (1980).

Intranasal capsaicin. A capsaicin suspension was applied 2 cm inside both nostrils in 45 cluster headache patients and 18 volunteers by Sicuteri *et al.* (1990), producing a burning sensation and rhinorrhoea. The procedure was repeated daily for 8 days, after which the number of attacks of cluster headache monitored over 10 days was reduced by 67 per cent. None of the 12 patients who received the vehicle only as a control group experienced any relief. This is a difficult procedure to blind and is very unpleasant for the patient. Unfortunately it is unlikely to affect intracranial pain-producing structures.

Treatment of acute attacks

Sumatriptan. The subcutaneous injection of sumatriptan 6 mg relieved the pain of cluster headache within 15 minutes in 74 per cent of cases in a crossover trial with placebo involving 39 patients (Ekbom, 1991). In this trial, 13 per cent of patients required oxygen as additional treatment after receiving sumatriptan, compared with 49 per cent of those given a placebo injection. Discomfort at the injection site was reported by 11 patients given sumatriptan and seven after placebo. Side-effects of dizziness, tiredness, numbness, paraesthesiae, a feeling of facial weakness or hot and cold sensations were noticed by 12 patients after sumatriptan and eight after placebo, but these were mild and transient.

The effect of sumatriptan by injection is rapid in onset and it is also effective in relieving the autonomic symptoms (Hardebo, 1993). Sumatriptan is generally well tolerated with longer term use (Ekbom *et al.*, 1992 ; Goadsby, 1994) but is not effective as a preventative when given at a dose of 100 mg three times daily (Monstad *et al.*, 1995).

Oxygen inhalation and ergotamine tartrate. The inhalation of 100 per cent oxygen relieves cluster headache within 15 minutes in most patients. Kudrow (1981) compared the inhalation of oxygen at 7 litres/minute through a face mask for 15 minutes with the sublingual administration of ergotamine tartrate 1 mg every 5 minutes, up to 3 mg in 15 minutes, in a crossover trial. Oxygen relieved 82 per cent and ergotamine tartrate was effective in 70 per cent of cases. The two methods can be combined with advantage, as the headache may recur some hours after oxygen inhalation alone. We sometimes recommend that the patient takes 1–2 mg of ergotamine tartrate orally at the first symptom of an attack, then inhales 100 per cent oxygen through a resuscitation mask (with no side-vents) at 7–10 litres/minute until the pain subsides. The oxygen cylinder, humidifier, reduction valve and mask can be rented from the supplier and installed in the home if the attacks are nocturnal or in the office or car if they recur during the day. The efficacy of inhaling oxygen rather than air was demonstrated by Fogan (1985) in a crossover trial. Of the 16 patients who breathed oxygen, nine experienced relief in 80 per cent or more of their cluster headaches, while only one of the 14 who breathed air was benefited.

Lidocaine nose drops. The intranasal installation of 1 ml of 4 per cent lidocaine with the body supine and the head extended over the head of a bed, inclined to the side of cluster headache, can be useful in shortening the duration of pain (Kittrelle, Grouse and Seybold, 1985). Although this technique has not been blessed by any controlled trial, we have found it useful in some resistant cases.

Chronic cluster headache

In those patients whose cluster attacks recur regularly without remission, ergotamine and methysergide may be used for prophylaxis as described above and observing reasonable limits. The following methods of management may also be helpful.

Lithium. Following a favourable report by Ekbom (1977), Kudrow (1980) evaluated the use of lithium carbonate in chronic cluster headache in doses of 300–600 mg daily, increasing to 900 mg daily after some weeks if necessary but maintaining a serum level of less than 1.2 mEq/litre. Serum levels were measured weekly for a month and monthly thereafter. Of 28 patients, 14 were more than 90 per cent improved, 11 were 60–90 per cent improved, and only one did not respond at all.

Ekbom (1981) described immediate partial remission in eight patients with chronic cluster headache, which was sustained for 2 years in one patient. Of 11 patients with episodic symptoms, only four responded to lithium therapy with almost complete suppression of cluster periods. In view of the widespread action of lithium on sodium and potassium exchange and amine metabolism it is not possible to be specific about its mode of action although its therapeutic action in bipolar disorder provides a common theme in terms of disorders that recur in cycles.

Side-effects of tremor, confusion, abdominal discomfort and weight loss may be experienced even though the serum level is within the normal therapeutic range, and may necessitate ceasing treatment. A recent negative trial emphasized the importance of measuring drug levels (Steiner *et al.*, 1997).

Calcium channel blocking agents. Verapamil has been used in the management of episodic and chronic cluster headache. In an open trial employing verapamil in large doses of 240–600 mg daily in episodic cluster headache and 120–1200 mg daily in chronic cluster headache, an improvement of more than 75 per cent was noted in 69 per cent of 48 patients (Gabai and Spierings, 1989). Since this early report verapamil has now established itself as being among the most effective preventative agents in cluster headache and is at least equal to lithium in effectiveness (Bussone *et al.*, 1990). It is generally true that the regular verapamil preparation is more useful than the slow-release preparations and that doses up to 480 mg or more daily may have to be used.

Occipital nerve injection. Anthony (1987) reported that injection of 1 per cent lidocaine into the region of the ipsilateral greater occipital nerve, followed by the injection of 160 mg of Depomedrol, relieved 18 of 20 patients for 5–73 (mean 20) days. We have found this helpful in some patients.

Antihistamines and histamine desensitization. Histamine desensitization has been used in the past but there is no evidence that it improves the natural history of cluster headache. A controlled clinical trial of the H_2 blocking agent, cimetidine, alone and in combination with the H_1 blocker, chlorpheniramine, demonstrated that these agents were ineffective in cluster headache (Anthony, Lord and Lance, 1978). A negative result for cimetidine has also been reported by Russell (1979).

Surgical treatment of chronic cluster headache

Occipital neurectomy

Three of seven patients subjected to ipsilateral occipital neurectomy obtained relief from chronic cluster headache for a period of 4–18 months (Anthony, 1987). The procedure is not a panacea for all cluster patients but can be a useful way to buy some time while trying other manoeuvres in the more intractable patients.

Section or decompression of the nervus intermedius and GSP nerve

The nervus intermedius (NI), the sensory component of the facial nerve, also contains those parasympathetic fibres that branch off as the GSP nerve. Surgical attacks on the NI began in the 1940s (Morgenlander and Wilkins, 1990). Sachs (1968) reported four cases of cluster headache relieved for up to 17 years by section of the NI, and later added three successes and two failures to this list (Sachs, 1970). Section of the GSP nerve relieved four out of five patients for periods of 1–5 years (Watson et al., 1983). Rowed (1990) divided the NI in eight patients with chronic cluster headache and found a loop or branch of the anterior inferior cerebellar artery in contact with the nerve in six out of eight cases, which he had not observed previously during 24 vestibular neurectomies for Ménière's disease. Of the eight patients operated on, two continued to have attacks without autonomic features and one had early post-operative recurrence with autonomic accompaniments before remitting. The other five patients experienced mild transient recurrence of headache with slight rhinorrhoea but no other autonomic disturbance. The results of combined NI and trigeminal section (Morgenlander and Wilkins, 1990) are discussed below. Solomon and Apfelbaum (1986) found compression of the facial nerve in 5 chronic cluster headache patients with partial relief in 2 after decompression. A variation on this approach is to use radio-frequency lesioning of one of the important outflow ganglia for the facial nerve, the sphenopalatine ganglion. This is reported to give complete or partial relief to 86% of 56 patients with episode cluster headache and 60% of 10 patients with chronic cluster headache (Sanders and Zuurmond, 1997). It should be compared with local anaesthetic injection at some future time.

Operations on the trigeminal nerve

Thermocoagulation of the Gasserian ganglion (ganglio-rhizolysis) relieved five out of eight patients with chronic cluster headache for follow-up periods of 7–59 months, although one continued to have episodes of flushing, lacrimation and nasal congestion without pain (Maxwell, 1982). The pains recurred in three patients but in two remained mild. Watson et al. (1983) reported 13 patients subjected to 27 radio-frequency lesions with significant relief in 12 for at least 5 months. The best improvement was obtained in those patients with post-operative anaesthesia in the previously most painful area. Onofrio and Campbell (1986) treated 16 patients by radio-frequency lesions with good or excellent results in 10, and 10 patients by trigeminal rhizotomy with excellent results in six. Surgical section of the first division of the trigeminal nerve provided pain relief in 12 of the patients operated on in the series described by Kirkpatrick, O'Brien and MacCabe (1993).

Morgenlander and Wilkins (1990) partially sectioned the trigeminal sensory root as well as cutting the NI in nine patients and performed one or the other procedure in another four patients. All but one suffered recurrence of headache after latencies of 2 days to 2 years. Curiously, the recurrent attacks of pain were associated with the usual autonomic symptoms. The authors commented that 'because of the variable and extensive branching of the nervus intermedius, it is difficult to identify and section all of its components'.

Four patients with cluster-tic syndrome (see below) underwent decompression surgery of the trigeminal nerve (and the facial nerve as well in two cases). The tic component disappeared in all four, but the cluster headache reappeared in modified form (Solomon, Apfelbaum and Guglielmo, 1985). Lesions of the Gasserian ganglion produced by glycerol injection relieved four out of seven patients with chronic cluster headache, improvement being correlated with the extent of sensory loss around the eye (Ekbom et al., 1987).

Conclusion

One must agree with Watson et al. (1983) that 'no one procedure gives consistent longlasting relief' from cluster headache. Surgical procedures should be reserved for patients unresponsive to a full trial of medical treatment, with radio-frequency lesions of the trigeminal ganglion giving the most satisfactory result. Success depends on producing anaesthesia in the affected area, which usually means loss of the corneal reflex with the resulting hazard of infection and ulceration of the cornea. Some patients (about 3 per cent) develop anaesthesia dolorosa after radio-frequency lesions or trigeminal root section. One of our patients lost his chronic cluster headache after trigeminal root section but developed an identical recurrent pain on the opposite side 3 days later. In those patients with tenderness over the greater occipital nerve on the symptomatic side, local steroid injections or occipital neurectomy are worth a trial as being the least invasive of surgical measures.

Conditions sharing clinical features with cluster headache

In recent times a number of rare but very characteristic clinical syndromes have been recognized which share some of the clinical features of cluster headache. These syndromes involve headache which is usually short-lasting with associated autonomic symptomatology (trigeminal autonomic cephalgias) and many have the characteristic of responding almost exclusively to treatment with indomethacin 25-50 mg three times daily (Goadsby and Lipton, 1997). It is not clear whether these syndromes share the same underlying pathogenetic mechanisms, although they seem to share a common final pathway of expression, the trigeminal-autonomic reflex that involves the facial (VIIth) cranial nerve (Goadsby and Duckworth, 1987). It has now been demonstrated that calcitonin gene-related peptide (CGRP) and vasoactive intestinal polypeptide (VIP) (see Chapter 8) are elevated in attacks of both cluster headache (Goadsby and Edvinsson, 1994) and chronic paroxysmal hemicrania (Goadsby and Edvinsson, 1996).

Episodic paroxysmal hemicrania

Attacks with the characteristics of cluster headache but of brief duration, recurring many times in each day and responding to indomethacin, were described by Sjaastad and Dale (1974) and named by them chronic paroxysmal hemicrania (CPH). More recently an episodic form has been recognized (Blau and Engel, 1990; Goadsby and Lipton, 1997; Kudrow, Esperanca and Vijayan, 1987; Newman et al., 1992a) in which the pain lasted a mean of 15 minutes, recurred 6–30 times daily for 3–16 weeks, and responded to indomethacin. Remissions varied from 3 months to 3 years.

Chronic paroxysmal hemicrania (CPH)

Sjaastad et al. (1980) reported eight definite cases of CPH, seven of whom were female, and 10 possible cases, eight female. The mean daily frequency of attacks varied from 7 to 22 with the pain persisting from 5 to 45 minutes on each occasion. The site and associated autonomic phenomena were similar to cluster headache, but the attacks of CPH were suppressed completely by indomethacin in doses ranging from 12.5 to 250 mg/24 hours. Antonaci and Sjaastad (1989) reviewed the 84 cases (59 females, 25 males) recorded in the literature to that time. A history of remission was obtained in 35 cases whereas 49 were truly 'chronic'. The headache had consistently affected the same side of the head in all but three patients.

Secondary CPH is well described and investigations are required to identify or exclude treatable underlying causes. A reasonably complete screen of a patient with CPH, considering the associated clinical problems reported, would include a blood count, looking for thrombocythemia (MacMillan and Nukada, 1989), ESR and vasculitic investigations (Medina, 1992), and a brain imaging procedure to look for an intracranial tumour such as a lesion in the region of the sella turcica (Gawel and Rothbart, 1992; Vijayan, 1992) or elsewhere (Medina, 1992). Other structural mimics of CPH include an arteriovenous malformation (Newman et al., 1992b) or cavernous sinus meningioma. Secondary CPH is more likely if the patient requires high doses (>200 mg per day) of indomethacin (Sjaastad et al., 1995). Should the pain become bilateral then a lumbar puncture should be carried out to look for intracranial hypertension, even in the face of a response to indomethacin (Hannerz and Jogestrand, 1993). When appropriate an electrocardiogram and Holter monitor should be considered to look for bundle branch block or atrial fibrillation (Russell and Storstein, 1984) and a chest X-ray should be considered to look for a Pancoast tumour (Delreux, Kevers and Callewaert, 1989).

Shortlasting unilateral neuralgiform headache attacks with conjunctival injection and tearing (SUNCT syndrome)

As the duration of the cluster-like syndromes becomes shorter, their names become longer. Sjaastad et al. (1989) reported three male patients whose brief attacks of pain in and around one eye were associated with sudden conjunctival injection and other autonomic features of cluster headache. Attacks lasted only 15–60 seconds and recurred 5–30 times per hour. One patient later had some involvement of the other eye. Attacks could be precipitated by chewing or eating certain foods, such as citrus fruits, and were not abolished by indomethacin or carbamazepine. Sjaastad *et al.* (1991) added the case history of another man with sporadic attacks of this sort in whom the diagnosis became clear only when he developed 20 or more such episodes in a day. Attacks could be brought on by touching his nose, eyelids or supraorbital area (including his hair in the trigeminally innervated area), as well as by certain movements, particularly of the neck. Of the patients recognized with this problem, males dominate with a ratio of 17 to 2 (Pareja and Sjaastad, 1994).

The paroxysms of pain usually last between 5 and 250 seconds (Pareja *et al.*, 1996) and one of us has witnessed attacks of 2 minutes duration, although longer, duller interictal pains have been recognized, as have attacks up to 2 hours in two patients (Pareja, Joubert and Sjaastad, 1996). Patients may have up to 30 episodes an hour, although more usually would have five to six per hour. The frequency may also vary in bouts. A frequency as low as once or twice in 1–4 weeks has been seen in a male patient who at other times had up to 20 attacks a day (Sjaastad *et al.*, 1991). A systematic study of attack frequency demonstrated a mean of 28 attacks per day with a range of six to 77 (Pareja *et al.*, 1996).

The conjunctival injection seen with SUNCT is often the most prominent autonomic feature and tearing may also be very obvious and has certainly been impressive in the patients that we have seen. Other less prominent autonomic stigmata include sweating of the forehead or rhinorrhoea. The attacks may become bilateral but the most severe pain remains unilateral. Most cases have some associated precipitating factors, particularly neck movements (Becser and Berky, 1995).

Secondary SUNCT and associations

There have been three reported patients with secondary SUNCT syndromes. The first two patients had homolateral cerebellopontine angle arteriovenous malformations diagnosed on MRI (Bussone *et al.*, 1991; De Benedittis, 1996). The third patient had a cavernous hemangioma of the brain stem seen only on MRI (Morales *et al.*, 1994). A posterior fossa lesion causing otherwise typical SUNCT has also been noted in HIV/AIDS (Graff-Radford, personal communication). These cases highlight the need for cranial MRI in investigating for secondary SUNCT. Just as there is a reported associated case of CPH and trigeminal neuralgia there is a single report of a patient with trigeminal neuralgia who developed a SUNCT syndrome (Bouhassira *et al.*, 1994). These cases suggest that the trigeminal pathways may be involved in the entire range of short-lasting headache syndromes.

Cluster-tic syndrome

Sudden jabs of pain resembling trigeminal neuralgia may be experienced by patients suffering from cluster headache or CPH and one of us has recently seen the coexistence in a patient with episodic paroxysmal hemicrania. Sjaastad (1992) called this the 'jabs and jolts syndrome'. Lance and Anthony (1971) commented on tic-like pains in three of their cluster headache patients and described an additional case where the typical lancinating pains of trigeminal neuralgia culminated in an attack of cluster headache. The stabbing pains in this case were felt in the right upper and lower jaw, and after 3 months radiated to the right temple. Pain then started in the right temple and persisted for 30 minutes, associated with watering of the right eye and nostril. These cluster-like episodes then recurred three times daily for some weeks. After 1 month, the pain spread from temple to vertex, appeared two or three times daily and persisted for 30–90 minutes on each occasion, These headaches then ceased but the jabbing pains persisted. The cluster-type headaches recurred for 5 days every 2 months for 3 years. When the tic-like pain was controlled by carbamazepine, the cluster headaches ceased.

In general the cluster headache component spans the range of typical cluster headache, attacks lasting 45 minutes with autonomic features such as lacrimation and nasal blocking, through to shorter attacks of 30 seconds at a frequency of 40 a day, more suggestive of a paroxysmal hemicrania (Alberca and Ochoa, 1994). There have been many other reports in the literature of a similar association (Diamond, Freitag and Cohen, 1984; Solomon, Apfelbaum and Guglielmo, 1985; Watson and Evans, 1985). We agree with these authors that the relationship is more than coincidental.

Other possibly related syndromes

Kudrow (1980), in his comprehensive monograph on cluster headache, recognizes 'cluster-migraine' as an entity in which migraine patients have some of the characteristics of cluster headache, and 'cluster-vertigo' for recurrent attacks of giddiness associated with bouts of cluster headache. The latter term has been criticized by Vijayan (1990) who pointed out that, when Ménière's disease and cluster headache affect the same patient, the conditions recur independently. Diamond, Mogabgab and Diamond (1982) put forward the concept of 'cluster headache variant', a combination of constant vascular headache with episodic exacerbations and sudden stabs of pain, mostly controlled by indomethacin. Does the response to indomethacin of chronic paroxysmal hemicrania, exertional headache and jabbing 'ice-pick' head pains (Mathew, 1981) imply a common underlying factor? Until the pathophysiology of headache is more clearly understood it is difficult to classify many of the variations seen in clinical practice.

Overview

Cluster headache must surely be mediated by paroxysmal discharge of central neurones that in turn permit trigeminal and parasympathetic nervous over-activity. Given the recent PET data it is most likely that the hypothalamic grey matter which contains the circadian or clock areas is the candidate for the fundamental driving or permissive area of the brain. The pain and autonomic phenomena usually develop together but one may precede the other or occur in isolation, as is particularly evident after section of the trigeminal root or nervus intermedius as described above. The fact that the pain of cluster headache may continue or recur after one or both of these surgical procedures further indicates its central origin. This does not deny the important contribution to pain made by the cerebral arteries or the efficacy of vasoconstrictor agents like sumatriptan and ergotamine in breaking the interaction between trigeminal nerves and blood vessels to relieve the pain. The ocular Horner's syndrome on the painful side is most readily explained as a post-ganglionic lesion of the cervical sympathetic nerves in the pericarotid plexus, which masks the effects of general sympathetic activation during the attack.

The distinctive clinical picture of cluster headache leaves no excuse for any delay in diagnosis or in applying the appropriate treatment. Most individual attacks respond well to oxygen inhalation or subcutaneous sumatriptan, if they have not already been helped by ergotamine. Most bouts of cluster headache can be brought under control by a course of steroids or prophylactic medication with verapamil, methysergide or ergotamine. Lithium and perhaps valproate have a place in the management of refractory cases. Rarely does one have to consider surgical intervention.

The challenge for future research is to understand the mechanism by which hypothalamic activation translates into pain and at what level in the central nervous system preventative drugs have their actions.

References

Alberca, R. and Ochoa, J. J. (1994). Cluster tic syndrome. *Neurology* **44**, 996–999

Anthony, M. (1987). The role of the occipital nerve in unilateral headache. In *Current Problems in Neurology: 4. Advances in Headache Research*, Ed. F. Clifford Rose. pp. 251–262. London, John Libbey

Anthony, M. and Lance J. W. (1971). Histamine and serotonin in cluster headache. *Arch. Neurol.* **25**, 225–229

Anthony, M., Lord, G. D. A. and Lance, J. W. (1978). Controlled trials of cimetidine in migraine and cluster headache. *Headache* **18**, 261–264

Antonaci, F. and Sjaastad, O. (1989). Chronic paroxysmal hemicrania (CPH): a review of the clinical manifestations. *Headache* **29**, 648–656

Appenzeller, O., Becker, W. J. and Ragaz, A. (1981). Cluster Headache. Ultrastructural aspects and pathogenic mechanisms. *Arch. Neurol.* **38**, 302–306

Becser, N. and Berky, M. (1995). SUNCT syndrome: a Hungarian case. *Headache* **35**, 158–160

Blau, J. N. and Engel, H. (1990). Episodic paroxysmal hemicrania: a further case and review of the literature. *J. Neurol. Neurosurg. Psychiat.* **53**, 343–344

Boiardi, A., Bussone, E., Martini, M. *et al.* (1983). Endocrinological responses in cluster headache. *J. Neurol. Neurosurg. Psychiat.* **46**, 956–958

Bouhassira, D., Attal, N., Esteve, M. and Chauvin, M. (1994). SUNCT syndrome. A case of transformation from trigeminal neuralgia. *Cephalalgia* **14**, 168–170

Broch, A., Horven, I., Nornes, H., Sjaastad, O. and Tonjum, A. (1970). Studies on cerebral and ocular circulation in a patient with cluster headache. *Headache* **10**, 1–8

Brooke, R. I. (1978). Periodic migrainous neuralgia: a cause of dental pain. *Oral Surg. Oral Med. Oral Pathol.* **46**, 511–516

Bussone, G., Leone, M., Peccarisi, C. *et al.* (1990). Double blind comparison of lithium and verapamil in cluster headache prophylaxis. *Headache* **30**, 411–417

Bussone, G., Leone, M., Volta, G. D., Strada, L. and Gasparotti, R. (1991). Short-lasting unilateral neuralgiform headache attacks with tearing and conjunctival injection: the first symptomatic case. *Cephalalgia* **11**, 123–127

Bussone, G., Leone, M., Zappacosta, B. M., Maltempo, C. and Parnti, A. E. (1992). A unifying concept of neuroendocrine dysfunctions in cluster headache. Paper presented at the *9th Migraine Trust International Symposium*, London, Sept. 7–10

Caviness, V. S. and O'Brien, P. (1980). Cluster headache: response to chlorpromazine. *Headache* **20**, 128–131

Cremer, P., Halmagyi, G. M. and Goadsby, P. J. (1995). Secondary cluster headache responsive to sumatriptan. *J. Neurol. Neurosurg. Psychiat.* **59**, 633–634

Curran, D. A., Hinterberger, H. and Lance, J. W. (1967). Methysergide. *Res. Clin. Studies Headache* **1**, 74–122

Cuypers, J. and Altenkirch, H. (1979). HLA antigens in cluster headache. *Headache* **19**, 228–229

Cuypers, J., Altenkirch, H. and Bunge, S. (1981). Personality profiles in cluster headache and migraine. *Headache* **21**, 21–24

Dahl, A., Russell, D., Nyberg-Hansen, R. and Rootwelt, K. (1990). Cluster headache: transcranial Doppler ultrasound and rCBF studies. *Cephalalgia* **10**, 87–94

D'Alessandro, R., Gamberini, G., Benassi, G., Morganti, G., Cortelli, P. and Lugaresi, E. (1986). Cluster headache in the Republic of San Marino. *Cephalalgia* **6**, 159–162

D'Andrea, G., Welch, K. M. A., Cananzi, A. R. *et al.* (1989). Reduced noradrenaline and adrenaline turnover in cluster headache: biochemical evidence for sympathetic hypofunction. In *New Advances in Headache Research*, Ed. F. Clifford Rose. pp. 199–202. London, Smith-Gordon

De Benedittis, G. (1996). SUNCT syndrome associated with cavernous angioma of the brain stem. *Cephalalgia* **16**, 503–506

Delepine, L., Bergerot, A., Henry, P. and Aubineau, P. (1996). Parasympathetic stimulation induces plasma protein extravasation in the rat dura mater. *Cephalalgia* **16**, 370

Delreux, V., Kevers, L. and Callewaert, A. (1989). Hemicranie paroxystique inaugurant un syndrome de Pancoast. *Rev. Neurolog.* **145**, 151–152

Diamond, S., Freitag, F. G. and Cohen, J. S. (1984). Cluster headache with trigeminal neuralgia. An uncommon association that may be more than coincidental. *Postgrad. Med.* **75**, 165–172

Diamond, S., Mogabgab, E. R. and Diamond, M. (1982). Cluster headache variant: spectrum of a new headache syndrome responsive to indomethacin. In *Advances in Migraine Research and Therapy*, Ed. F. Clifford Rose. pp. 57–65. New York, Raven Press

Dimitriadou, V., Henry, P., Brochet, B., Mathiau, P. and Aubineau, P. (1990). Cluster headache: ultra-structural evidence for mast cell degranulation and interaction with nerve fibres in the human temporal artery. *Cephalalgia* **10**, 221–228

Drummond, P. D. (1988). Autonomic disturbance in cluster headache. *Brain* **111**, 1199–1209

Drummond, P. D. and Lance, J. W. (1984). Thermographic changes in cluster headache. *Neurology* **34**, 1292–1298

Drummond, P. D. and Lance, J. W. (1985). Clinical symptoms and thermographic asymmetry in cluster headache. In *Migraine: Clinical and Research Advances*, Ed. F. Clifford Rose. pp. 155–161. Basel, Karger

Drummond, P. D. and Lance, J. W. (1992). Pathological sweating and flushing accompanying the trigeminal lacrimation reflex in patients with cluster headache and in patients with a confirmed site of cervical sympathetic deficit. Evidence for parasympathetic crossinnervation. *Brain* **115**, 1429–1445

Ekbom, K. (1970). A clinical comparison of cluster headache and migraine. *Acta Neurol. Scand.* **46** (Suppl. 41), 1

Ekbom, K. (1975). Some observations on pain in cluster headache. *Headache* **14**, 219–225

Ekbom, K. (1977). Lithium in the treatment of chronic cluster headache. *Headache* **17**, 39–40

Ekbom, K. (1981). Lithium for cluster headache: review of the literature and preliminary results of long-term treatment. *Headache* **21**, 132–139

Ekbom, K. (1991). Treatment of acute cluster headache with sumatriptan. *N. Eng. J. Med.* **325**, 322–326

Ekbom, K., Ahlborg, B. and Schele, R. (1978). Prevalence of migraine and cluster headache in Swedish men of 18. *Headache* **18**, 9–19

Ekbom, K. and Greitz, T. (1970). Carotid angiography in cluster headache. *Acta Radio. (Diagn.)* **10**, 177–186

Ekbom, K., Hardebo, J. E. and Waldenlind, E. (1988). Mechanisms of cluster headache. In *Basic Mechanisms of Headache*, Eds J. Olesen and L. Edvinsson. pp. 463–476. Amsterdam, Elsevier

Ekbom, K., Lindgren, L., Nilsson, B. Y., Hardebo, J. E. and Waldenlind, E. (1987). Retro-Gasserian glycerol injection in the treatment of chronic cluster headache. *Cephalalgia* **7**, 21–27

Ekbom, K., Waldenlind, E., Cole, J. A., Pilgrim, A. J. and Kirkham, A. (1997). Sumatriptan in chronic cluster headache: results of continuous treatment for eleven months. *Cephalalgia* **12**, 254–256

Evers, S., Soros, P., Brilla, R., Gerding, H. and Husstedt, I.-W. (1997). Cluster headache after orbital exenteration. *Cephalalgia* **17**, 680–682

Fanciullacci, M., Pietrini, U., Gatto, G., Boccuni, M. and Sicuteri, F. (1982). Latent dysautonomic pupillary lateralization in cluster headache: a pupillometric study. *Cephalalgia* **2**, 135–144

Fanciullacci, M., Alessandri, M., Figini, M., Geppetti, P. and Michelacci, S. (1995). Increases in plasma calcitonin gene-related peptide from extracerebral circulation during nitroglycerin-induced cluster headache attack. *Pain* **60**, 119–123

Fogan, L. (1985). Treatment of cluster headache: a double blind comparison of oxygen vs. air inhalation. *Arch. Neurol.* **42**, 362–363

Gabai, I. J. and Spierings, E. L. H. (1989). Prophylactic treatment of cluster headache with verapamil. *Headache* **29**, 167–168

Gawel, M., Krajewski, A., Luo, Y. M. and Ichise, M. (1990). The cluster diathesis. *Headache* **30**, 652–655

Gawel, M. J. and Rothbart, P. (1992). Chronic paroxysmal hemicrania which appears to arise from either third ventricle pathology or internal carotid artery pathology. *Cephalalgia* **12**, 327

Goadsby, P. J. (1994). Cluster headache and the clinical profile of sumatriptan. *Eur. Neurol.* **34** (Suppl.), 35–39

Goadsby, P. J. and Duckworth, J. W (1987). Effect of stimulation of trigeminal ganglion on regional cerebral blood flow in cats. *Am. J. Physiol.* **253**, R270–R274

Goadsby, P. J. and Edvinsson, L. (1994). Human *in vivo* evidence for trigeminovascular activation in cluster headache. *Brain* **117**, 427–434

Goadsby, P. J. and Edvinsson, L. (1996). Neuropeptide changes in a case of chronic paroxysmal hemicrania – evidence for trigemino-parasympathetic activation. *Cephalalgia* **16**, 448–450

Goadsby, P. J. and Hoskin, K. L. The distribution of trigeminovascular afferents in the non-human primate brain *Macaca nemestrina*: a c-fos immunocytochemical study. *J. Anatomy* **190**, 367–375

Goadsby, P. J., Hoskin, K. L. and Knight, Y. E. (1997). Stimulation of the greater occipital nerve increases metabolic activity in the trigeminal nucleus caudalis and cervical dorsal horn of the cat. *Pain* **73**, 23–28

Goadsby, P. J. and Lance, J. W. (1988). Brainstem effects on intra- and extracerebral circulations. Relation to migraine and cluster headache. In *Basic Mechanisms of Headache*, Eds J. Olesen and L. Edvinsson. pp. 413–427. Amsterdam, Elsevier Science Publishers

Goadsby, P. J. and Lipton, R. B. (1997). A review of paroxysmal hemicranias, SUNCT syndrome and other short-lasting headaches with autonomic features, including new cases. *Brain* **120**, 193–209

Graham, J. R. (1972). Cluster headache. *Headache* **11**, 175–185

Hannerz, J. and Jogestrand, T. (1993). Intracranial hypertension and sumatriptan efficacy in a case of chronic paroxysmal hemicrania which became bilateral. (The mechanism of indomethacin in CPH). *Headache* **33**, 320–323

Hardebo, J. E. (1993). Subcutaneous sumatriptan in cluster headache: A time study in the effect of pain and autonomic symptoms. *Headache* **33**, 18–21

Harris, W. (1936). Ciliary (migrainous) neuralgia and its treatment. *Br. Med. J.* **1**, 457–460

Headache Classification Committee of The International Headache Society (1988). Classification and diagnostic criteria for headache disorders, cranial neuralgias and facial pain. *Cephalalgia* **8** (Suppl. 7), 1–96

Heidegger, S., Mattfeldt, T., Rieber, A. *et al.* (1997). Orbito-sphenoidal aspergillus infection mimicking cluster headache: a case report. *Cephalalgia* **17**, 676–679

Hering, R., Couturier, E. G. M., Davies, P. T. G. and Steiner, T. J. (1991). ^{99m}Tc-HMPAO study during cluster headache period and in acute attacks. In *Migraine and Other Headaches. The Vascular Mechanisms*, Ed. J. Olesen, pp. 297–299. New York, Raven Press

Horton, B. T., MacLean, A. R. and Craig, W. M. (1939). A new syndrome of vascular headache; results of treatment with histamine; a preliminary report. *Proc. Mayo Clinic* **14**, 250–257

Hørven, I. and Sjaastad, O. (1977). Cluster headache syndrome and migraine: ophthalmological support for a two-entity theory. *Acta Ophthalmol. (Cophenhagen)* **55**, 35–51

Hunter, C. R. and Mayfield, F. H. (1949). Role of the upper cervical roots in the production of pain in the head. *Am. J. Surg.* **78**, 743–749

Jammes, J. L. (1975). The treatment of cluster headaches with prednisone. *Dis. Nerv. Syst.* **36**, 375–376

Kirkpatrick, P. J., O'Brien, M. D. and MacCabe, J. J. (1993). Trigeminal nerve section for chronic migrainous neuralgia. *Br. J. Neurosurg.* **7**(5), 483–490

Kittrelle, J. P., Grouse, D. S. and Seybold, M. (1985). Cluster headache: local anesthetic abortive agents. *Arch. Neurol.* **42**, 496–498

Koenigsberg, A. D., Solomon, G. D. and Kosmorsky, D. O. (1994). Pseudoaneurysm within the cavernous sinus presenting as cluster headache. *Headache* **34**, 111–113

Krabbe, A. A., Henriksen, L. and Olesen, J. (1984). Tomographic determination of cerebral blood flow during attacks of cluster headache. *Cephalalgia* **4**, 17–23

Kudrow, L. (1980). *Cluster Headache: Mechanisms and Management.* Oxford, Oxford University Press

Kudrow, L. (1981). Response of cluster headache attacks to oxygen inhalation. *Headache* **21**, 1–4

Kudrow, L., Esperanca, P. and Vijayan, N. (1987). Episodic paroxysmal hemicrania? *Cephalalgia* **7**, 197–201

Kudrow, L. and Sutkus, B. J. (1979). MMPI pattern specificity in primary headache disorders. *Headache* **19**, 18–24

Kunkel, R. S. (1981). Eleven clues to cluster headache – and tips on drug therapy. *Mod. Med. Aust.* September, 14–21

Kunkle, E. C. (1959). Acetylcholine in the mechanism of headaches of the migraine type. *Arch. Neurol. Psychiat.* **84**, 135–140

Kunkle, E. C. and Anderson, W. B. (1961). Significance of minor eye signs in headache of migraine type. *Arch. Ophthalmol. Chicago* **65**, 504–508

Kunkle, E. C., Pfieffer, J. B., Wilhoit, W. M. and Hamrick, L. W. (1952). Recurrent brief headache in cluster pattern. *Trans. Am. Neurol. Assoc.* **27**, 240–243

Kuritzky, A. (1984). Cluster headache-like pain caused by an upper cervical meningioma. *Cephalalgia* **4**, 185–186

Lance, J. W. and Anthony, M. (1966). Some clinical aspects of migraine: a prospective survey of 500 patients. *Arch. Neurol.* **15**, 356–361

Lance, J. W. and Anthony, M. (1971). Migrainous neuralgia or cluster headache? *J. Neurol. Sci.* **13**, 401–414

Lance, J. W. and Drummond, P. D. (1987). Horner's syndrome in cluster headache. In *Current Problems in Neurology: 4. Advances in Headache Research*, Ed. F. Clifford Rose. pp. 169–174. London, John Libbey

Leone, M., Attanasio, A., Croci, D. *et al.* (1997). The *m*-chlorophenylpiperazine test in cluster headache: a study on central serotoninergic activity. *Cephalalgia* **17**, 666–672

Leone, M., Maltempo, C., Parati, E. A. and Bussone, G. (1994). A unifying concept of neuroendrocrine dystunction in cluster headache. In *New Advances in Headache Research: 3*, Ed. F. Clifford Rose. pp. 207–211. London, Smith Gordon

MacMillan, J. C. and Nukada, H. (1989). Chronic paroxysmal hemicrania. *N.Z. Med. J.* **102**, 251–252

Mani, S. and Deeter, J. (1982). Arteriovenous malformation of the brain presenting as a cluster headache – a case report. *Headache* **22**, 184–185

Manzoni, G. C., Terzano, M. G., Bono, G., Micieli, G., Martucci, N. and Nappi, G. (1983). Cluster headache – clinical findings in 180 patients. *Cephalalgia* **3**, 21–30

Mathew, N. T. (1981). Indomethacin-responsive headache syndromes. *Headache* **21**, 147–150

Maxwell, R. E. (1982). Surgical control of chronic migrainous neuralgia by trigeminal ganglio-rhizolysis. *J. Neurosurg.* **57**, 459–466

May, A., Bahra, A., Büchel, C., Frackowiak, R. S. J. and Goadsby, P. J. (1998a). Hypothalamic activation in cluster headache attacks. *Lancet* **351**, 275–278

May, A., Kaube, H., Büchel, C., Eichten, C., Rijntjes, M., Jueptner, M., *et al.* (1998b). Experimental cranial pain elicited by capsaicin: a PET-study. *Pain* **74**, 61–66.

May, A., Shepheard, S., Wessing, A., Hargreaves, R. J., Goadsby, P. J. and Diener, H. C. (1998c). Retinal plasma extravasation can be evoked by trigeminal stimulation in rat but does not occur during migraine attacks. *Brain* **121**, 1231–1237.

Medina, J. L. (1992). Organic headaches mimicking chronic paroxysmal hemicrania. *Headache* **32**, 73–74

Medina, J. L., Diamond, S. and Fareed, J. (1979). The nature of cluster headache. *Headache* **19**, 309–322

Medina, J. L., Fareed, J. and Diamond, S. (1980). Lithium carbonate therapy for cluster headache. Changes in number of platelets and serotonin and histamine levels. *Arch. Neurol.* **37**, 559–563

Meyer, J. S., Kawamura, J. and Terayama, Y. (1991). CT-CBF and ^{133}Xe inhalation cerebral blood flow studies in cluster headache. In *Migraine and Other Headaches. The Vascular Mechanisms*, Ed. J. Olesen. pp. 305–310. New York, Raven Press

Monstad, I., Krabbe, A., Micieli, G. *et al.* (1995). Preemptive oral treatment with sumatriptan during a cluster period. *Headache* **35**, 607–613

Morales, F., Mostacero, E., Marta, J. and Sanchez, S. (1994). Vascular malformation of the cerebello-pontine angle associated with SUNCT syndrome. *Cephalalgia* **14**, 301–302

Morgenlander, J. C. and Wilkins, R. H. (1990). Surgical treatment of cluster headache. *J. Neurosurg.* **72**, 866–871

Nappi, G. and Martignoni, E. (1988). Significance of hormonal changes in primary headache disorders. In *Basic Mechanisms of Headache*, Eds J. Olesen and L. Edvinsson. pp. 287–298. Amsterdam, Elsevier

Newman, L. C., Gordon, M. L., Lipton, R. B., Kanner, R. and Solomon, S. (1992a). Episodic paroxysmal hemicrania: two new cases and a literature review. *Neurology* **42**, 964–966

Newman, L. C., Herskovitz, S., Lipton, R. and Solomon, S. (1992b). Chronic paroxysmal headache: two cases with cerebrovascular disease. *Headache* **32**, 75–76

Nieman, E. A. and Hurwitz, L. J. (1961). Ocular sympathetic palsy in periodic migrainous neuralgia. *J. Neurol. Neurosurg. Psychiat.* **24**, 269–373

Onofrio, B. M. and Campbell, J. K. (1986). Surgical treatment of chronic cluster headache. *Proc. Mayo Clinic* **61**, 537–541

Pareja, J. A., Joubert, J. and Sjaastad, O. (1996). SUNCT syndrome. Atypical temporal patterns. *Headache* **36**, 108–110

Pareja, J. A., Ming, J. M., Kruszewski, P., Caballero, V., Pamo, M. and Sjaastad, O. (1996). SUNCT syndrome: duration, frequency and temporal distribution of attacks. *Headache* **36**, 161–165

Pareja, J. A. and Sjaastad, O. (1994). SUNCT syndrome in the female. *Headache* **34**, 217–220

Procacci, P., Zoppi, M., Maresca, M., Zamponi, A., Fanciullacci, M. and Sicuteri, F. (1989). Lateralisation of pain in cluster headache. *Pain* **38**, 275–278

Romberg, M. H. (1840). *A Manual of Nervous Diseases of Man.* Trsl. E. G. Sieveking. p. 56. London, Sydenham Society, 1853

Rowed, D. W. (1990). Chronic cluster headache managed by nervus intermedius section. *Headache* **30**, 401–406

Russell, D. (1979). Cluster headache: trial of a combined histamine H1 and H2 treatment. *J. Neurol. Neurosurg. Psychiat.* **42**, 668–669

Russell, D. and Storstein, L. (1983). Cluster headache: a computerized analysis of 24 h Holter ECG recordings and description of ECG rhythm disturbances. *Cephalalgia* **3**, 83–107

Russell, D. and Storstein, L. (1984). Chronic paroxysmal hemicrania: heart rate changes and ECG rhythm disturbances. A computerized analysis of 24 h ambulatory ECG recordings. *Cephalalgia* **4**, 135–144

Russell, M. B., Andersson, P. G. and Iselius, L. (1996). Cluster headache is an inherited disorder in some families. *Headache* **36**, 608–612

Russell, M. B., Andersson, P. G., Thomsen, L. L. and Iselius, L. (1995). Cluster headache is an autosomal dominantly inherited disorder in some families: a complex segregation analysis. *J. Med. Genet.* **32**, 954–956

Sachs, E. J. (1968). The role of the nervus intermedius in facial neuralgia. Report of four cases with observations on the pathways for taste, lacrimation, and pain in the face. *J. Neurosurg.* **28**, 56–60

Sachs, E. J. (1970). Further observations on surgery of the nervus intermedius. *Headache* **9**, 159–161

Salvesen, R., Bogucki, A., Wysocka-Bakowska, M. M., Antonaci, F., Fredriksen, T. A. and Sjaastad, O. (1987). Cluster headache pathogenesis: a pupillometric study. *Cephalalgia* **7**, 273–284

Salvesen, R., Sand, T. and Sjaastad, O. (1988). Cluster headache: combined assessment with pupillometry and evaporimetry. *Cephalalgia* **8**, 211–218

Sanders, M. and Zuurmond, W. (1997). Efficacy of sphenopalatine ganglion blockade in 66 patients suffering from cluster headache: A 12- to 70-month follow-up evaluation. *J. Neurosurg.* **87**, 876–880

Sandrini, G., Alfonso, E., Ruiz, L. *et al.* (1991). Impairment of corneal pain perception in cluster headache. *Pain* **47**, 299–304

Saunte, C. (1984). Autonomic disorders in cluster headaehe, with special referenee to salivation, nasal secretion and tearing. *Cephalalgia* **4**, 57–64

Sianard-Gainko, J., Milet, J., Ghuysen, V. and Schoenen, J. (1994). Increased parasellar activity on gallium SPECT is not specific for active cluster headache. *Cephalalgia* **14**, 132–133

Sicuteri, F., Fanciullacci, M., Nicolodi, M. *et al.* (1990). Substance P theory: a unique focus on the painful and painless phenomena of cluster headache. *Headache* **30**, 69–79

Sjaastad, O. (1992). *Cluster Headache Syndrome*. London, Saunders

Sjaastad, O., Apfelbaum, R., Caskey, W. *et al.* (1980). Chronic paroxysmal hemicrania (CPH). The clinical manifestations. A review. *Uppsala J. Med. Sci.* **31** (Suppl.), 27–33

Sjaastad, O. and Dale, I. (1974). Evidence for a new (?) treatable headache entity. *Headache* **14**, 105–108

Sjaastad, O. and Rinck, P. (1990). Cluster headache. MRI studies of the cavernous sinus and base of the brain. *Headache* **30**, 350–351

Sjaastad, O., Saunte, C., Salvesen, R. *et al.* (1989). Shortlasting unilateral neuralgiform headache attacks with conjunctival injection, tearing, sweating, and rhinorrhea. *Cephalalgia* **9**, 147–156

Sjaastad, O., Stovner, L. J., Stolt-Nielsen, A., Antonaci, F. and Fredriksen, T. A. (1995). CPH and hemicrania continua: requirements of high dose indomethacin dosages – an ominous sign? *Headache* **35**, 363–367

Sjaastad, O., Zhao, J. M., Kruszewski, P. and Stovner, L. J. (1991). Short-lasting unilateral neuralgiform headache attacks with conjunctival injection, tearing, etc. (SUNCT): III. Another Norwegian case. *Headache* **31**, 175–177

Sluder, G. (1910). The syndrome of sphenopalatine ganglion neurosis. *Am. J. Med.* **140**, 868–878

Solomon, S., Apfelbaum, R. I. and Guglielmo, K. M. (1985). The cluster-tic syndrome and its surgical therapy. *Cephalalgia* **5**, 83–89

Solomon, S. and Apfelbaum, R. I. (1986). Surgical decompression of the facial nerve in the treatment of chronic cluster headache. *Arch. Neurol.* **43**, 479–482

Steiner, T. J., Hering, R., Couturier, E. G. M., Davies, P. T. G. and Whitmarsh, T. E. (1997). Double-blind placebo controlled trial of lithium in episodic cluster headache. *Cephalalgia* **17**, 673–675

Sutherland, I. M. and Eadie, M. J. (1972). Cluster headache. *Res. Clin. Studies Headache* **3**, 92–125

Suzuki, N. and Hardebo, J. E. (1991). Anatomical basis for a parasympathetic and sensory innervation of the intracranial segment of the internal carotid artery in man. Possible implications for vascular headache. *J. Neurol. Sci.* **104**, 19–31

Swanson, J. W., Yanagihara, T., Stang, P. E. *et al.* (1994). Incidence of cluster headaches: a population-based study in Olmsted County, Minnesota. *Neurology* **44**, 433–437

Symonds, C. P. (1956). A particular variety of headache. *Brain* **79**, 217–232

Tfelt-Hansen, P., Paulson, O. B. and Krabbe, A. E. (1982). Invasive adenoma of the pituitary gland and chronic migrainous neuralgia. A rare coincidence or a causal relationship? *Cephalalgia* **2**, 25–28

Vail, H. H. (1932). Vidian neuralgia. *Ann. Otol. Rhinol. Laryngol.* **41**, 837–856

Vijayan, N. (1990). Cluster headache and vertigo. *Cephalalgia* **10**, 67–76

Vijayan, N. (1992). Symptomatic paroxysmal hemicrania. *Cephalalgia* **12**, 111–113

Vijayan, N. and Watson, C. (1985). Corneal sensitivity in cluster headache. *Headache* **25**, 104–106

Vincent, M. B., Ekman, R., Edvinsson, L., Sand, T. and Sjaastad, O. (1992). Reduction of calcitonin gene-related peptide in the jugular blood following electrical stimulation of rat greater occipital nerve. *Cephalalgia* **12**, 275–279

Waldenlind, E. and Gustafson, S. A. (1987). Prolactin in cluster headache: diurnal secretion, response to thyrotropin-releasing hormone, and relation to sex steroids and gonadotropins. *Cephalalgia* **7**, 43–54

Waldenlind, E., Gustafsson, S. A., Ekbom, K. and Wetterberg, L. (1987). Circadian secretion of cortisol and melatonin in cluster headache during active cluster periods and remission. *J. Neurol. Neurosurg. Psychiat.* **50**, 207–213

Watson, C. P., Morley, T. P., Richardson, J. C., Schutz, H. and Tasker, R. R. (1983). The surgical treatment of chronic cluster headache. *Headache* **23**, 289–299

Watson, P. and Evans, R. (1985). Cluster-tic syndrome. *Headache* **25**, 123–126

West, P. and Todman, D. (1991). Chronic cluster headache associated with a vertebral artery aneurysm. *Headache* **31**, 210–212

Chapter 12

Other headaches without any structural abnormality

Many otherwise normal people may have a headache when challenged by some sudden change in their internal or external environment or exposure to vasodilator agents. Others may experience transient jabs of pain in the head without apparent reason. Headache may be a symptom of an epileptic discharge and may follow complex partial seizures as well as tonic–clonic attacks. This miscellaneous group of headaches can be mediated by peripheral nerve irritability, dilatation of cranial blood vessels or discharge of central pain pathways without any pathological change being demonstrable in these structures.

Rasmussen and Olesen (1992) assessed the life-time prevalence of headache in 1000 people between the ages of 25 and 64 years. Idiopathic stabbing headache was reported by 2 per cent, external compression headache by 4 per cent and cold stimulus headache by 15 per cent. Hangover headache had been experienced by 72 per cent, fever headache by 63 per cent and benign cough headache, benign exertional headache and headaches associated with sexual activity each by 1 per cent in this survey.

The exploding head syndrome

This term was coined by Pearce (1988) to describe the night start that may awaken healthy individuals from sleep with the sensation of a loud bang in the head, like an explosion, sometimes associated with the perception of a flash of light. Patients may initially describe this inaccurately as a headache. It is probably a quasi-epileptic experience like the nocturnal myoclonic jerk that occurs in normal people on drifting off to sleep.

Idiopathic stabbing headache

Three varieties of stabbing headache have been described: 'ice-pick pains', 'jabs and jolts syndrome' and ophthalmodynia.

Ice-pick pains

Raskin and Schwartz (1980) described sharp jabbing pains in the head resembling a stab from an ice-pick, nail or needle. They compared the prevalence of such pains in 100 migraine patients (20 men, 80 women) and 100 headache-free controls (53 men, 47 women). Only three of the control subjects had experienced ice-pick pains compared with 42 of the migraine patients, of whom 60 per cent had more than one attack each month. The pains affected the temple or orbit more often than the parietal and occipital areas and often occurred before or during migraine headaches. Drummond and Lance (1984) obtained a history of ice-pick pains in 200 of 530 patients with recurrent headache (migraine and tension headache). The site of the ice-pick pains was recorded for 92 patients and coincided with the site of the patient's habitual headache in 37 (19 unilateral and 18 bilateral). This was most apparent when the ice-pick pains were restricted to one eye or temple.

Ice-pick pains have also been described in conjunction with cluster headaches, experienced in the same area as the cluster pain. Three out of 60 patients studied by Lance and Anthony (1971) and 11 of 33 patients examined by Ekbom (1975) described ice-pick pains during the cluster attack, becoming more frequent as the attack abated. Similar lancinating pains have been reported with temporal arteritis (Raskin and Schwartz, 1980), but we have not encountered this.

Jabs and jolts syndrome

Sjaastad (1992) first referred to sharp pains associated with chronic paroxysmal hemicrania (CPH) in 1979. He describes 'jabs and jolts' as sharp knife-like pains less than 1 minute in duration, occurring in patients with tension headache, migraine or cluster headache as well as in headache-free individuals. It is probable that these sensations are a variation on ice-pick pains but last longer and must be distinguished from episodes of CPH, which have a minimum duration of 3 minutes. Medina and Diamond (1981) reported multiple jabbing pains with episodic headaches, which they regarded as a cluster variant.

Ophthalmodynia

Sudden stabbing pain in the eye has been described as 'ophthalmodynia periodica'. Lansche (1964) reported that over 60 per cent of patients with this syndrome were migraine sufferers.

Pathophysiology and treatment of idiopathic stabbing headache

Although the mechanism of these transient pains is unknown, the lancinating quality of the pain resembles that of trigeminal neuralgia and suggests a paroxysmal neuronal discharge. The localization of stabbing pains to the habitual site of migraine or cluster headache may be a pointer to the pathophysiology of these conditions. While it is possible that there is a source of irritation in the peripheral branches of the trigeminal nerve, it would seem more likely that there is an intermittent deficit in central pain control mechanisms that permits the spontaneous synchronous discharge of neurones receiving impulses from the area to which headache is referred.

Mathew (1981) reported that five patients with this syndrome improved substantially while treated with indomethacin 50 mg 3 times daily and did not respond to aspirin or placebo. Medina and Diamond (1981) found that 20 patients who were subject to frequent jabbing pains (unilateral in 13 cases) in association with atypical vascular headaches responded well to indomethacin whereas Sjaastad (1992) stated that the response of 'jabs and jolts' to indomethacin was partial or lacking.

External compression

A tight hat, a band around the head, the wearing of a protective helmet by construction workers or the use of tight swimming goggles (Pestronk and Pestronk, 1983) may induce headache.

Exposure to cold

Exposure of the bare head to sub-zero temperatures or diving into cold water will cause headache, presumably from excessive stimulation of temperature-sensitive receptors in the face and scalp. Pain induced by dipping the top of the head into cold water ($<18°C$) reaches a peak in 60 seconds and spreads from the vertex to temples and occiput (Wolff and Hardy, 1941). The only areas of the body from which these authors could not provoke pain by exposure to cold were the ear lobes and the glans penis.

Ice-cream headache
Drake (1850) commented on the possible injurious effects of eating ice-cream: 'first, swallowing it before the ice has dissolved in the mouth, when it sometimes raises an acute pain in the pharynx, and gives a sense of coldness and sinking in the stomach; second, eating it when the stomach is torpid and inactive from dyspepsia, and the individual is inclined, at the time, to sick headache'.

Holding ice or ice-cream in the mouth, or swallowing a cold food or drink as a bolus, may cause discomfort in the palate and throat. It may also refer pain to the forehead or temple by the trigeminal nerve and to the ears by the glossopharyngeal nerve. Raskin and Knittle (1976) found that 15 of 49 subjects not normally prone to headache had experienced infrequent mild ice-cream headaches at some time of their lives. In contrast, 55 of 59 migraine patients were subject to such headaches, which were frequent and severe in 46. Most patients felt the pain in the midfrontal region but eight reported pain in the temporal and maxillary regions and two in the occiput.

Drummond and Lance (1984) reported that 189 (36.7 per cent) of 530 patients attending a headache clinic had experienced ice-cream headache. The prevalence of such headaches increased in direct proportion to the number of migrainous symptoms associated with the patient's customary headache (Figure 12.1). Although the headache was usually midline or bilateral, the pain was localized to one side of the head for 18 of the 90 patients in whom the site had been documented. In 13 of these 18, and in 17 of the 72 patients with bilateral headache, the site of the ice-cream headache coincided with the area habitually affected by their headaches.

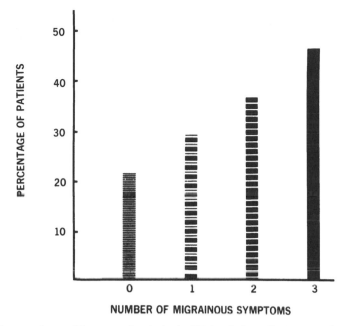

Figure 12.1 The prevalence of ice-cream headache in 530 headache patients grouped according to the number of migrainous characteristics (unilateral headache, focal neurological symptoms and gastrointestinal disturbance) experienced by each. It can be seen that the prevalence increases progressively from 20 per cent in tension-type headache (no migrainous symptoms) to almost 50 per cent in typical migraine headache (all three groups of migrainous symptoms). (From Drummond and Lance, 1984, by permission of the publishers, ADIS Health Science Press)

Wolff (1963) found that applying ice to the palate referred pain to the frontal region and cooling the posterior pharynx caused pain behind the ears. Odell-Smith (1968) reported on his own sensations. Discomfort in the temples appeared 20–30 seconds after the application of ice to the palate and ceased 10–20 seconds after the stimulus was removed.

The fact that ice-cream headache is more common in migraine patients and is often referred to the part of the head afflicted by the patient's customary headache suggests that there may be a segmental disinhibition of central pain pathways in migraine patients which is responsible for undue susceptibility to an afferent volley of impulses from the excitation of cold receptors in the oropharynx.

Benign cough headache

Sharp pain in the head on coughing, sneezing, straining, laughing or stooping has long been regarded as a symptom of organic intracranial disease, commonly associated with obstruction of the CSF pathways. Symonds (1956) presented the case histories of six patients in whom cough headache was a symptom of a space-occupying lesion in the posterior fossa or of basilar impression from Paget's disease.

He then described 21 patients with the same symptom in whom no intracranial disease became apparent. Cough headache disappeared in nine patients and improved spontaneously in another six patients. Two patients died of heart disease and four were lost to follow-up. Symonds concluded that there was a syndrome of benign cough headache, which he attributed to the stretching of a pain-sensitive structure in the posterior fossa, possibly the result of an adhesive arachnoiditis. Of Symonds' 21 patients, 18 were males and ages ranged from 37 to 77 years, with an average age of 55.

Ekbom (1986) cites an earlier description in the French literature by Tinel in 1932 concerning four patients whose headaches were brought on by coughing, nose-blowing, breath-holding and bending the head forwards. He also quotes observations by Nick on 15 patients, 12 of whom were men, ranging in age from 19 to 73 years.

Rooke (1968) considered cough headache to be a variety of exertional headache and recorded his experience with 103 patients who developed transient headaches on running, bending, coughing, sneezing, lifting or straining at stool, in whom no intracranial disease could be detected and who were followed for 3 years or more. During the follow-up period, reinvestigation discovered structural lesions such as Arnold–Chiari malformation, platybasia, subdural haematoma, and cerebral or cerebellar tumour in 10 patients. Of the remaining 93, 30 were free of headache within 5 years and 73 were improved or free of headache after 10 years. This type of headache was found in men more often than women in the ratio 4 : 1. Rooke observed that this form of headache may appear for the first time after a respiratory infection with cough, and that some patients reported an abrupt recovery after the extraction of abscessed teeth, which had also been noted by Symonds.

We would prefer to maintain the separation between 'benign cough headache' and 'benign exertional headache' (which is more common in a younger age group), although there is an obvious overlap between the two.

Williams (1976) recorded CSF pressure from the cisterna magna and lumbar region during coughing. He found that there was a phase in which lumbar pressure exceeded cisternal pressure followed by a phase in which the pressure gradient was reversed. He postulated that cough headache may be caused by a valve-like blockage at the foramen magnum which interferes with the downward or rebound pulsation. Williams (1980) followed up this observation by studying two patients with cough headache whose cerebellar tonsils descended below the foramen magnum without any obvious obstruction, and confirmed a severe craniospinal pressure dissociation during the rebound after a Valsalva manoeuvre. Decompression of the cerebellar tonsils relieved the headache and eliminated the steep pressure gradient on coughing. He commented that coughing led to an increase in intrathoracic and intra-abdominal pressure, which was transmitted to the epidural veins thereby creating a pressure wave and causing CSF to move rostrally. The headache was presumably caused by temporary impaction of the cerebellar tonsils when the subject relaxed and the pressure gradient then reversed. Whether this explanation applies to those patients without an Arnold–Chiari type I malformation remains uncertain. The possibility of a sudden increase in venous pressure being sufficient by itself to cause headache must be considered. Lance (1991) reported the case of a man with a goitre sufficiently large to cause sudden headache when his arms were elevated and the jugular veins distended (see Figure 14.1).

The presence of an Arnold–Chiari malformation or any lesion causing obstruction of CSF pathways or displacing cerebral structures must be excluded before cough headache is assumed to be benign. In cases where cough headache is unilateral, stenosis of the internal carotid artery should be considered (Britton and Guiloff, 1988).

Mathew (1981) reported two patients with benign cough headache (one of whom had proved unresponsive to ergotamine, propranolol and methysergide) who improved with indomethacin 50 mg three times daily. When this therapy was compared with placebo, the reduction of cough headache on the active drug was 95 per cent in one case and 85 per cent in the other, while the reduction on placebo medication was 0 and 18 per cent, respectively. Raskin (1995) found that lumbar puncture relieved six out of 14 patients with cough headaches. Six of the remainder and 14 of 16 patients in a comparison group responded to indomethacin.

Benign exertional headache

Headache may be precipitated by any form of exercise and often has the pulsatile quality of migraine. Credit must be given to Hippocrates for first recognizing this syndrome, as he wrote: 'one should be able to recognize those who have headaches from gymnastic exercises, or running, or walking, or hunting, or any other unseasonable labour, or from immoderate venery' (Adams, 1848).

Dalessio (1971) drew attention to this form of headache in an editorial in which he cited running, rowing, tennis and wrestling as possible causes, and mentioned that heat, high humidity, lack of training and performance at high altitudes (such as the Olympic games in Mexico City) were contributing factors. Massey (1982) presented three cases of headaches resembling migraine, one with visual disturbance and mild hemiparesis, precipitated by running short or long distances. Sudden severe headache can also be precipitated by swimming (Indo and Takahashi, 1990) and weightlifting (Paulson, 1983). Paulson considered strain or stretch of cervical ligaments as a possible cause of weight-lifters' headaches, but the sudden onset and persisting sensitivity to coughing, sneezing and straining suggests acute venous distension as a possible mechanism. The development of headache after sustained exertion, particularly on a hot day, is more likely to be caused by arterial dilatation but objective evidence is lacking.

Cardiac ischaemia may present as unilateral or bilateral exertional headache, relieved promptly by rest, as an unusual referral pattern of angina which may precede chest pain (Grace et al., 1997; Lance and Lambros, 1998). Stress testing (exercise on a treadmill) will confirm the diagnosis as ST changes develop in the ECG at the onset of headache (Figure 12.2). Coronary angiography followed by angioplasty or bypass surgery relieves the symptom.

Phaeochromocytoma may occasionally be responsible for exertional headache (Paulson, Zipf and Beekman, 1979). Intracranial lesions or stenosis of the carotid arteries may have to be excluded as discussed for benign cough headache.

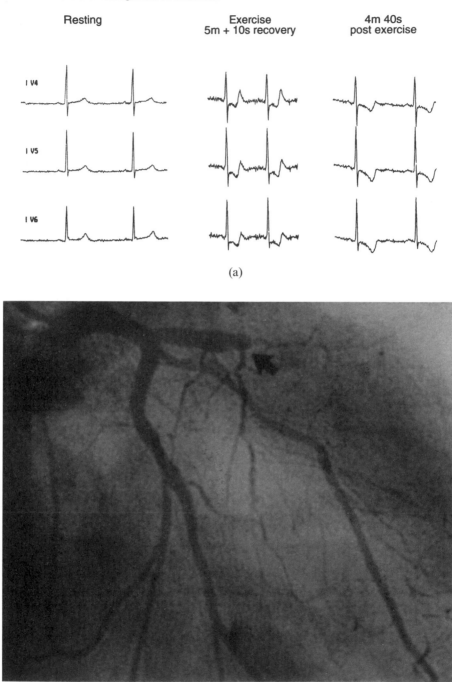

(a)

(b)

Figure 12.2 (a) Anginal headache, appearing at the same time as ST changes in the ECG during stress testing. (b) Occlusion of the left anterior descending branch of the coronary artery. Anginal headache was cured by coronary artery bypass grafting. Reproduced by permission from the Editor of *Headache*

The most logical form of treatment is to take exercise gradually and progressively whenever possible. Lambert and Burnet (1985) described how a prescribed warm-up period prevented 'swimmers headache'. Diamond and Medina (1979) reported that nine out of 11 patients were relieved of exertional headache by the administration of indomethacin over a follow-up period of 3–18 months. A similar successful outcome with indomethacin 50 mg three times daily (with an antacid) was recorded by Mathew (1981). Diamond (1982) described 15 patients, aged 8–54 years, with exertional headaches lasting for an average of 4 hours. Indomethacin in daily doses varying from 25 to 150 mg controlled the headaches almost completely in 13. Ergotamine tartrate 1–2 mg orally or methysergide 1–2 mg orally given 30 minutes before exercise begins is also a useful prophylactic measure.

Headache associated with sexual activity

Hippocrates included immoderate venery (defined as 'the practice or pursuit of sexual pleasure' or 'indulgence of sexual desire' by the Oxford English Dictionary) as a cause of exertional headache (Adams, 1848) but this is not necessarily the case since 'benign sex headache' can arise with little or no physical exertion by the participant.

Headaches developing at the time of orgasm are not always benign. Subarachnoid haemorrhage was precipitated by sexual intercourse in three (4.5 per cent) of 66 cases reported by Fisher (1968) and six (12 per cent) of 50 cases studied by Lundberg and Osterman (1974). Cerebral or brain stem infarction has also been reported. One young man developed a brain stem thrombosis (Lance, 1976) and another a left hemisphere infarction (Levy, 1981). Martinez, Roig and Arboix (1988) described three patients whose neurological deficits began at the moment of orgasm. A 50-year-old woman developed confusion and amnesia lasting three days with a right Babinski sign for 20 days; a man aged 40 years had a right hemisensory defect for 24 hours, and a 36-year-old man had a left homonymous hemianopia, which cleared over 2 weeks. Cerebral angiography was normal in the first two patients but showed poor filling of the right posterior cerebral artery in the third. These authors cite another three cases described by Nick and Bakouche in 1980.

The recognition that most headaches occurring during sexual activity are not associated with an underlying vascular malformation and have a benign prognosis probably belongs to Wolff (1963), but Kriz later reported 25 cases from Czechoslovakia in 1970, cited by Martin (1973). Martin related the histories of five male patients subject to severe headache toward the end of intercourse, three of whom had a past history of migraine. Paulson and Klawans (1974) reported 14 patients with this condition as having 'benign orgasmic cephalgia' but this term does not cover those patients whose headache begins before orgasm.

Sex headache affects men more than women and may occur at any time during the years of sexual activity. It is capricious in that it may develop on several occasions in succession then not trouble the patient again, although there is no obvious change in sexual technique. In a description of 21 patients (Lance, 1976) 16 were male and five female, aged from 18 to 58 years. Three patients experienced headache with masturbation, two of whom also complained of similar headaches during sexual intercourse. The headaches of the remaining patients were confined to sexual intercourse. Those patients who desisted from sexual activity when headache was first noticed found that it subsided within a period of 5 minutes to 2 hours. Those who proceeded to orgasm reported that a severe headache persisted for 3 minutes to 4 hours and a milder headache lingered for 1–48 hours afterwards. Only four patients had previously suffered from migraine and two had experienced exertional headaches. Seven were hypertensive.

The headaches were more likely to occur when intercourse was attempted for a second time after a brief interval. One young man complained of headaches at orgasm while he was on holiday for a month, indulging in sexual intercourse two or three times daily. When the holiday was over and the frequency of intercourse declined to once daily he remained free of headache. Carotid or vertebral angiography was performed in nine of the patients with this syndrome and was completely normal. As familiarity with the syndrome increases, investigation can be reserved for those patients in whom there is suspicion of an underlying lesion.

There are three kinds of headache associated with sexual activity. The first is a dull headache, commonly bilateral and occipital in site, that comes on as sexual excitement mounts. It is probably related to excessive contraction of head and neck muscles, because it can be prevented or relieved by deliberate relaxation of these muscle groups. The second type of headache, more severe and explosive in onset, appears immediately before or at the moment of orgasm, presumably caused by the increase in blood pressure at this time. A third type, which we have now encountered, was described by Paulson and Klawans (1974) in three of their 14 patients with headaches arising during coitus. This form of headache was worse on standing up and thus resembles the low pressure headache following lumbar puncture, leading the authors to postulate that a dural leak may have developed during enthusiastic sexual intercourse.

What is the relationship between sex headaches and physical exertion? Silbert *et al.* (1991) found that 18 of their 45 patients subject to acute vascular headaches during sexual intercourse had also experienced headaches on exertion. Nine patients described a close link between the two sorts of headache, with one following the other within a few days and a dull generalized headache persisting between the two acute events. During follow-up for an average of 6 years, two-fifths of these patients had recurrences of their sex headaches, usually at times of fatigue or stress. Selwyn (1985) reported that, of 32 patients with headaches related to coitus who replied to a questionnaire, 11 had experienced similar headaches after both exercise and sexual intercourse. Nine of these had a history of hypertension and 15 a background of migraine. Of another 10 patients whose headaches developed at the time of orgasm, five had previously suffered from migraine. Taking all 32 patients, 21 had a history of migraine and 11 of hypertension. Two patients had experienced such headaches with masturbation and one after a nocturnal emission following dreaming during sleep. Pascual *et al.* (1996) found a relationship between sex headaches and exertional headaches, but not with cough headaches.

Johns (1986) summarized 110 cases recorded in the literature at that time, 86 male and 24 female. Five had a low CSF pressure syndrome after intercourse, 17 had a muscle contraction type of headache and the remaining headaches had vascular features with 40 occurring at orgasm. He also described four sisters with this syndrome. Ostergaard and Kraft (1992) followed 26 patients for up to 14 years. Half of the patients lost their headaches after periods of 6 weeks to 6 months but half had recurrences after freedom for up to 6 years.

Pathophysiology

The possible relationship of sex headaches with migraine, hypertension and exertional headaches has been mentioned above.

Muscle contraction appears to be a major feature in the milder headache that becomes more severe as sexual excitement increases. Of 21 patients (Lance, 1976), 10 stated that they were subject to headaches at times of emotional tension unrelated to sexual activity. The tension headache was similar but milder than the headache experienced with intercourse in seven patients. Five patients stated that they were aware of excessive muscle contraction, particularly involving the jaw and neck muscles, and found that they could reduce the intensity of the headache by deliberately relaxing those muscles while continuing with intercourse or masturbation. The headache seemed to be related to the degree of sexual excitement and not to physical exertion. If patients with such 'muscle contraction headaches' continued to orgasm, the headache usually became very intense and persisted for up to 48 hours afterwards. Masters and Johnson (1966) have commented on the excessive contraction of facial, jaw and neck muscles as sexual excitement mounts.

The vascular aspect of sex headaches may be superimposed on the tension-type headache or may occur without warning at orgasm. It is abrupt in onset, occipital or generalized, frequently throbbing and sometimes associated with palpitations, resembling the headache of phaeochromocytoma (Lance and Hinterberger, 1976). Masters and Johnson observed that blood pressure rose by 40–100 mmHg systolic and 20–50 mmHg diastolic during orgasm, figures quite comparable with the paroxysms caused by phaeochromocytoma. Littler, Honour and Sleight (1974) recorded similar increases of up to 214/135 mmHg. One of our patients experienced a headache comparable in severity with her sex headache after taking a tablet of the sympathomimetic drug pseudephedrine, supporting the concept that a sudden increase in blood pressure at orgasm may be responsible for the explosive nature of these headaches. An interesting example of a pressor response causing coital cephalgia was provided by Staunton and Moore (1978). A patient with obstruction of the lower aorta who presented with this problem developed a blood pressure of 250/130 mmHg after 3 minutes exercise on a bicycle ergometer. After a successful aortic-iliac bypass his coital headaches disappeared.

Multiple areas of cerebral arterial spasm were found in a 30-year-old man after a coital headache exacerbated by exertion (Silbert et al., 1989). If cerebral arterial spasm is a feature of the explosive orgasmic headache, it is not surprising that strokes have resulted on some occasions.

It may be concluded that an acute pressor response with or without pre-existing hypertension and arterial disease is responsible for the 'thunderclap headache' that may occur at the moment of orgasm.

Management

Benign sex headaches are usually irregular and infrequent in recurrence so that management can often be limited to reassurance and advice about ceasing sexual activity if a milder warning headache develops. When the condition recurs regularly or frequently, it can be prevented by the administration of propranolol but the dosage required varies from 40 to 200 mg daily (Porter and Jankovic, 1981). Beta-blockers presumably act by limiting the surge of blood pressure at orgasm. One patient was successfully treated by the calcium-channel blocking agent diltiazem 60 mg three times daily (Akpunonu and Ahrens, 1991). Ergotamine tartrate or methysergide administered before sexual activity may also prevent this unfortunate sequel.

Differential diagnosis of 'thunderclap headache'

Headaches of explosive onset may be caused by the ingestion of sympathomimetic drugs or tyramine-containing foods while a patient is taking monoamine oxidase inhibitors, and can also be a symptom of phaeochromocytoma.

This type of headache was called 'thunderclap headache' by Day and Raskin (1986) who reported a woman with three such episodes who was found to have an unruptured aneurysm of the internal carotid artery with adjacent areas of segmental vasospasm. The relationship between thunderclap headache and aneurysm in the absence of CT scan or CSF evidence of subarachnoid haemorrhage was questioned by Abbott and Van Hille (1986) who described 14 patients, six of whom had normal four-vessel cerebral angiography. Wijdicks, Kerkhoff and Van Gijn (1988) followed up 71 patients, whose CT scan and CSF findings were negative, for an average of 3.3 years. Twelve patients had further such headaches and 31 (44 per cent) later had regular episodes of migraine or tension headache. Factors identified as precipitating the headaches were sexual intercourse in three cases, coughing in four and exertion in 12, while the remainder had no obvious cause. A history of hypertension was obtained in 11 and of previous headache in 22.

Markus (1991) compared the presentation of 37 patients with subarachnoid haemorrhage and 18 with a similar thunderclap headache but normal CSF examination and could not discern any characteristic to distinguish the two conditions on clinical grounds. Four patients with thunderclap headache in whom subarachnoid haemorrhage had been excluded were found to have diffuse segmental arterial vasospasm by Slivka and Philbrook (1995) who considered this as an entity distinct from the acute onset of migraine.

It may be concluded that the investigations of thunderclap headache unrelated to coitus should include a CT scan and CSF examination but that cerebral angiography is usually unnecessary. When a typical explosive headache occurs at orgasm, particularly if it is preceded by an escalating tension-type headache, investigation could be limited to CT scanning unless other features, such as neck stiffness, make a CSF examination mandatory.

Headache as a symptom of epilepsy

Young and Blume (1983) examined the seizure pattern of 358 epileptic patients and found 24 who experienced pain during their attacks, including 11 with headache as a symptom. Unilateral or bilateral headache was the first indication of a seizure in seven and followed other ictal symptoms in four patients. Eight out of 11 had a temporal lobe origin for their epilepsy but the area affected by their headache bore no relation to the site of the epileptogenic focus. In some of these patients, headaches were migrainous in which case the epileptic manifestations may have been precipitated by diminished cerebral blood flow during an aura but, in others, the headache was clearly a part of the ictal discharge. Two patients with ictal headaches were discovered by Laplante, Saint-Hilaire and Douvier (1983) to have a right temporal origin for their attacks, which vanished after right temporal lobectomy. The headaches were paroxysmal, lasting for less than a minute and 'not like any headache before'.

Headaches caused by vasoactive substances

Headaches resulting from dilatation of intracranial vessels are characteristically throbbing in nature and made worse by jarring of the head or any sudden movement.

Alcohol

Ethyl alcohol is of course a vasodilator agent and may trigger migraine or cluster headache in this way. The cause of 'hangover headache', which happens the day after excessive alcohol intake, is still uncertain. The average rate at which a normal-sized adult metabolizes alcohol is about 10 ml/hour (Ritchie, 1970). It is first oxidized to acetaldehyde by alcohol dehydrogenase, and acetaldehyde is then converted to acetyl-coenzyme A, which is oxidized or used in the synthesis of cholesterol and fatty acids. Disulfiram, administered to discourage the intake of alcohol, increases the blood acetaldehyde concentration five to 10 times and produces the 'aldehyde syndrome'. The face becomes flushed and a throbbing headache may develop, which is associated with nausea, vomiting and giddiness followed by hypotension and pallor. Whether the headache of a hangover can be attributed solely to acetaldehyde or other breakdown products of alcohol remains unknown. The subject is reviewed by Raskin and Appenzeller (1980) who conclude by stating that 'the performance of experiments that very often must take place on Sunday mornings may be an important factor in perpetuating our ignorance'.

Marijuana

Dryness of the mouth, paraesthesiae, a sensation of warmth and suffusion of the conjunctivae are common after the ingestion of 60 mg of *Cannabis sativa*. Five out of 10 subjects studied by Ames (1958) complained of mild frontal headache, presumably related to vasodilatation. Some tension headaches are relieved by smoking marijuana so that its relaxing and vasodilator properties may combine to help this form of headache just as alcohol does.

Cocaine

The complaint of headache in cocaine abusers should be taken seriously because intracranial haemorrhage, ischaemic stroke, endocarditis and brain abscess have been reported (Dhuna, Pascual-Leone and Belgrade, 1991). Dhuna *et al.* described headaches with migrainous features during cocaine intoxication. Some developed acutely, some during the course of a cocaine binge, and others on withdrawal. Associated neurological symptoms and signs were attributed to the sympathomimetic effect of cocaine causing cerebral vasoconstriction.

Monosodium glutamate: 'the Chinese-restaurant syndrome'

Headache has been reported as part of the Chinese restaurant syndrome (Schaumburg *et al.*, 1969) – a symptom complex of pressure and tightness in the face, burning over the trunk, neck and shoulders, and a pressing pain in the chest, which may follow 20–25 minutes after eating a Chinese meal. The headache, a pressure or throbbing over the temples and a band-like sensation around the forehead, has been attributed to monosodium glutamate (MSG), which is used abundantly in Chinese cooking. About 3 g of MSG, contained in 200 ml of wonton ('short') soup, may provoke headache in those sensitive to it.

Nitrites and nitrates: 'hot dog headache'

When the inhalation of amyl nitrite was used for the treatment of angina pectoris it often caused a sudden bilateral throbbing headache as a complication of its vasodilator action. Glyceryl trinitrate may have the same effect in patients who are not usually subject to headache and it is a reliable precipitating agent of cluster headache during a bout.

An uncommon but interesting variation on this theme is a headache that afflicts some unfortunate people after eating cured-meat foods. Nitrites are added to salt to give a uniform red appearance to cured meat. The concentration of nitrite in the meat when cooked is only 50–130 parts per million but this is sufficient to cause headache in some susceptible individuals after eating hot dogs, bacon, ham or salami. Henderson and Raskin (1972) described such a patient who developed headache on most occasions after ingesting 10 mg of sodium nitrite but not after a placebo of sodium bicarbonate.

Histamine headache

Pickering and Hess (1933) found that the intravenous infusion of histamine caused flushing of the face followed by a generalized throbbing headache. Wolff (1963) and his colleagues showed that headache came on after the scalp arteries had returned to their normal calibre whereas CSF pulsation was still increased by 250 per cent while histamine headache was in progress. Increasing intracranial pressure to 1000 mm CSF relieved histamine headache immediately, confirming the idea that it was caused by dilatation of intracranial vessels rather than scalp arteries. The intravenous infusion of histamine, in doses which did not cause headache in normal subjects, evoked headache in 24 of 25 migraine patients and five out of 10 patients susceptible to tension headache (Krabbe and Olesen, 1980).

Rebound headache – nicotine and caffeine

Unlike vasodilators, vasoconstrictor agents do not in themselves induce headache, but a rebound dilatation may follow the constriction induced by nicotine as the result of excessive tobacco smoking or the vasoconstrictor effect of caffeine contained in tea, coffee or commercial analgesic preparations. As the effect of the last dose wears off, a dull headache may become apparent, which is relieved by repeating the dose, one of the factors in habituation (Greden et al., 1980).

Regional cerebral blood flow was shown to decrease after the ingestion of 250 mg of caffeine and to increase in the frontal areas during abstinence in a group with high habitual caffeine consumption, involving more than six cups of coffee daily for at least 3 years (Mathew and Wilson, 1985).

Peptide-secreting tumours

Lance (1991) reported the rare association of episodic flushing and headache with an abdominal tumour (renal oncocytoma). The vacuoles of some cells stained for calcitonin gene-related peptide. Headaches and flushing ceased after the tumour was removed.

Drug-induced headaches

Headache may be a side-effect of some drugs other than vasodilators, possibly by interference with 5-HT mechanisms. Zemelidine, indomethacin, cimetidine and ranitidine were commonly reported to the WHO as being responsible for headaches (Askmark, Lundberg and Olsson, 1989). Agents that lower serum cholesterol, such as gemfibrozil and bezafibrate, may cause generalized pulsatile headaches (Hodgetts and Tunnicliffe. 1989). Simvastatin has also been reported as being a cause of headache and muscle pains. Cyclosporin was held responsible for headache in six out of 24 patients after liver transplants (Steiger et al. 1994). The frequent consumption of analgesics or ergotamine tartrate is now considered to be a cause of chronic daily headache. Lane and Routledge (1983) list a large number of drugs that have been reputed to induce headaches.

Headache associated with systemic infections

Most febrile illnesses are accompanied by headache, presumably because bacterial or viral toxins dilate the cerebral circulation. Neck stiffness (meningismus) may be present even in the absence of aseptic or bacterial meningitis but warrants immediate investigation – and urgent treatment if bacterial meningitis is suspected. Injections of typhoid and other vaccines may induce a febrile reaction with headache.

Hypnic headache

Raskin (1988) reported six patients over the age of 65 years who were awakened by bilateral headaches, often associated with nausea, that persisted for 30–60 minutes. These headaches were relieved by taking a bedtime dose of 300–600 mg of lithium carbonate. Further reports of the syndrome have appeared (Newman *et al.*, 1990) and from our experience it is a distinct, recognizable syndrome.

Metabolic causes of headache

Hypoxia and hypercapnia

Carbon dioxide is the most efficient cerebral vasodilator and the headache caused by prolonged exposure to an overcrowded, underventilated room presumably owes its origin to this effect. Conversely, oxygen constricts cerebral vessels which dilate under conditions of hypoxia. Headache may be a symptom of sleep apnoea, mountain sickness or chronic pulmonary insufficiency. Carbon monoxide poisoning may induce headache by hypoxia. In 1931, Charles Kingsford Smith set out to fly from Australia to England in an Avro Avian named Southern Cross Minor in an attempt to break the record. The plane developed a leak in the exhaust pipe, allowing carbon monoxide to leak into the cockpit. Before the defect was remedied, he wrote in his diary that he felt awful: 'a rotten night .... my head bashed away like a bloody drum' (McNally, 1966).

Sleep apnoea
Sleep apnoea commonly affects overweight men and is characterized by snoring during sleep and long pauses without respiration followed by a loud inspiratory gasp, producing a restless night followed by daytime drowsiness. Pocera and Dalessio (1995) found that morning headache was not more frequent after sleep apnoea than in other sleep disorders but 30 per cent of patients did improve with the use of intranasal positive air pressure (CPAP) treatment. The relationship of headache to sleep disorders is discussed by Ramadan (1997).

Mountain sickness
Headache is the most frequent and severe symptom of acute mountain sickness (Appenzeller, 1972; King and Robinson, 1972). Of 30 young men subjected for 30 hours to simulated altitudes of 14,000–15,000 feet in a hypobaric chamber, 28 developed headache. This was usually bilateral but was localized to one side in 25 per cent. The headache was relieved by compression of the superficial temporal arteries more completely than by the Valsalva manoeuvre, suggesting that the extracranial arteries

were of more importance for the production of headache than intracranial vasodilatation.

The cause of the headache is not necessarily hypoxia because the inhalation of oxygen does not provide relief and similar headaches resembling migraine have been reported after exposure to a hyperbaric chamber. Other factors such as fluid and electrolyte changes may play a part. Spironolactone, an aldosterone antagonist, has been reported as preventing the headache of mountain sickness if taken prophylactically. Acetazolamide 500 mg daily proved to be an effective preventive agent in a double-blind crossover trial, the crossing over taking place between Mount Kenya and Mount Kilimanjaro! (Greene *et al.*, 1981). Diuretics such as frusemide are used for the treatment of altitude headache.

Hypoglycaemia

Hypoglycaemia may produce a vascular headache in some people who miss a regular mealtime or in those with carbohydrate intolerance, in which case headache appears several hours after meals. The relationship of hypoglycaemia to migraine is discussed by Amery (1987). Fasting enforced by religious practices may be responsible, exemplified by 'Yom Kippur headache' (Mosek and Korczyn, 1995), although dehydration may also play a part as these headaches may be eased by lying down.

Headache during haemodialysis

Bana, Yap and Graham (1972) reported that 70 per cent of 44 patients had experienced headache during haemodialysis. Six patients described typical muscle contraction headaches and 11 of 12 migraine patients had their usual headache precipitated by dialysis. The authors described a new entity of 'dialysis headache', which started a few hours after the procedure as a mild bifrontal ache and later became throbbing, sometimes accompanied by nausea and vomiting. The severity of the headache was related to hypertension, longer intervals between each dialysis, fall in blood pressure during dialysis, decrease in serum sodium and decrease in osmolality. Headaches were relieved by bilateral nephrectomy and successful renal transplant. Dialysis headache appears to be of vascular origin, associated with the release of vasodilator peptides, and is responsive to small doses of ergotamine.

Headache following epileptic seizures

Cerebral vasodilatation is probably responsible for the headache that follows a major (tonic–clonic) epileptic seizure. Plum, Posner and Troy (1968) have analysed the effects on the monkey's cerebral circulation of the direct metabolic changes resulting from the seizure discharge itself and the indirect effects from alterations in respiration and muscle metabolism. Although the animals were anaesthetized, paralysed and adequately ventilated with oxygen, cerebral blood flow increased during an induced seizure to a mean of 264 per cent over the resting level. This was caused by increased carbon dioxide production and loss of autoregulation of the cerebral blood vessels, so that flow increased passively with the neurogenic elevation of blood pressure accompanying a seizure. In spite of an increase in cerebral metabolism of 60 per cent, venous oxygen tension actually rose and there was no demonstrable cerebral acidosis. Similar findings in man have been reported by the same group of workers. In a spontaneous epileptic seizure, hypoxia from respiratory arrest is an added factor.

Post-ictal headaches were suffered by 51 of 100 epileptic patients studied by Schon and Blau (1987). In eight out of nine previously migrainous patients, the postictal headache resembled a mild attack of their usual migraine and half of the remainder had migrainous symptoms such as nausea and photophobia associated with their headaches. Of the 51 patients, 13 were subject only to 'minor seizures', which throws doubt on metabolically induced changes in cerebral blood being the sole causative factor. Following this line of thought, D'Alessandro *et al.* (1987) examined 174 patients with non-convulsive epileptic attacks and found that the 23 patients who were prone to postictal headache all suffered from complex partial seizures. There was no greater tendency for these patients to suffer inter-ictal headaches than those who had simple partial seizures or generalized non-convulsive attacks (absences with or without myoclonic jerks). The authors postulated that neuronal discharges originating in the locus coeruleus and brain stem raphe nuclei might trigger the vascular changes responsible for postictal headaches.

Conclusion

The syndromes described in this chapter are 'benign' in the sense that no structural lesion can be held responsible and the prognosis is favourable. Because of the association of similar symptoms with the presence of space-occupying intracranial lesions, aneurysms, cerebral atherosclerosis or cardiac ischaemia in some instances, clinical judgement is required to determine the extent of investigation required in each individual.

References

Abbott, R. J. and van Hille. P. (1986). Thunderclap headache and unruptured cerebral aneurysm. *Lancet* **ii**, 1459

Adams, F. (1848). *The Genuine Works of Hippocrates.* p. 94. London, Sydenham Society (reprint: Baltimore, Williams and Wilkins, 1939)

Akpunonu, S. E. and Ahrens. J. (1991). Sexual headaches: case report, review, and treatment with calcium blocker. *Headache* **31**, 141–145

Amery ,W. K. (1987) The oxygen theory of migraine. In *Migraine, Clinical and Research Aspects,* Ed. J. N. Blau. pp. 411–412. Baltimore, Johns Hopkins Press

Ames. F. (1958). A clinical and metabolic study of acute intoxication with *Cannabis sativa* and its role in the model psychoses. *J. Ment. Sci.* **104**, 977–999

Appenzeller, O. (1977). Altitude headache. *Headache* **12**, 126–179

Askmark, H., Lundberg, P. O. and Olsson, S. (1989) Drug-related headache. *Headache* **29**, 441–444

Bana, D. S., Yap, A. U. and Graham, J. R. (1972) Headache during hemodialysis. *Headache* **2**, 1–14

Britton, T. C. and Guiloff, R. J. (1988). Carotid artery disease presenting as cough headache. *Lancet* **i**, 1406–1407

D'Alessandro, R., Sacquegna, T., Pazzaglia, P. and Lugaresi, E. (1987). Headache after partial complex seizures. In *Migraine and Epilepsy*, Eds F. Andermann and E. Lugaresi. pp. 273–278. Boston, Butterworths

Dalessio, D. J. (1974). Editorial. Effort migraine. *Headache* **14**, 53

Day, J. W. and Raskin, N. H. (1986). Thunderclap headache: symptom of unruptured cerebral aneurysm. *Lancet* **ii**, 1247–1248

Dhuna, A., Pascual-Leone, A. and Belgrade, M. (1991). Cocaine-related vascular headaches. *J. Neurol. Neurosurg. Psychiat.* **54**, 803–806

Diamond, S. (1982). Prolonged benign exertional headache: its clinical characteristics and response to indomethacin. *Headache* **22**, 96–98

Diamond, S. and Medina, J. L. (1979). Benign exertional headache: successful treatment with indomethacin. *Headache* **19**, 249

Drake, D. (1850). *A Systematic Treatise, Historical, Epidemiological and Practical, on the Principal Diseases of the Interior Valley of North America, as May Appear in the Caucasian, African and Indian and Esquimaux Varieties of its Population.* Cincinnati, W. B. Smith & Co.

Drummond. P. D. and Lance, J. W. (1984). Neurovascular disturbances in headache patients. *Clin. Exp. Neurol.* **20**, 93–99

Ekbom, K. (1975). Some observations on pain in cluster headache. *Headache* **14**, 219–225

Ekbom, K. (1986). Cough headache. In *Handbook of Clinical Neurology*, Vol. 4(48): *Headache*, Ed. F. Clifford Rose. pp. 367–371. Amsterdam, Elsevier

Fisher, C. M. (1968). Headache in cerebrovascular disease. In *Handbook of Clinical Neurology*, Vol. 5, *Headaches and Cranial Neuralgias*, Eds P. J. Vinken and G. W. Bruyn. pp. 124–156. Amsterdam, Elsevier

Grace, A., Horgan, J., Breathnach, K. and Staunton, H. (1997). Anginal headache and its basis. *Cephalalgia* **17**, 195–196

Greden, J. F., Victor, B. S., Fontaine, P. and Lubelsky, M. (1980). Caffeine-withdrawal headache: a clinical profile. *Psychosomatics* **21**, 411–418

Greene, M. K., Kerr, A. M., McIntosh, I. B. and Prescott, R. J. (1981). Acetazolamide in prevention of acute mountain sickness: a double-blind controlled cross-over study. *Br. Med. J.* **283**, 811–813

Henderson, W. R. and Raskin, N. H. (1972). Hot-dog headache: individual susceptibility to nitrite. *Lancet* **ii**, 1162–1163

Hodgetts, T. J. and Tunnicliffe, C. (1989). Bezafibrate-induced headache. *Lancet* **i**, 163

Indo, T. and Takahashi, A. (1990). Swimmer's migraine. *Headache* **30**, 485–487

Johns, D. R. (1986). Benign sexual headache within a family. *Arch. Neurol.* **43**, 1158–1160

King, A. B. and Robinson, S. M. (1972). Vascular headaches of acute mountain sickness. *Aerospace Med.* August, 849–851

Krabbe, A. A. and Olesen, J. (1980). Headache provocation by continuous intravenous infusion of histamine. Clinical results and receptor mechanisms. *Pain* **8**, 253–259

Lambert, R. W. and Burnet, D. L. (1985). Prevention of exercise-induced migraine by quantitative warmup. *Headache* **25**, 317–319

Lance, J. W. (1976). Headaches related to sexual activity. *J. Neurol. Neurosurg. Psychiat.* **39**, 1226–1230

Lance, J. W. (1991). Solved and unsolved headache problems. *Headache* **31**, 439–445

Lance, J. W. and Anthony, M. (1971). Migrainous neuralgia or cluster headache? *J. Neurol. Sci.* **13**, 401–411

Lance, J. W. and Hinterberger, H. (1976). Symptoms of phaeochromocytoma with particular reference to headache, correlated with catecholamine production. *Arch. Neurol.* **33**, 281–288

Lance, J.W. and Lambros, J. (1998). Headache associated with cardiac ischaemia. *Headache* **38**, 315–316

Lane, J. M. R. and Routledge, P. A. (1983). Drug-induced neurological disorders. *Drugs* **26**, 124–147

Lansche, R. K. (1964). Ophthalmodynia periodica. *Headache* **4**, 247–249

Laplante. P., Saint-Hilaire, J. M. and Bouvier, G. (1983). Headache as an epileptic manifestation. *Neurology* **33** 1493–1495

Levy, R. L. (1981). Stroke and orgasmic cephalalgia. *Headache* **21**, 12–13

Littler, W. A., Honour, A. J. and Sleight, P. (1974). Direct arterial pressure, heart rate and electrocardiogram during human coitus. *J. Reprod. Fertil.* **40**, 321–331

Lundberg, P. O. and Osterman, P. O. (1974). The benign and malignant forms of orgasmic cephalgia. *Headache* **14**, 164–165

Markus, H. S. (1991). A prospective follow-up of thunderclap headache mimicking subarachnoid hae-morrhage. *J. Neurol. Neurosurg. Psychiat.* **54**, 1117–1125

Martin, E. A. (1973). Severe headache accompanying orgasm. *Br. Med. J.* **4**, 44

Martinez, J. M., Roig, C. and Arboix, A. (1988). Complicated coital cephalalgia. Three cases with benign evolution. *Cephalalgia* **8**, 265–268

Massey, E. W. (1982). Effort headache in runners. *Headache* **22**, 99–100

Masters, W. H. and Johnson, V. E. (1966). *Human Sexual Response.* pp. 278–294. Boston, Little Brown

Mathew, N. T. (1981). Indomethacin-responsive headache syndromes. *Headache* **21**, 147–150

Mathew, R. J. and Wilson, W. H. (1985). Caffeine consumption, withdrawal and cerebral blood flow. *Headache* **25**, 305–309

McNally, W. (1966). *Smithy: The Kingsford Smith Story.* London, Robert Hale

Medina, J. L. and Diamond, S. (1981). Cluster headache variant: spectrum of a new headache syndrome. *Arch. Neurol.* **38**, 705–709

Mosek, A. and Korczyn, A.D. (1995). Yom Kippur headache. *Neurology* **45**, 1953–1955

Newman, L. C., Lipton, R. B. and Soloman, S. (1990). The hypnic headache syndrome: a benign headache disorder of the elderly. *Neurology* **40**, 1904–1905

Odell-Smith, R. (1968). Ice-cream headache. In *Handbook of Clinical Neurology, Volume 5, Headaches and Cranial Neuralgias*, Eds P. J. Vinken and G. W. Bruyn. pp. 188–191. Amsterdam, Elsevier

Ostergaard, J. R. and Kraft, M. (1992). Natural history of benign coital headache. *Brit. Med. J.* **305**, 1129

Pascual, J., Iglesias, F., Oterino, A., Vasquez-Barquero, A. and Berciano, J. (1996). Cough, exertional and sexual headaches. *Neurology* **46**, 1520–1524

Paulson, G. W. (1983). Weightlifter's headache. *Headache* **23**, 193–194

Paulson, G. W. and Klawans, H. L. (1974). Benign orgasmic cephalalgia. *Headache* **13**, 181–187

Paulson, G. W., Zipf, R. E. and Beekman, J. F. (1979). Phaeochromocytoma causing exercise-related headache and pulmonary edema. *Ann. Neurol.* **5**, 96–99

Pearce, J. M. S. (1988). Exploding head syndrome. *Lancet* **ii**, 270–271

Pestronk, A. and Pestronk, S. (1983). Goggle migraine. *New Engl. J. Med.* **308**, 226

Pickering, G. W. and Hess, W. (1933). Observations on the mechanism of headache produced by hista-mine. *Clin. Sci.* **1**, 77–101

Plum, F., Posner, J. B. and Trov, B. (1968). Cerebral metabolic and circulatory responses to induced convulsions in animals. *Arch. Neurol.* **18**, 1–13

Pocera, J. S. and Dalessio, D. J. (1995). Identification and treatment of sleep apnea in patients with chronic headache. *Headache* **35**, 586–589

Porter, M. and Jankovic, J. (1981). Benign coital cephalalgia. Differential diagnosis and treatment. *Arch. Neurol.* **38**, 710–712

Ramadan, N. M. (1997). Unusual causes of headache. *Neurology* **48**, 1494–1499

Raskin, N. H. (1988). The hypnic headache syndrome. *Headache* **28**, 534–536

Raskin, N. H. (1995). The cough headache syndrome: treatment. *Neurology* **46**, 1784

Raskin, N. H. and Appenzeller, O. (1980). *Headache. Major Problems in Internal Medicine*, Vol. 19, Ed. J. H. Smith, Jr. p. 16. Philadelphia, Saunders

Raskin, N. H. and Knittle, S. C. (1976). Ice-cream headache and orthostatic symptoms in patients with migraine. *Headache* **16**, 222–225

Raskin, N. H. and Schwartz. R. K. (1980). Icepick-like pain. *Neurology* **30**, 203–205

Rasmussen, B. K. and Olesen, J. (1992). Symptomatic and non-symptomatic headaches in a general population. *Neurology* **42**, 1225–1231

Ritchie, J. M. (1970). The aliphatic alcohols. In *The Pharmacological Basis of Therapeutics*, 4th Edition, Eds L. S. Goodman and A. Gilman. p. 135. London, Collier-Macmillan

Rooke, E. D. (1968). Benign exertional headache. *Med. Clin. N. Amer.* **52**, 801–808

Schaumburg, H. H., Byck, R., Gerstl, R. and Mashman, J. H. (1969). Monosodium L-glutamate. Its pharmacology and role in the Chinese restaurant syndrome. *Science N.Y.* **163**, 826–828

Schon, F. and Blau, J. N. (1987). Post-epileptic headache and migraine. *J. Neurol. Neurosurg. Psychiat.* **50**, 1148–1152

Selwyn, D. L. (1985). A study of coital related headaches in 32 patients. *Cephalalgia* **5** (Suppl. 3), 300–301

Silbert, P. L.. Edis, R. H., Stewart-Wynne, E. G. and Gubbay, S. S. (1991). Benign vascular sexual headache and exertional headache: interrelationships and long term prognosis. *J. Neurol. Neurosurg. Psychiat.* **54**, 417–421

Silbert, P. L., Hankey, G. J., Prentice, D. A. and Apsimon, H. T. (1989). Angiographically demonstrated arterial spasm in a case of benign sexual headache and benign exertional headache. *Aust. N.Z. J. Med.* **19**, 466–468

Sjaastad, O. (1992). *Cluster Headache Syndrome.* pp. 310–312. London, W. B. Saunders

Slivka, A. and Philbrook, B. (1995). Clinical and angiographic features of thunderclap headache. *Headache* **35**, 1–6

Staunton, H. P. and Moore, J. (1978). Coital cephalgia and ischaemic muscle work of the lower limbs. *J. Neurol. Neurosurg. Psychiat.* **41**, 930–933

Steiger, M. J., Farrah, T., Rolles, K., Harvey, P. and Burrows, A. K. (1994). Cyclosporin associated with headache. *J. Neurol. Neurosurg. Psychiat.* **57**, 1258–1259

Symonds, C. (1956). Cough headache. *Brain* **79**, 557–568

Wijdicks, E. F. M., Kerkhoff, H. and van Gijn, J. (1988). Long-term follow-up of 71 patients with thunderclap headache, mimicking subarachnoid haemorrhage. *Lancet* **ii**, 68–70

Williams, B. (1976). Cerebrospinal fluid changes in response to coughing. *Brain* **99**, 331–346

Williams, B. (1980). Cough headache due to craniospinal pressure dissociation. *Arch. Neurol.* **37**, 226–230

Wolf, S. and Hardy, J. D. (1941). Studies on pain. Observations on pain due to local cooling and on factors involved in the 'cold pressor' effect. *J. Clin. Invest.* **20**, 521–533

Wolff, H. G. (1963). *Headache and Other Head Pain.* New York, Oxford University Press

Young, G. B. and Blume, W. T. (1983). Painful epileptic seizures. *Brain* **106**, 537–554

Chapter 13

Post-traumatic headache

Definition

The Headache Classification Committee of the International Headache Society (IHS) (1988) considered post-traumatic headache in two categories. The first follows significant head trauma documented by loss of consciousness, post-traumatic amnesia of greater than 10 minutes or objective signs of neurological deficit; the second category did not fulfil these criteria, but nevertheless started within 14 days of injury and continued for at least 8 weeks afterwards. Young and Packard (1996) commented that the 2-week period selected by the Committee may not have physiological validity but may be an arbitrary compromise in order to establish causality for disability, compensation, litigation and insurance purposes.

Incidence

Estimates of the frequency of post-traumatic headache vary widely. At the lower end of the scale, Wilkinson and Gilchrist (1977) reported that only 12 per cent of 84 patients admitted by a rehabilitation unit 4–146 weeks after a severe head injury (with loss of consciousness for at least 24 hours) had complained of headache at any time. Other authors have found an incidence ranging from 28 per cent to 70 per cent (Scherokman and Massey, 1983; Appenzeller, 1987). Brenner et al. (1944) found that post-traumatic headache lasting more than 2 months was uncommon in patients who were only dazed and not disorientated after the injury, and in those without post-traumatic amnesia. It was significantly higher in patients with laceration of the scalp, and in those of a nervous disposition before the accident, with symptoms of anxiety after the accident or with occupational difficulties or pending litigation. There was no correlation with the duration of coma, disorientation or post-traumatic amnesia when these were present, or with EEG abnormalities during the first week, skull fracture or the finding of blood in the CSF.

Pathophysiology

People may become subject to headaches after what seems to be a relatively minor head injury, with or without loss of consciousness. Povlishock *et al.* (1983) studied the effect of head injury in anaesthetized cats, administered by the impact of a 4.8 kg pendulum swinging through 12 degrees. Axonal function was studied by the application of horse-radish peroxidase to the motor cortex and cerebellar nuclei 24 hours before the injury. Axonal swelling and, eventually, disruption was found without parenchymal or vascular damage, indicating that axonal changes could result from minor head injury.

Taylor and Kakulas (1991) examined the cervical spine in 43 patients who died after trauma. Only 28 per cent had fractures whereas disc injuries were found in 96 per cent and soft tissue injuries of the facet joints in 72 per cent. They reported two cases of extension neck injury with persisting pain in the neck, shoulder or arm in individuals who had no convincing radiographic abnormality but were found to have disc pathology at autopsy. They observed that clefts in the cervical discs of trauma patients persist for a year or more in the innervated parts of the anterior annulus and commented 'that it is unreasonable to assume that chronic pain in such cases has a psychosomatic basis'.

These histological studies make it clear that injury to the head and neck can produce changes that are not detectable by our present methods of investigation and should caution clinicians against leaping to the conclusion that symptoms without signs indicate a psychosomatic origin; this is not surprising because no structural basis has yet been demonstrated for migraine and cluster headache.

Brenner *et al.* (1944) quote earlier work by Friedman and Brenner showing that patients with localized post-traumatic headache were very sensitive to intravenous histamine, which reproduced the characteristic headache. They suggested that some post-traumatic headache is of vascular origin (worsened by histamine), some is of extracranial origin (following laceration of the scalp), and some is of psychosomatic origin (worsened by anxiety and concern about litigation).

Simons and Wolff (1946) found that the intravenous injection of 0.1–0.2 mg histamine in 16 patients with post-traumatic headache gave rise to a deep ache, sometimes throbbing, which was most intense in the occipital and frontal regions. The sensitivity of the patients to histamine was no greater than that of normal subjects but in three cases the headache was most severe at the site of head injury.

Ramadan, Norris and Shultz (1995) demonstrated abnormal asymmetry of cerebral blood flow in patients with chronic post-traumatic headache by xenon inhalation single-photon emission computed tomography (SPECT). Changes correlated with the severity of headache and could provide an objective assessment of abnormality in patients who usually lack CT or MRI support for their complaint of continuing headache. These findings were confirmed by Gilkey *et al.* (1997).

Classification

Simons and Wolff (1946) divided post-traumatic headache into three groups. The first was a dull pressure sensation associated with nervous tension and depression, in which EMG recordings from the scalp muscles correlated with the severity of headache. The injection of local anaesthetic into areas of deep tenderness reduced or abolished the headache. They concluded that this form resulted from sustained contraction of skeletal muscle. The second variety of headache was local pain and tenderness in an area of scarring, and which was superimposed on a generalized dull headache of the first type. The third variety was a unilateral throbbing headache with nausea, accompanied by dilatation of arteries and veins, and relieved by ergotamine. This is referred to below as extracranial vascular headache or post-traumatic migraine. With the present state of knowledge, headache following injury cannot be classified with certainty. It is probable that there are at least six distinct types of post-traumatic headache, with overlap between the groups.

1. Intracranial vascular headache

It is generally accepted that concussion is followed by dilatation of intracranial vessels, giving rise to a pulsating headache that is made worse by head movement, jolting, coughing, sneezing and straining. Tubbs and Potter (1970) found that 83 of 200 patients admitted to hospital had a headache in the day or so after head injury. Headache was complained of spontaneously by 22 patients (11 per cent), of whom three required an analgesic. The remainder admitted to headache only on questioning. Sensitivity to jolting, coughing or straining may persist in some patients without any obvious neurological signs being present. It may be associated with other symptoms of organic origin, such as giddiness on looking upwards or on lying down with the head on one side or the other (benign positional vertigo). The same type of headache may develop, or intensify, if extradural or subdural haematoma complicates head injury.

2. Extracranial vascular headache

It is not uncommon for patients who have experienced local damage to the scalp overlying a main extracranial vessel to become subject to periodic headache in the distribution of that vessel. Such headaches may recur with the periodicity of migraine and be associated with nausea and photophobia. Jabbing pains may also arise from any scalp nerve damaged by the blow, or subsequent development of scar tissue. Ligation and section of the affected nerve and vessel may be helpful in abolishing this syndrome. Apart from surgical measures, the management is the same as for migraine.

3. Post-traumatic migraine

Migraine with aura may be precipitated in children or adults by a sharp blow to the head ('footballer's migraine'; see Chapter 7). It is not uncommon for migrainous headaches to begin after open or closed head injury, which poses the medicolegal question: was migraine caused by the injury or would it have started spontaneously? To examine this problem, Russell and Olesen (1996) looked at the family histories of 29 patients with no past history of migraine who developed migrainous headaches after head injury, fulfilling IHS criteria for significant trauma in 11 cases and minor trauma in 18 cases. Three patients had migraine with aura and 26 had migraine-type headaches without aura. The first-degree relatives of patients with post-traumatic migraine had a significantly lower prevalence of migraine than migrainous patients without any history of head trauma. The authors concluded that it is very likely that head trauma, even a minor one, can cause migraine without aura. The number of patients with aura was too small for conclusions to be drawn. Haas (1996) examined 48 patients with chronic post-traumatic headache concluding that, in 21 per cent, the headaches had the characteristics of migraine without aura, indistinguishable from the histories of migrainous patients without any previous head injury.

4. Post-traumatic dysautonomic cephalalgia

Vijayan and Dreyfus (1975) described five patients with a distinctive syndrome that followed injury to the anterior triangle of the neck, presumably involving the carotid artery sheath. All patients complained of pain and tenderness in this area for some weeks after the injury. Some weeks or months after the injury the patients began to suffer from severe unilateral episodic headaches on the side previously injured. The headaches were frontotemporal in site, and associated with severe sweating over the same side of the face, dilatation of the pupil on that side, blurring of vision and photophobia in the ipsilateral eye, and nausea. The headaches recurred several times each month and lasted from 8 hours to 3 days. After the headache subsided, three patients were said to have ptosis and miosis on the affected side. The attacks were attributed to a paroxysmal excess of sympathetic activity followed by a period of diminished activity, as a result of trauma to the pericarotid sympathetic plexus. Partial sympathetic denervation was confirmed by the fact that the pupil on the affected side dilated in response to a 1 : 1000 solution of adrenaline. The headaches did not improve with ergotamine but responded promptly to propranolol, 40 mg daily. We have never encountered this syndrome.

5. Pain in the neck and occipital region from injury to the upper cervical spine

The part played by whiplash injury of the cervical spine is difficult to assess in the absence of definite radiological changes. Recently, PET and SPECT scanning have demonstrated hypoperfusion and hypometabolism in both parieto-occipital regions in patients with neck pain and headache after whiplash injury in comparison with normal subjects used as controls (Otte *et al.* 1997). These studies give objective support to the existence of an organic syndrome in patients with no obvious structural basis for continuing headache. Balla (1980) analysed the symptoms attributed to whiplash injury in 300 patients, two-thirds of whom were female, examined 6 months or more after the accident which was considered to be responsible. Daily aching in the neck was a complaint of 219 patients and 58 had aching in the arms. Headache recurred daily in 176 patients (59 per cent), every week or so in 42 patients (14 per cent), and occasionally or not at all in 82 patients (27 per cent). The daily headaches were described as a generalized ache, worse toward the back of the head. Occasional or weekly headaches resembled migraine without aura.

When a stationary car is hit in the rear by a vehicle travelling at about 15 miles (24 km) per hour, the neck of any person sitting in the stationary car is subjected to hyperextension, well beyond the normal range of movement. Anatomical studies after such acceleration injuries in monkeys have demonstrated apophyseal joint damage that was not visible on radiological examination (La Rocca, 1978). Similar evidence was produced for human whiplash injuries by Taylor and Kakulas (1991). In reviewing the problems of whiplash injury, La Rocca pointed out that degenerative changes in the cervical spine in patients who have experienced whiplash injury are six times as common as would be expected for that age group.

After cervical disc injury, the neck may be held in a slightly tilted or rigidly fixed position. Points of referred tenderness are often found, not only in the suboccipital and cervical regions, but over the upper part of the medial edge of the scapula, the deltoid muscle and around the elbow on the affected side (Raney and Raney, 1948). Ryan et al. (1993) analysed the symptoms of 32 individuals with neck strain after a car accident in relation to the dynamics of the impact. Some 80 per cent complained of pain in the back of the neck, head and shoulders while others experienced pain in the upper back or arms. The initial severity of neck symptoms correlated with the severity of the crash. Tenderness, spasm or pain was evoked on examination more often over the middle segments of the cervical spine than the upper and lower ends. Those people who had been aware of the impending crash had a greater range of neck movement and fewer adverse responses to palpation than those who were taken unaware.

Lord et al. (1994) studied 100 patients with neck pain persisting more than 3 months after whiplash injury. Headache was the main complaint in 40 per cent and a secondary problem in 31 per cent. They assessed the part played by trauma to the upper cervical facet joints by blocking the third occipital nerve. This technique provided temporary relief to 27 per cent of patients, increasing to 53 per cent of those patients with associated headache. Tenderness over the C2–3 facet joint was more common in those who responded. The same group (Lord et al., 1996) completed a double-blind controlled study of radio-frequency neurotomy in 24 patients. Of 12 submitted to the genuine procedure, the mean duration of pain relief before returning to 50 per cent of baseline level was 263 days compared with 8 days for those having a placebo procedure.

Neck injury can cause dissection of a vertebral artery with resulting infarction of the brain stem and occipital cortex at the time of the accident or even 2 or 3 months later (Tulyapronchote et al., 1994). Basilar artery migraine has also been reported after whiplash injury (Jacome, 1986).

Some patients respond to the application of heat, cervical traction, mobilization of the neck, the temporary use of a surgical collar or to the injection of a local anaesthetic agent and long-acting corticosteroids, such as Depomedrol, into tender areas of the suboccipital region. Transcutaneous electrical nerve stimulation (TENS) may relieve pain and thus restore mobility more rapidly (Nordemar and Thorner, 1981). Relaxation training is a useful adjunct to other forms of treatment because excessive muscle contraction is commonly present. Psychological management and the use of antidepressants may be equally important (Tyler, McNeely and Dick, 1980). Release of the occipital nerve in 13 patients with occipital neuralgia after a whiplash injury caused improvement but not complete pain relief in most (Magnusson et al., 1966). In a few patients resistant to other forms of therapy, division of the posterior rami or radio-frequency lesions of the facet joints or dorsal root ganglia may be considered (Sluijter and Koetsveld-Baart, 1980).

More work is required to establish which components of the whiplash syndrome are caused by damage to cervical discs, ligaments or soft tissues, and which are caused by excessive muscle contraction associated with anxiety and depression.

6. Muscle-contraction ('tension') headache

It has been amply pointed out in the medical literature that multiple symptoms may follow minor head injuries where compensation or litigation is involved, that self-employed or professional men return to work more rapidly than employees after head injury, and that sporting injuries are not usually followed by disability. Any tendency to anxiety or depression appears to be accentuated by head injury, and the personality of the patient before the accident plays a large part in the way that he or she reacts to injury. Some post-traumatic headaches have all the qualities of tension-type headache and respond, at least in part, to the use of tranquillizing and anti-depressant drugs. This form of headache is often engendered by that natural worry which attaches to the possibility of brain damage and is reinforced by some legal advisers who instruct their clients not to resume work or normal activities until the case is settled.

7. Other post-traumatic headaches

Cluster-like headache has been described after head injury and is more usual after injury near the eye or forehead. Newman *et al.* (1996) recently reported three patients with hemicrania continua after head injury.

Psychological aspects

A strong case for the concept of accident neurosis being the most important factor in post-traumatic symptoms was made by Miller (1961). Certainly, cases of 'functional overlay' and even frank malingering are encountered. Ellard (1970) has summarized the psychological reactions that he has encountered in patients with a compensatable injury.

Attitudinal pathosis. A patient who does not seek to be healed but to be justified. He is not incapacitated by symptoms but has a grievance and believes that he cannot work because he has been dealt with unjustly.

Schizophrenic reaction. This is commonly paranoid with feelings of persecution by doctors, solicitors and even the law courts.

Bizarre hypochondriasis. A group of patients who before injury were fitness fanatics, narcissistic and preoccupied with health foods and sporting activities. They commonly describe their headache in an exaggerated manner and are often diagnosed as hysterical.

Traumatic neurosis. Here the accident may have symbolic significance but more commonly the patient's anxiety is conditioned by the accident. Such patients may respond to behaviour therapy.

Depression. Many patients who become depressed are of compulsive personality in whom work has become an important defence mechanism. Typical depressive symptoms follow deprivation of their normal working pattern.

Compensation neurosis. Depressive symptoms are usually overshadowed by those of anxiety. The patient often becomes aggressive at work as well as at home. Hysterical manifestations may become superimposed. The total amount of disability is usually greater than the sum of its parts.

Malingering. The paradox of the man who remains sick because of the hope of financial reward.

Ellard stresses the need to assess each patient in the light of his racial, cultural and educational background as well as his premorbid personality. The patient with an excessive psychological reaction to injury looks well in spite of his description of suffering. There is a lack of motivation to get well and his attitude to treatment is unusual and may be resentful.

Not all patients with head and neck pain following injury have a psychological disorder and not all have their eye fixed on financial gain. McKinlay, Brooks and Bond (1983) compared two groups of patients after a blunt head injury, those with and those without a claim for financial compensation. Post-concussional symptoms, intellectual performance and behavioural changes were similar in the two groups, although claimants did report more symptoms than the control group. There was no significant difference between the two groups in the time taken to return to work. Radanov *et al.* (1991) found that psychosocial factors, negative affect and personality traits were not helpful in predicting the outcome of whiplash injury. Young and Packard (1997) recently summarized the extensive literature on post-traumatic headache, helping to dispel the 'myth of non-organicity'.

Prognosis

The settlement of the legal aspects of the matter does not always lead to disappearance of symptoms and return to work. Balla and Moraitis (1970) followed up 82 patients, 41 of whom suffered from headache, after industrial or traffic accidents. They found that 21 patients had not returned to work 2 years after financial settlement. Those who did return to work usually did so within a year. Mendelson (1982) reviewed follow-up studies of litigants to ascertain the effect of legal settlement on symptoms that were attributed to injuries relating to compensation claims. Up to 75 per cent failed to return to gainful employment 2 years after the legal case was concluded. Cartlidge and Shaw (1981) distinguished between those patients whose headaches had persisted since discharge from hospital, dropping from about 36 per cent at the time of discharge to about 20 per cent of patients at 1- and 2-year follow-up, and 'late-acquired' headaches that had developed in 20 per cent of cases during the 6 months since the accident. Of the latter group, 83 per cent were pursuing compensation claims, compared with only 20 per cent of the 'persisting group'. Depression was a feature in 44 per cent and 12 per cent, respectively, at the 6-month follow up. McKinlay, Brooks and Bond (1983) could find no significant difference in the time taken to return to work after blunt head injury between those who were claiming compensation and those who were not.

Of 78 patients who suffered a whiplash injury of the neck, 57 had recovered fully within 6 months, while 21 had persisting symptoms (Radanov et al., 1991). A poor prognosis was related to the initial intensity of neck pain, injury-related cognitive impairment and age.

As a late sequel of head injury, a meningioma may develop at the site of a previous skull injury (Walshe, 1961). The evidence is anecdotal but, as Walshe commented: 'The perpetually "open mind" is not an effective instrument of thought, and may too easily become a euphemism for the mind closed to the lessons of experience'.

Treatment

The early management of head injury may be important in reducing the disability which so often follows. Relander, Troupp and Bjorkesten (1972) compared the result of an active treatment programme with the routine treatment of comparable patients in the same hospital. The active treatment group were visited daily and the nature of the injury was explained to them. They were encouraged to get out of bed and start physiotherapy. When they attended the follow-up clinic, they were seen by the same doctors who had looked after them in hospital. The active treatment group returned to work in an average of 18 days compared with 32 days for other patients.

Symptomatic treatment depends on the variety of post-traumatic headache. The vascular forms of headache are best treated with the medications used for the management of migraine and cluster headache. Specific forms of treatment for whiplash injury are considered above under that heading and also in Chapter 16. The tension-type headaches may respond to psychological counselling, relaxation therapy and antidepressant agents.

Conclusion

The great difficulty in handling patients with post-traumatic headache is to differentiate the organic from the psychogenic components. It seems undeniable that many post-traumatic headaches are of organic origin, in the sense that the control of cranial vessels has become more unstable and cranial arteries have become more susceptible to painful dilatation since injury (Taylor, 1967). The probability of a headache being caused by head or neck injury depends upon a comparison of the patient's susceptibility to headache before and after head injury, the latent period between injury and the onset of headache or aggravation of any pre-existing symptoms, and the site and nature of the headache. It requires an unbiased approach on the part of the physician and a careful assessment of each patient's personality and his or her headache pattern to ensure that justice is done to any legal claim and that treatment is appropriate to the variety of headache.

References

Appenzeller, O. (1987). Post-traumatic headaches. In *Wolff's Headache and Other Head Pain*, 5th Edition, Ed. D. J. Dalessio. pp. 289–303. New York, Oxford University Press

Balla, J. I. (1980). Late whiplash syndrome. *Aust. N. Z. J. Surg.* **50**, 610–614

Balla, J. I. and Moriatis. S. (1970). Knights in armour. A follow-up study of injuries after legal settlement. *Med. J. Aust.* **2**, 355–361

Brenner, C., Friedman. A. P., Merritt, H. H. and Denny-Brown, D. E. (1944). Post-traumatic headache. *J. Neurosurg.* **6**, 379–392

Cartlidge, N. E. F. and Shaw, D. A. (1981). *Head Injury.* pp. 95–115. London, W. B. Saunders

Ellard, J. (1970). Psychological reactions to compensatable injury. *Med. J. Aust.* **2**, 349–355

Gilkey, S. J., Ramadan, N. M., Aurora, T. K. and Welch, K. M. A. (1997). Cerebral blood flow in chronic post-traumatic headache. *Headache* **37**, 583–587

Haas, D. C. (1996). Chronic post-traumatic headaches classified and compared with natural headaches. *Cephalalgia* **16**, 486–493

Headache Classification Committee of the International Headache Society (1988). Classification and diagnostic criteria for headache disorders, cranial neuralgias and facial pain. *Cephalalgia* **8** (Suppl. 7), 9–96

Jacome, D. E. (1986). Basilar artery migraine after uncomplicated whiplash injuries. *Headache* **26**, 515–516

La Rocca, H. (1978). Acceleration injuries of the neck. *Clin. Neurosurg.* **25**, 209–217

Lord, S. M., Barnsley, L., Wallis, B. J. and Bogduk, N. (1994). Third occipital nerve headache: a prevalence study. *J. Neurol. Neurosurg. Psychiat.* **57**, 1187–1190

Lord, S. M., Barnsley, L., Wallis, B. J., McDonald, G. J. and Bogduk, N. (1996). Percutaneous radio-frequency neurotomy for chronic cervical zygapophyseal-joint pain. *New Eng. J. Med.* **335**, 1721–1726

Magnusson, T., Ragnarsson, T. and Bjornsson, A. (1996). Occipital nerve release in patients with whiplash trauma and occipital neuralgia. *Headache* **36**, 32–36

McKinlay, W. W., Brooks, D. N. and Bond, M. R. (1983). Post-concussional symptoms, financial compensation and the outcome of severe blunt head injury. *J. Neurol. Neurosurg. Psychiat.* **46**, 1084–1091

Mendelson, G. (1982). Not 'cured by a verdict'. Effect of legal settlement on compensation claims. *Med. J. Aust.* **2**, 132–134

Miller, H. (1961). Accident neurosis. *Br. Med. J.* **1**, 919–925, 992–998

Newman, L. C., Solomon, S. and Lipton R. B. (1997). Post-traumatic hemicrania continua. *Neurology* **48** (Suppl.), A123

Nordemar, R. and Thorner, C. (1981). Treatment of acute cervical pain – a comparative group study. *Pain* **10**, 93–101

Otte, A., Ettlin, T. M., Nitzsche, E. U., Wachter, K., Hoegerle, S., Simon, G. H., Fierz, L., Moser, E. and Mueller-Brand, J. (1997). PET and SPECT in whiplash syndrome: a new approach to a forgotten brain. *J. Neurol. Neurosurg. Psychiat.* **63**, 368–372.

Povlishock, J. T., Becker, D. P., Cheng, C. L. Y. and Vaughan, G. W. (1983). Axonal change in minor head injury. *J. Neuropath. Exp. Neurol.* **42**, 725–742

Radanov, B. P., Di Stefano, G., Schnidrig, A. and Ballarini, P. (1991). Role of psychosocial stress in recovery from common whiplash. *Lancet* **338**, 712–715

Ramadan, N. M., Norris, L. L. and Schulz, L. R. (1995). Abnormal cerebral blood flow correlates with disability due to chronic post-traumatic headache. *J. Neuroimaging* **5**, 68

Raney, A. A. and Raney, R. B. (1918). Headache: a common symptom of cervical disk lesions. *Arch. Neurol. Psychiat., Chicago* **59**, 603–621

Relander, M., Troupp, H. and Bjorkesten, G. (1972). Controlled trial of treatment for cervical concussion. *Br. Med. J.* **2**, 777–779

Russell, M. D. and Olesen, J. (1996). Migraine associated with head trauma. *Eur. J. Neurol.* **3**, 424–428

Ryan, G. A., Taylor, G. W., Moore, V. M. and Dolinis, J. (1993). Neck strain in car occupants. The influence of crash-related factors on initial severity. *Med. J. Aust.* **159**, 651–656

Scherokman, B. and Massey, W. (1983). Post-traumatic headaches. In *Neurologic Clinics, Volume 1, No. 2. Symposium on Headache*, Ed. R. C. Packard. pp. 457–463. Philadelphia, Saunders

Simons, D. J. and Wolff, H. G. (1946). Studies on headache: mechanisms of chronic post-traumatic headache. *Psychosom. Med.* **8**, 227–242

Sluijter, M. E. and Koetsveld-Baart, C. C. (1980). Interruption of pain pathways in the treatment of the cervical syndrome. *Anaesthesia* **35**, 302–307

Taylor, A. R. (1967). Post-concussional sequelae. *Br. Med. J.* **2**, 67

Taylor, J. R. and Kakulas, B. A. (1991). Neck injuries. *Lancet* **338**, 1343

Tubbs, O. N. and Potter, J. M. (1970). Early post-concussional headache. *Lancet* **ii**, 128–129

Tulyapronchote, R., Selhorst, J. B., Malkoff, M. D. and Gomez, C. R. (1994). Delayed sequelae of vertebral artery dissection and occult cervical fractures. *Neurology* **44**, 1397–1399

Tyler, G. S., McNeely, H. E. and Dick, M. L. (1980). Treatment of post-traumatic headache with amitriptyline. *Headache* **20**, 213–216

Vijayan, N. and Dreyfus, P. M. (1975). Post-traumatic dysautonomic cephalagia, clinical observations and treatment. *Arch. Neurol.* **32**, 649–652

Walshe, F. (1961). Head injuries as a factor in the aetiology of intracranial meningioma. *Lancet* **ii**, 993–996

Wilkinson, M. and Gilchrist, E. (1977). The incidence of headache in patients with severe head injuries. In *Cephalees Post-Traumatiques, Colloque de Bordeaux*. p. 41. Laboratories Sandoz, Rueil Malmaison

Young, W. B. and Packard, R. D. (1997). Post-traumatic headache and post-traumatic syndrome. In *Headache*. Eds P. J. Goadsby and W. D. Silberstein. pp. 253–277. Boston, Butterworth-Heinemann

Chapter 14

Vascular disorders

Acute ischaemic cerebrovascular disease

Transient ischaemic attacks

Fisher (1968) reported that seven out of 20 patients with vertebrobasilar ischaemic attacks experienced headache, usually occipital or occipito-frontal in distribution. He described the headache that accompanied transient ischaemic attacks (TIAs) in six patients who subsequently developed a complete internal carotid occlusion. The ache was mild, commonly frontal but sometimes radiating to the occiput, and lasted only for the duration of the neurological deficit. He also questioned 58 patients with transient monocular blindness (amaurosis fugax) but found none who felt pain or discomfort with the attack.

In contrast to this experience, Grindal and Toole (1974) noted that four out of five patients with amaurosis fugax complained of pain behind the eye or in the temple, severe and stabbing in two cases, following the episode. These authors reviewed the case histories of 240 patients with TlAs and selected 58 in whom a definite history of headache had been recorded. They concluded that headache was a prominent symptom in about 25 per cent of patients and was the presenting complaint in nearly one-third. A negative history of headache was recorded for only 50 of the 240 patients, so the prevalence of headache in TIAs may have been underestimated. Of 33 patients with carotid insufficiency, the headache was ipsilateral to the diseased carotid in nine, contralateral in two and bilateral in the remainder, commonly affecting the frontal region. Headache in vertebrobasilar insufficiency was more consistently associated with the ischaemic attacks and affected the occiput or neck in 15 out of 23 cases.

Portenoy et al. (1984) found that 10 out of 28 patients (36 per cent) had complained of headache before, during or after their TIAs. Medina, Diamond and Rubino (1975) commented on late onset vascular headaches starting in middle age or later in 18 of their 34 patients and recurring independently of their TIAs. These headaches began several years before the onset of TIAs in 13 and some months after in five cases. There was no association with hypertension or a previous history of migraine.

The cause of headaches in transient ischaemia remains obscure. As the site of headache is related to the site of origin of the TIA some local factor is presumably involved. Edmeads (1979) investigated 58 patients with TIAs by cerebral angiography and cortical blood flow studies. The frequency of headache in those TIAs with a carotid origin was 26 per cent and for those of vertebrobasilar origin 17 per cent. There was no evidence that collateral circulation was any greater in those with headache than those without. Possibly a transient reflex vascular dilatation in response to ischaemia or the passage of a platelet embolus may be responsible.

Thromboembolic stroke

Occlusion of a major cerebral vessel usually takes place without pain. Fisher (1968) recorded some pain or discomfort in 35 of 109 cases (31 per cent) with internal carotid occlusion. Two had experienced neck pain. Pain in the neck overlying the carotid artery (carotidynia) may signal the presence of a long intraluminal clot, particularly if associated with headache and symptoms of vascular insufficiency (Donnan and Bladin, 1980).

The incidence of headache with middle cerebral artery occlusion was determined by Fisher (1968) to be 21 per cent, and for the posterior cerebral artery 50 per cent, whereas nine patients with anterior cerebral artery thrombosis were not aware of headache. Of 94 patients with basal artery occlusion, 41 (44 per cent) had headache or head pain. Lacunar infarcts were not accompanied by pain. Edmeads (1979) found similar figures for headaches with infarction in carotid (25 per cent) and vertebrobasilar (27 per cent) territories. Gorelick et al. (1986) reported a warning ('sentinel') headache days or weeks before stroke in 10 per cent of patients and a headache at onset in 17 per cent.

The size of the infarct and attendant oedema is usually not sufficient to account for headache by displacement of intracranial structures. It is unlikely that 5-HT or other vasoactive agents could be released from platelet emboli in quantities sufficient to cause significant vascular changes. Possibly ischaemia of the brain or brain stem may trigger vascular changes or migrainous phenomena. Collateral circulation does not appear to be a factor (Edmeads, 1979).

The combination of mitochondrial myopathy, encephalopathy, lactic acidosis and stroke-like episodes (MELAS syndrome) has episodic headache as one of the main features (Goto et al., 1992).

Thrombosis of the posterior inferior cerebellar artery is demonstrated by vertebral arteriography in Figure 18.2.

Intracranial haematoma

Intracerebral haematoma

The most important cause of intracerebral haemorrhage is chronic hypertension and the most common sites are the putamen (60 per cent), thalamus (10 per cent), pons (10 per cent) and cerebellum (10 per cent). Fisher (1968) reported the frequency of headache as varying from 13 per cent for putaminal haemorrhage to 50 per cent in the case of the cerebellum. Gorelick et al. (1986) found that 55 per cent of patients with intraparenchymal haemorrhage suffered headache, usually unilateral and severe, at the onset. Bleeding into one lobe of the cerebrum is less common than into basal ganglia or thalamus but gives rise to a more localized referral of pain. Pain is felt around the ipsilateral eye if the haemorrhage is in the occipital lobe, anterior to the ear for the temporal lobe, in the temporal region for the parietal lobe and in the forehead in the case of the frontal lobe (Ropper and Davis, 1980).

As would be expected, headache is a presenting feature in those patients with signs of meningeal irritation or CT evidence of intraventricular or subarachnoid bleeding, hydrocephalus, transtentorial herniation or midline shift (Melo, Pinto and Ferro, 1996). In most patients with cerebral haemorrhage, the headache is overshadowed by the rapid onset of a devastating neurological deficit, drowsiness or vomiting. Progressive deterioration or the CT finding of hydrocephalus may dictate urgent evacuation of an intracerebellar haematoma but, contrary to earlier belief, many patients recover well with conservative management (Melamed and Satya-Murti, 1984).

Subdural and extradural haematoma

Extradural (epidural) haematomas are nearly always the result of head injury with a fracture line extending across the middle meningeal artery. Headache and impairment of consciousness following head injury should arouse the suspicion of an extradural bleed before dilatation of the ipsilateral pupil indicates impending tentorial herniation. Urgent removal of the haematoma is required as the patient may die within a matter of hours.

On the other hand, subdural haematoma generally runs a slow course as bleeding takes place from small veins bridging the gap between cortex and venous sinuses. There may be a latent period of weeks or months between a minor head injury and the onset of symptoms. Subdural haematomas may present acutely if the source of bleeding is rupture of small arteries on the surface of the cortex. Headache and drowsiness usually antecede neurological signs.

Subarachnoid haemorrhage

Bleeding into the subarachnoid space may take place after head injury, or secondary to an intracerebral haemorrhage or 'spontaneously' in patients with a cerebral aneurysm or angioma. Less commonly, bleeding may be a result of blood dycrasias, haemorrhage from a cerebral tumour or some form of arteritis. The ratio of aneurysm to angioma as a cause of subarachnoid haemorrhage varies in different Western series from 5 : 1 to 25 : 1. The pattern is quite different in Asia, where angioma is more common. The headache of subarachnoid haemorrhage follows exertion in about one-third of patients. It usually starts suddenly and dramatically, 'like a blow on the head'. There may be a poorly localized sensation of something giving way inside the head, followed by unilateral headache that rapidly becomes generalized and spreads to the back of the head and neck, accompanied by photophobia. The patient may lose consciousness, with or without an epileptic seizure. The neck is usually rigid, and focal neurological signs are found if the aneurysm has compressed cranial nerves in enlarging or has bled into the brain substance. Pain in the back and legs may follow a subarachnoid haemorrhage after some hours or days, because of blood irritating the lumbosacral nerve roots. Haemorrhages may be seen in the fundi, spreading out from the optic discs, in some 7 per cent of patients, and papilloedema is found in 13 per cent (Walton, 1956). Fever, albuminuria, glycosuria, hypertension and electrocardiographic changes may be present in the acute phase.

One or more brief severe headaches may precede subarachnoid haemorrhage by several months. Such 'sentinel' headaches have been reported in 31 per cent (Gorelick *et al.*, 1986), 43 per cent (Verweij, Wijdicks and van Gijn, 1988) and 50 per cent (Østergaard, 1991) of patients who later developed subarachnoid haemorrhage. The headaches are usually bioccipital, bifrontal or unilateral and are unlike anything the patient has ever experienced before. They may be associated with vomiting, neck stiffness and blurred or double vision, suggesting that they are caused by a small preliminary leak.

The initial investigation for suspected subarachnoid haemorrhage is computerized tomography (CT scanning), which is positive in about 95 per cent of patients in the first 24 hours (Adams *et al.*, 1983). If the CT scan is negative but the index of suspicion is high, a lumbar puncture should be done, which usually demonstrates uniformly bloodstained fluid.

After 4–12 hours, xanthochromia of the cerebrospinal fluid becomes apparent and it disappears from 12–40 days after the haemorrhage. A lymphocytic cellular reaction and increase in CSF protein to 70–130 mg/100 ml (0.7–1.3 g/litre) usually follows subarachnoid haemorrhage (Walton, 1956). Cerebral angiography in patients with proven subarachnoid haemorrhage demonstrates an aneurysm in most cases (Duffy, 1983) and this is clipped whenever possible. If no aneurysm or angioma can be found, the patient is confined to bed for 4–6 weeks, and resumes normal activities gradually.

Unruptured aneurysm or vascular malformation

Of 220 patients with arteriovenous malformations diagnosed by carotid angiography at the National Hospital for Nervous Diseases, London, 12 (5 per cent) were found to have a history of migraine (Blend and Bull, 1967). Other studies have reported a migraine history in 15 per cent of 110 patients (Paterson and McKissock, 1956) and 31 per cent of 48 patients (Waltimo, Hokkanen and Piiskanen, 1975) with arteriovenous malformations. The last figure was derived after careful questioning of all patients about their previous headache pattern.

In Walton's series of 312 cases of subarachnoid haemorrhage, 16 (5 per cent) gave a definite history of migraine. Six of his patients lost their migraine attacks after the episode of haemorrhage. Davis (1967) found that 6 per cent of 431 patients presenting with subarachnoid haemorrhage had a migrainous history. Wolff (1963) found that seven out of 46 patients with subarachnoid haemorrhage had suffered from migraine and another 12 had periodic recurrent headaches. However, the side of the aneurysm did not always relate to the side of the headache, and Wolff considered that the headache was independent of the presence or absence of aneurysm.

It seems to be quite clear that unruptured aneurysms are not associated with migraine or other recurrent headaches, but it remains uncertain whether arteriovenous malformations are found in migraine patients more than would be expected by chance. Bruyn (1984) argues for such an association. We remain doubtful because cerebral angiography is undertaken in migraine patients only when the habitual occurrence of neurological symptoms has alerted the clinician to the possibility of an underlying lesion. It is more probable that the presence of an arteriovenous malformation reduces local cortical perfusion to the point that it produces focal neurological symptoms when cerebral blood flow is further reduced during the aura, and is thus responsible for the nature of the aura but not for the initiation of the migrainous process.

Certainly carotid arteriography is not indicated solely because migraine attacks habitually affect the same side of the head. If the patient also has a loud intracranial bruit, focal fits, an equivocal CT scan or has had a subarachnoid haemorrhage, then the likelihood of a positive result from carotid angiography is greatly increased. Some patients with cerebral angiomas have repeated small subarachnoid haemorrhages which are confused with migraine attacks or are thought to be episodes of 'encephalitis'.

Arteritis

Granulomatous angiitis, as an intracranial manifestation of herpes zoster, causes neurological deficit that is not usually accompanied by headache (MacKenzie, Forbes and Karnes, 1981). Systemic lupus erythematosus (SLE) may be associated with headache and papilloedema that respond to corticosteroid administration (Silverberg and Laties, 1973). Montalbán et al. (1992) found that, of 103 patients with SLE, 32 suffered from migraine headaches. The presence of anticardiolipin antibodies in SLE was 29 per cent but showed no correlation with a tendency to migraine. In the absence of other neurological symptoms and signs, the presence of headache in this condition does not indicate involvement of the central nervous system (Atkinson and Appenzeller, 1975). By way of contrast, a related disorder known as temporal or giant-cell arteritis has headache as its most important presenting symptom.

Giant-cell arteritis (temporal arteritis)

Temporal arteritis is a rare form of chronic daily headache but assumes clinical importance because it is a preventable cause of blindness. It usually affects people over 50 years of age but patients as young as 35 years of age have been reported. The prevalence in the over-fifties is 133 per 100,000 but rises to 843 per 100,000 in those over 80 years of age (Huston et al., 1978). The female to male ratio is 2 : 1.

Headache is the presenting complaint in about half the patients and is a feature in about 85 per cent during the course of the illness. It is commonly bitemporal but may be unilateral or generalized as a constant dull ache. Sudden loss of vision in one eye was the first symptom in eight of 35 patients examined in our own hospital group

(Koorey, 1984). In this series the temporal artery was clinically abnormal in 24 cases, with tenderness, thickening or nodularity of the vessel wall and diminished pulsation being found on examination (Figure 14.1a). A low grade fever and other indications of systemic disturbance, such as muscle and joint pain (polymyalgia rheumatica), are a feature in about 25–40 per cent of patients. Temporal artery biopsy shows the typical appearance of giant-cell arteritis in about half of the patients with this condition (Murray, 1977) (Figure 14.1b).

Inflammation may spread to arteries other than the temporal and other extracranial vessels. The cause of blindness is involvement of the posterior ciliary artery supplying the optic disc, which produces ischaemic papillopathy and consecutive optic atrophy. Double vision may result from ischaemia of the oculomotor nerve, in which case the pupil is usually spared, or from damage to the extra-ocular muscles themselves. Diplopia is reported by about 15 per cent of patients at some stage of the illness. Pain in the temporal and masseter muscles on chewing (jaw claudication) is virtually pathognomonic of temporal arteritis but occurs in only 25–40 per cent of patients in reported series. A rare complication is gangrene of the tongue (Davis and Davis, 1966; Dare, Byrne and Robertson, 1981). A patient of ours developed this unpleasant condition while on steroid therapy for temporal arteritis (Figure 14.1c and d). The aorta, vertebral, coronary, renal and iliac arteries may become affected. Transient ischaemic attacks, vertigo, ischaemic neuropathies and myelopathy have also been reported.

The erythrocyte sedimentation rate (ESR) ranged from 40 to 140 mm/hour (mean 82 mm/hour) in the case histories analysed by Koorey (1984). A normal value may be found early in the disease, even at a time when biopsy shows the process to be active. If the index of suspicion is high, a temporal artery biopsy should be arranged as a matter of urgency. Steroid therapy should be started as soon as the diagnosis is made on clinical grounds because blindness can strike suddenly while the patient is awaiting biopsy and subsequent histological confirmation. Temporal artery biopsy is not always positive because the disease process may be patchy with unaffected 'skip lesions' (Klein *et al.*, 1976). Selective extracranial angiography may help to identify the affected areas and thus guide the hand of the surgeon. The removal of a long segment of temporal artery for examination improves the success rate. Even with these precautions, the biopsy may still prove negative. Hall *et al.* (1983) followed up 134 patients who had undergone temporal artery biopsies. Of 46 patients with positive biopsies, polymyalgia rheumatica was a feature in 38 per cent and jaw claudication in 54 per cent. Temporal arteries were palpable in 67 per cent and the ESR was 50 mm/hour or more in all cases. The 88 patients with negative biopsies had almost equal frequencies of polymyalgia rheumatica, malaise, fever and weight loss, but jaw claudication was rare and the temporal arteries were palpable in only 31 per cent. Only eight of the biopsy-negative patients required long-term steroid therapy. Non-specific abnormalities in giant-cell arteritis include mild anaemia, neutrophil leucocytosis, low serum albumin, increased alpha-2 globulin, and abnormal liver enzyme levels. Hyperthyroidism is an occasional association.

Biopsy demonstrates a thickened arterial wall and intima, and often a thrombus in the lumen (Figure 14.1b). The elastic lamellae are disrupted, the media is infiltrated with round cells and giant cells may be seen. The condition appears to belong

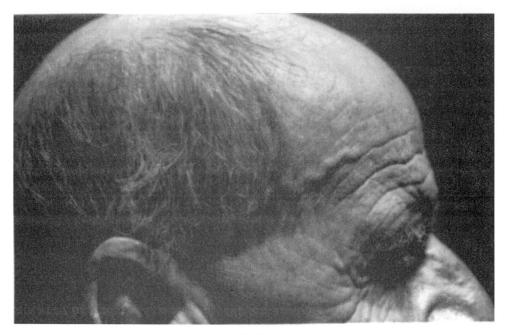

14.1(a)

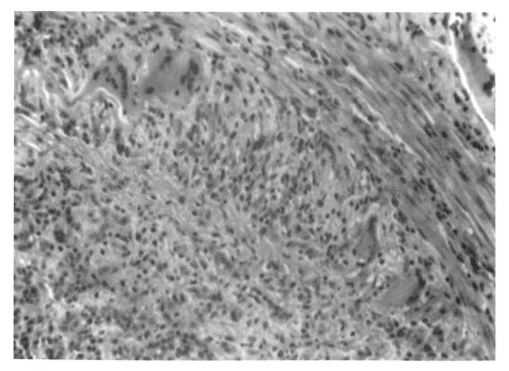

14.1(b)

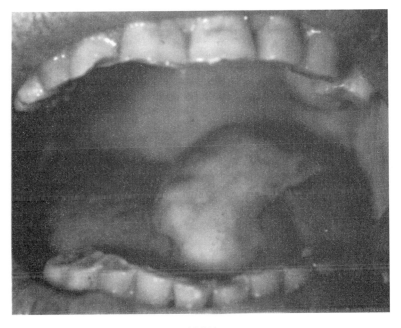

14.1(c)

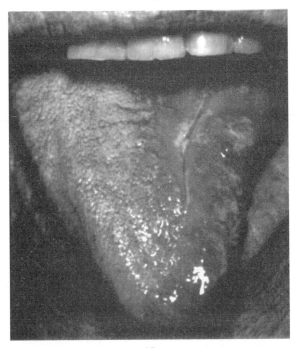

(d)

Figure 14.1 Temporal arteritis: (a) a prominent tender temporal artery; (b) biopsy appearance of giant-cell arteritis; (c) gangrene of one-half of the tongue caused by occlusion of the lingual artery; (d) after resolution of the tongue lesion

somewhere between acute auto-immune vasculitis and chronic non-caseating granuloma such as sarcoid. Immunoglobins demonstrated in the arterial wall may represent antibodies to elastin or may be taken up from circulating immune complexes (Liang, Simkin and Mannik, 1974).

Temporal arteritis is usually a self-limited inflammatory disease that generally runs a course of 1–2 years (Caselli, Hunder and Whisnant, 1988). The prognosis was worse in those patients reported by Graham et al. (1981) from Moorfield's Eye Hospital and neurological centres in London. Of 90 patients, 44 presented with visual loss and 32 patients died. Of the surviving patients, the disease 'burnt out' in a period ranging from 6 months to 7 years in one-third, was stabilized on low dosage of steroids in one-third, and ran a relapsing and remitting course in the remainder. Visual loss in one or both eyes has been reported in up to 50 per cent of untreated cases but is reduced to about 13 per cent by the early introduction of steroid therapy (Klein et al., 1976). The late incidence of stroke is probably no greater than that of age-matched control patients (Caselli et al., 1988) but Graham et al. (1981) described four patients out of 90 with proven disease who died in the acute phase of a brain stem stroke, with vertebral arteritis or thrombosis being demonstrated in the three autopsied cases. Life expectancy is diminished in women, but not men (Dare, Byrne and Robertson, 1981; Graham et al., 1981). The outlook is worse if vision has been lost or maintenance dosage of prednisone exceeds 10 mg daily.

Prednisone 75 mg daily should be started as soon as the condition is diagnosed clinically, pending histological confirmation. The dosage is usually reduced in stages every third day down to 30 mg daily. The daily dose can then usually be reduced by 5 mg each week to a maintenance of about 10 mg daily, which is then continued for 3 months. Further reduction depends upon the clinical response and the ESR. Steroid therapy can be ceased in most patients after a period of 12–14 months. Side-effects of prolonged therapy include Cushingoid features, osteoporosis and avascular necrosis of the hip. Intravenous heparin and dextran may be given if there is fluctuating visual impairment.

Although the symptoms of temporal arteritis are readily recognizable, their duration before diagnosis in two series was a mean of five and a half months (Koorey, 1984; Dare and Byrne, 1980). The headache may lack distinctive features and be mistaken for tension headache. Muscle and joint pains are common in the elderly and are often treated symptomatically without investigation.

Early diagnosis is of great importance. A tragic example of a missed opportunity was a patient presenting when she was totally blind. She had consulted her medical practitioner 6 months previously for generalized muscular aching, and she had noted pain in the jaws on chewing at that time. A blood count was done, but not an ESR. She was treated with a series of antirheumatic drugs without relief until she went blind in one eye. She was admitted to hospital where steroid treatment was started immediately but the next day she lost her vision in the other eye. Probably the most common reason for the diagnosis being missed is that a normal ESR is mistakenly considered to exclude temporal arteritis. It must be borne in mind that up to 30 per cent of biopsy-confirmed patients may have an ESR of 40 mm/hour or less (Kansu et al., 1977). When the condition is suspected on the basis of the clinical history, whether or not the ESR is elevated, it is a good policy to have one temporal artery biopsied. Treatment can be started immediately, before the biopsy is taken. Steroid therapy may have to be continued for years and it is reassuring to have a firm histological diagnosis at the outset.

Carotid or vertebral artery pain

Carotid or vertebral dissection

West, Davies and Kelly (1976) reported a distinctive headache syndrome in eight patients with narrowing or occlusion of one internal carotid artery, shown to be caused by a dissecting aneurysm of the arterial wall in one operated case. The pain was unilateral and was associated with a Horner's syndrome on the same side and with contralateral neurological symptoms or signs in half the patients. The pain involved the head, neck or face and had a burning or throbbing quality. It subsided over a period of 2 months. Mokri et al. (1986) studied 36 patients with carotid dissection in whom headache, commonly periorbital and frontal, was a presenting symptom in 33, as was neck pain in seven and focal cerebral ischaemic symptoms in 24. An ocular Horner's syndrome was present in 21. Follow-up angiography demonstrated that the stenosis had resolved or diminished in 85 per cent of patients, associated with a good clinical recovery. A similar clinical picture was described by Bogousslavsky, Despland and Regli (1987) in 30 patients in whom headache was a feature in 17, associated with monocular blindness in four and some other neurological deficit in two. Two patients had an isolated neck pain (carotidynia). An ocular Horner's syndrome was observed in only 20 per cent in this series. Fisher (1982) emphasized that the pain usually occurs in the forequarter of the head, but may also involve the cheek, side of the nose, teeth and jaw. Of his 21 patients with carotid dissection, 12 had neck pain as well.

Dissection of the vertebral arteries causes pain in the upper neck and occiput, associated with a lateral medullary syndrome or cerebellar infarction (Caplan, Zarins and Hemmati, 1985). One patient developed a severe pain in one side of the occiput and upper neck after being struck by the boom of his yacht. The pain became much worse after chiropractic manipulation of his neck and angiography showed a localized dissection of the vertebral artery at the craniospinal junction (Figure 14.2). Caplan et al. (1985) cite 11 instances in which vertebral artery dissection has followed manipulation of the neck.

Carotidynia

There are many causes of carotidynia, a syndrome of neck pain associated with tenderness of the carotid artery (Roseman, 1968). One form is of acute onset in young or middle-aged adults in which the pain persists for an average of 11 days and does not usually recur. The pain radiates to the side of the face in about half the cases. Tenderness is maximal over the carotid bifurcation. There are usually no signs of systemic infection although some patients feel unwell and complain of nasal blockage and lacrimation. The ESR remains normal. The cause is unknown but

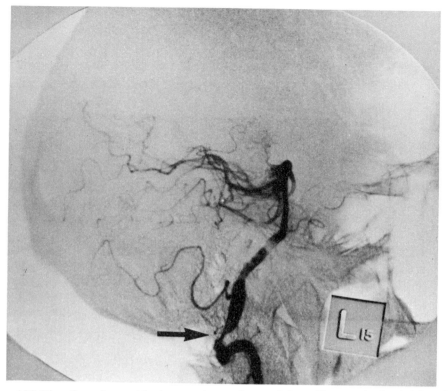

Figure 14.2 Dissection of a vertebral artery (arrowed) caused by a blow to the head followed by manipulation of the neck

the short course of the disorder suggests a viral infection. Treatment is symptomatic with analgesics. Prednisolone therapy has not proven helpful.

Another form of carotidynia may appear at any stage of adult life and recurs in attacks lasting minutes to hours, daily or weekly, often in conjunction with throbbing headache (Raskin and Prusiner, 1977). This form responds to ergotamine or substances such as methysergide used in the prophylaxis of migraine. Tenderness of the carotid artery is not uncommon in migraine and carotidynia may be an extreme form of this vascular sensitivity. (See also 'Recurrent neck pain' in Chapter 6.)

Carotidynia has also been reported with temporal arteritis, fibrosis around the carotid sheath, long intraluminal clots in the internal carotid artery (Donnan and Bladin, 1979) and dissecting aneurysm involving the arterial wall (Chambers *et al.*, 1981, and other references cited in the section above). An elongated styloid process may give rise to pain in the cheek, chin or neck along the area of distribution of the carotid artery (Eagle's syndrome) (Massey and Massey, 1979).

Post-endarterectomy headache

There have been reports of an intense vascular headache, localized to the fronto-temporal area of the affected side, following carotid endarterectomy (Leviton,

Caplan and Salzman, 1975; Pearce, 1976; Messert and Black, 1978). The headache comes on after a latent period of 36–72 hours and recurs intermittently for 1–6 months. It seems unlikely that the headache could be caused simply by the restoration of normal cerebral perfusion pressure. It is presumably triggered by afferent impulses from the carotid arterial wall.

Venous thrombosis

Of 38 patients described by Bousser *et al.* (1985) with thrombosis of cerebral veins or venous sinuses, 74 per cent presented with headache, 45 per cent with increased intracranial pressure, 34 per cent with hemiplegia and 29 per cent with seizures. Nine of the 38 patients were eventually found to have Behçet's disease, and five had underlying malignant disorders. Four cases followed mild head injury and four developed after infections of the ear or throat.

The lateral sinus may thrombose following infection of the middle ear and mastoid bone, causing cerebral oedema, termed 'otitic hydrocephalus' (Figure 14.3). There is no internal hydrocephalus since the ventricles are normal or small in size. The patient, usually a child, develops headache and papilloedema after an ear infection. The sixth nerve may be paralysed on the side of the lesion, or on both sides because of the nerves being stretched by the expanded brain. Radiographs commonly show opacity of the mastoid air cells. Treatment is directed to the infected ear and mastoid (which may include mastoidectomy and removal of the clot from the lateral sinus) and to reducing cerebral oedema.

Benign intracranial hypertension may be associated with a partial thrombosis of the superior sagittal sinus and is discussed in Chapter 15.

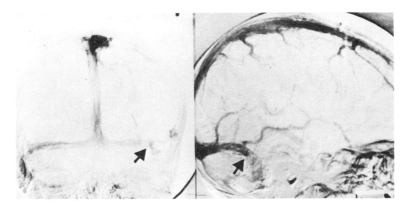

Figure 14.3 Thrombosis of the lateral sinus at the apex of the petrous temporal bone

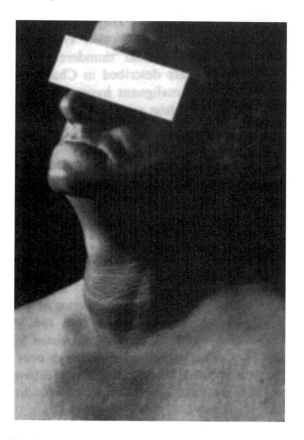

Figure 14.4 Increased jugular venous pressure caused by a large goitre. (From Lance, 1991, by permission of the editor of *Headache*)

Increased venous pressure

Mediastinal obstruction and emphysema can increase venous pressure sufficiently to interfere with cerebral venous drainage and cause papilloedema. Hypoxia associated with these conditions probably increases the tendency to oedema of the brain and optic nerve.

A patient of ours experienced a severe headache, at first right-sided and later generalized, which developed on lying down, flexing his neck or lifting his arms above his head. On coughing or sneezing he felt a sharp pain in and behind both eyes often followed by aching in the right temple (Lance, 1991). He was seen to have a large goitre (Figure 14.4), which proved to be Riedel's thyroiditis. After removal of the goitre, which was obstructing his jugular venous flow, he became completely free of headache. A similar increase in jugular venous pressure may be the basis of 'weightlifter's headache'. The mechanism of headache in thoracic outlet syndrome (Raskin, Howard and Ehrenfeld, 1985) is unknown but could well be related to venous compression in the neck.

Arterial hypertension

There is no doubt that a sudden rise of systemic blood pressure can cause headache. Acute pressor reactions caused by phaeochromocytoma and MAO inhibitors are described below. Such headaches are usually bilateral, affecting the occipital or frontal areas, and may involve the whole head. They are commonly severe, bursting or throbbing in quality, and associated with other symptoms of catecholamine release, such as tremor or palpitations. Similar 'thunderclap' headaches developing at the climax of sexual intercourse are described in Chapter 12. The increase in blood pressure in acute nephritis or malignant hypertension may also take place rapidly enough to cause headache (Healton *et al.*, 1982).

Whether the insidious onset of hypertension can be responsible for headache is less certain. The typical headache ascribed to hypertension by various writers over the past 60 years is bilateral, usually occipital in site, present on waking and easing as the patient gets up and about. Wolff (1963) pointed out that the headache associated with hypertension may respond to rest and relaxation without any material change in blood pressure. Symptoms of anxiety are common in hypertensive patients once they know that their blood pressure is elevated and muscle contraction headache may be a manifestation of this anxiety.

A community survey (Waters, 1971) involving 414 people, of whom 36 had a systolic pressure greater than 195 mmHg and 13 a diastolic pressure higher than 115 mmHg, disclosed no difference in the prevalence of headache between the small hypertensive group and the control subjects. On the other hand, Bulpitt, Dollery and Carne (1976) found that 31 per cent of untreated hypertensive patients complained of headaches on waking compared with 15 per cent of normal subjects and treated hypertensive patients, a statistically significant difference. The headache improved more often in those patients whose blood pressure dropped substantially on treatment.

Badran, Weir and McGuiness (1970) studied a group of 100 patients with a blood pressure of 150/95 mmHg or more and 100 matched normotensive controls. Headache was a symptom in 50 hypertensive patients and 39 controls. Headache was significantly more common in hypertensive patients only when the diastolic pressure was 140 mmHg or more. Eight of 12 patients with papilloedema had headache. Of the 11 patients in the grossly hypertensive group only two experienced occipital headache, the remainder being bitemporal or diffuse. Oddly enough, occipital headache was more common in the control group, affecting 20 of the 39 patients. The headache of gross hypertension did indeed occur in the mornings, eased after several hours and improved in those whose blood pressure responded to treatment. Bauer (1976), in a retrospective survey of 400 patients, could not find any significant correlation between the height of blood pressure and the incidence of headache. A follow-up extending to 15 years showed that there was no difference in mortality between those with headache and those without.

It may be tentatively concluded that hypertension by itself is not a common cause of headache but that there is an association between these disorders which may lead to improvement in headache with control of hypertension.

What of the relationship between hypertension and migraine? Walker (1959) found that hypertension was significantly more common in migraine patients over the age of 50 years. Leviton, Malvea and Graham (1974) compared the frequency of hypertension and vascular disease in migrainous and nonmigrainous parents of patients with migraine. 'High blood pressure' was significantly more common in the migrainous parents (whether men or women) in a ratio of 1.7 : 1 ($P < 0.05$). The incidence of heart attacks under the age of 70 years was almost three times higher in the migrainous parents ($P < 0.05$), irrespective of whether or not they were hypertensive. Curiously, the tendency to stroke was not increased.

Pressor reactions

Medication with MAO inhibitors

There have been many reports of patients under treatment with monoamine oxidase (MAO) inhibitors who have experienced sudden severe headache, often occipital in site, following the administration of sympathomimetic agents, drinking red wine or eating cheeses with a high tyramine content. The headaches are associated with a rapid increase in blood pressure and are relieved by the alpha-noradrenergic blocking agent, phentolamine. Some cases of subarachnoid and intracerebral haemorrhage have occurred at the height of the pressor reaction. Foods which contain large amounts of tyramine, excessive intake of caffeine (which is present in cola-flavoured drinks as well as in tea and coffee) and any sympathomimetic drugs must be avoided by patients taking MAO inhibitors. We issue a sheet of instructions to all patients prescribed MAO inhibitors stating that they must not take cheese, meat extracts such as Marmite, red wines, broad beans, chicken livers (pâté) or pickled herrings (rich in tyramine). They are prohibited from having any injections or tablets other than those prescribed specifically for headache, such as ergotamine, aspirin or codeine. The use of nasal decongestant sprays or tablets for sinusitis containing sympathomimetic agents must be avoided (see Figure 8.2).

Phaeochromocytoma

A rare but interesting cause of acute pressor reactions is phaeochromocytoma. Thomas, Rooke and Kvale (1966) reviewed the clinical histories of 100 patients with proven phaeochromocytoma seen at the Mayo Clinic in the preceding 20 years. Episodic headache was a feature of the attacks in 80 per cent of cases. It was usually of rapid onset, bilateral, severe, throbbing and was associated with nausea in about half the cases. The headache lasted less than 1 hour in 70 per cent and was accompanied by other symptoms of catecholamine release in 90 per cent.

Lance and Hinterberger (1976) analysed the case histories of 27 patients in whom the content of adrenaline (A) and noradrenaline (NA) had been assayed in blood, urine and in the tumour after it had been removed. We were unable to find any distinctive syndrome for tumours producing predominantly one of these amines. Sustained hypertension was more common in the NA-secreting group while pallor and tremor were more common when adrenaline was produced by the tumour as well. Other symptoms such as palpitations, sweating and anxiety were present in both groups. Headaches, which appeared to be related to a rapid increase in blood pressure, were a symptom in 20 of the 27 patients and had the same characteristics as those previously described by Thomas, Rooke and Kvale (1966). Blood pressure recorded during a headache ranged from 200/100 mmHg to 300/160 mmHg. However, blood pressures as high as 260/100 mmHg had been recorded in some patients who were not subject to headache. Two patients with bladder phaeochromocytoma experienced severe headache starting 15–20 seconds after micturition and lasting 1–3 minutes. Others described the headache as lasting for a few seconds or minutes only at the onset of their paroxysmal symptoms, but mostly the headache persisted for 5 minutes to 2 hours, subsiding gradually with the other symptoms of the attack. Nausea and vomiting accompanied the headache in seven patients and two complained of blurred vision. Six patients had collapsed, lost consciousness or developed focal neurological signs during the episodes. Attacks were provoked by exertion, straining, emotional upsets, worry or excitement. High levels of circulating catecholamine cause uptake and storage in other adrenergic tissue including the adrenal medulla, from which they are released on nervous stimulation. This accounts for paroxysmal symptoms being triggered by anxiety and excitement as well as by compression of the tumour.

The diagnosis depends on clinical suspicion being aroused when the history is first taken and is confirmed by finding increased excretion of catecholamines in three 24-hour specimens of urine, or elevated blood levels during an attack. Care must be taken that the patient has not taken any sympathomimetic drugs preceding the urine collection, nasal decongestant sprays being the most consistent offender. Blood sugar is usually elevated at the time of the attack, a useful distinction from hypoglycaemic attacks which may simulate phaeochromocytoma because of the secondary release of adrenaline in hypoglycaemia. The tumour is localized by ultrasound, CT or MR imaging or by aortic angiography if it is present in the characteristic suprarenal site. It must be borne in mind that phaeochromocytomas may arise at any point along the line of development of the sympathetic chain, extending downwards from the neck to the pelvis and scrotum. (See also 'Thunderclap headache' in Chapter 6.)

References

Adams, H. P., Kassell, N. F., Torner, J. C. and Sahs, A. L. (1983). CT and clinical correlations in recent aneurysmal subarachnoid haemorrhage: a preliminary report of the cooperative aneurysm study. *Neurology* **33**, 981–988

Atkinson, R. A. and Appenzeller, O. (1975). Headache in small vessel disease of the brain: a study of patients with systemic lupus erythematosus. *Headache* **15**, 198–201

Badran, R. H. Al., Weir, R. J. and McGuiness, J. B. (1970). Hypertension and headache. *Scott. Med. J.* **15**, 48–51

Bauer, G. E. (1976). Hypertension and headache. *Aust. N.Z. J. Med.* **6**, 492–497

Blend, R. and Bull, J. W. D. (1967). The radiological investigation of migraine. In *Background to Migraine*, Ed. R. Smith. pp. 1–10. London, Heinemann

Bogousslavsky, J., Despland, P.A. and Regli, F. (1987). Spontaneous carotid dissection with acute stroke. *Arch. Neurol.* **44**, 137–140

Bousser, M. G., Chiras, J., Bories, J. and Castaigne, P. (1985). Cerebral venous thrombosis – a review of 35 cases. *Stroke* **16**, 199–213

Bruyn, G. W. (1984) Intracranial arteriovenous malformation and migraine. *Cephalalgia* **4**, 191–207

Bulpitt, C. J., Dollery, C. T. and Carne, S. (1976). Change in symptoms of hypertensive patients after referral to hospital clinic. *Br. Heart J.* **38**, 121–128

Caplan, L. R., Zarins, C. K. and Hemmati, M. (1985). Spontaneous dissection of the extracranial vertebral arteries. *Stroke* **16**, 1030–1038

Caselli, R. J., Hunder, G. G. and Whisnant, J. P. (1988). Neurologic disease in biopsy-proven giant cell (temporal) arteritis. *Neurology* **38**, 352–359

Chambers, S. R. Donnan, G. A., Riddell, R. J. and Sladin, P. F. (1981). Carotidynia: aetiology, diagnosis and treatment. *Clin. Exp. Neurol.* **17**, 113–123

Dare, B. and Byrne, E. (1980). Giant cell arteritis. A five-year review of biopsy-proven cases in a teaching hospital. *Med. J. Aust.* **1**, 372–373

Dare, B., Byrne, E. and Robertson, A. (1981). Acute lingual ischaemia complicating temporal arteritis. *Med. J. Aust.* **1**, 534

Davis, E. (1967). Subarachnoid haemorrhage. *Med. J. Aust.* **2**, 12–14

Davis, A. E. and Davis, T. P. (1966). Gangrene of the tongue caused by temporal arteritis. *Med. J. Aust.* **2**, 459–460

Donnan, G. A. and Bladin, P. F. (1980) The stroke syndrome of long intraluminal clots with incomplete vessel obstruction. *Clin. Exp. Neurol.* **16**, 41–47

Duffy, G. P. (1983). The warning leak in spontaneous subarachnoid haemorrhage. *Med J. Aust.* **1**, 514–516

Edmeads, J. (1979). The headaches of ischemic cerebrovascular disease. *Headache* **19**, 345–349

Fisher, C. M. (1968). Headaches in cerebrovascular disease. In *Handbook of Clinical Neurology*, Vol. 5, Eds P. J. Vinken and G. W. Bruyn. pp. 124–151. Amsterdam, North Holland

Fisher, C. M. (1982). The headache and pain of spontaneous carotid dissection. *Headache* **22**, 60–65

Gorelick, P. B., Hier, D. B., Caplan, L. R. and Langenberg, P. (1986). Headache in acute cerebrovascular disease. *Neurology* **36**, 1445–1450

Goto, Y., Horai, S., Matsuoka, T. *et al.* (1992). Mitochondrial myopathy, encephalopathy, lactic acidosis, and stroke-like episodes (MELAS): a correlative study of the clinical features and mitochondrial DNA mutation. *Neurology* **42**, 545–550

Graham, E., Holland, A., Avery, A. and Ross Russell, R. W. (1981). Prognosis in giant-cell arteritis. *Br. Med. J.* **282**, 269–271

Grindal, A. B. and Toole, J. F. (1974). Headache and transient ischemic attacks. *Stroke* **5**, 603–606

Hall, S., Persellin, S., Lie, J. T., O'Brien, P. C., Kurland, C. T. and Hunder, G. G. (1983). The therapeutic impact of temporal artery biopsy. *Lancet* **ii**, 1217–1220

Healton, E. B., Brust. J. C., Feinfeld, D. A. and Thomson, G. E. (1982). Hypertensive encephalopathy and the neurological manifestations of malignant hypertension. *Neurology* **32**, 127–132

Huston, K. A., Hunder, G. G., Lie, J. T., Kennedy, R. H. and Elveback, L. R. (1978). Temporal arteritis. A 25 year epidemiologic, clinical and pathologic study. *Ann. Int. Med.* **88**, 162–167

Kansu, T., Corbett, J. J., Savino, P. and Schatz, N. J. (1977). Giant cell arteritis with normal sedimentation rate. *Arch. Neurol.* **34**, 624–625

Klein, R. G., Campbell, R. J., Hunder, G. G. and Carney, J. A. (1976). Skip lesions in temporal arteritis. *Mayo Clin. Proc.* **51**, 504–510

Koorey, D. J. (1984). Cranial arteritis. A twenty year review of cases. *Aust. N.Z. J. Med.* **14**, 143–147

Lance, J. W. (1991). Solved and unsolved headache problems. *Headache* **31**, 439–445

Lance, J. W. and Hinterberger, H. (1976). Symptoms of pheochromocytoma, with particular reference to headache, correlated with catecholamine production. *Arch. Neurol.* **33**, 281–288

Leviton, A., Caplan, L. and Salzman, E. (1975). Severe headache after carotid endarterectomy. *Headache* **15**, 207–210

Leviton, A., Malvea, B. and Graham, J. R. (1974). Vascular diseases, mortality, and migraine in the parents of migrainous patients. *Neurology* **24**, 669–672

Liang, C. G., Simkin, P. A. and Mannik, M. (1974). Immunoglobulins in temporal arteries. An immunofluorescent study. *Ann. Int. Med.* **81**, 19–24

MacKenzie, R. A., Forbes, G. S. and Karnes, W. E. (1981). Angiographic findings in herpes zoster arteritis. *Ann. Neurol.* **10**, 458–464

Massey, E. W. and Massey, J. (1979). Elongated styloid process (Eagle's syndrome) causing hemicrania. *Headache* **19**, 339–344

Medina, J. L., Diamond, S. and Rubino, R. A. (1975). Headache in patients with transient ischemic attacks. *Headache* **15**, 194–197

Melamed, N. and Satya-Murti, S. (1984). Cerebellar haemorrhage. A review and reappraisal of benign cases. *Arch. Neurol.* **41**, 425–428

Melo, T.P., Pinto, A.N. and Ferro, J.M. (1996). Headache in intracerebral hematoma. *Neurology* **47**, 494–500

Messert, B. and Black, J. A. (1978). Cluster headache, hemicrania and other head pains: morbidity of carotid endarterectomy. *Stroke* **9**, 559–562

Mokri, B., Sundt, T. M., Houser, O. W. and Piepgras, D. G. (1986). Spontaneous dissection of the cervical internal carotid artery. *Ann Neurol.* **19**, 126–138

Montalbán, J., Cervera, R., Font, J. *et al.* (1992). Lack of association between anticardiolipin antibodies and migraine in systemic lupus erythematosus. *Neurology* **42**, 681–682

Murray, T. J. (1977). Temporal arteritis. *J. Am. Geriat. Soc.* **25**, 450–453

Østergaard, T. R. (1991). Headache as a warning symptom of impending aneurysmal subarachnoid haemorrhage. *Cephalalgia* **11**, 53–55

Paterson, J. H. and McKissock, W. (1956). A clinical survey of intracranial angiomas with special reference to their mode of progression and surgical treatment: a report of 110 cases. *Brain* **79**, 233–266

Pearce, J. (1976). Headache after carotid endarterectomy. *Br. Med. J.* **3**, 85–86

Portenoy, R. K., Abissi, C. J., Lipton, R. B. *et al.* (1984). Headache in cerebrovascular disease. *Stroke* **15**, 1009–1012

Raskin, N. H., Howard, M. W. and Ehrenfeld, W. K. (1985). Headache as the leading symptom of the thoracic outlet syndrome. *Headache* **25**, 208–210

Raskin, N. H. and Prusiner, S. (1977). Carotidynia. *Neurology* **27**, 43–46

Roseman, D. M. (1968). Carotidynia. In *Handbook of Neurology*, Vol. 5, Eds P. J. Vinken and G. W. Bruyn. pp. 375–377. Amsterdam, North Holland

Ropper, A. H. and Davis, K. R. (1980). Lobar cerebral hemorrhages: acute clinical syndromes in 26 cases. *Ann. Neurol.* **8**, 141–147

Silberberg, D. H. and Laties, A. M. (1973). Increased intracranial pressure in disseminated lupus erythematosus. *Arch. Neurol.* **29**, 88–90

Thomas, J. E., Rooke, E. D. and Kvale, W. F. (1966). The neurologist's experience with pheochromocytoma: a review of 100 cases. *J. Am. Med. Assoc.* **197**, 751–758

Verwei, R. D., Wijdicks, E. F. M. and van Gijn, J. (1988). Warning headache in aneurysmal subarachnoid haemorrhage. *Arch. Neurol.* **45**, 1019–1020

Walker, C. H. (1959). Migraine and its relationship to hypertension. *Br. Med. J.* **2**, 1430–1433

Waltimo, O., Hokkanen, E. and Pirskanen, R. (1975). Intracranial arteriovenous malformations and headache. *Headache* **15**, 133–135

Walton, J. N. (1956). *Subarachnoid Haemorrhage*. Edinburgh, Livingstone

Waters, W. E. (1971). Headache and blood pressure in the community. *Br. Med. J.* **1**, 142–143

West, T. E. T., Davies, R. J. and Kelly, R. E. (1976) Horner's syndrome and headache due to carotid artery disease. *Br. Med. J.* **i**, 818–821

Wolff, H. G. (1963). *Headache and Other Head Pain*. London, Oxford University Press

Chapter 15

Non-vascular intracranial disorders

High cerebrospinal fluid pressure

Internal (obstructive) hydrocephalus

Any lesion that obstructs the flow of cerebrospinal fluid (CSF) from the lateral ventricles through the foramen of Monro, third ventricle, aqueduct and/or fourth ventricle and its exit foramina, or prevents the passage of CSF over the cortex to its absorption site (Figure 15.1) will cause a rapid increase in intracranial pressure so that headache becomes the main presenting symptom. The headache is commonly bilateral and is made worse by coughing, sneezing or head movement.

A tumour in the vicinity of the third ventricle or within it (such as a colloid cyst) (Figure 15.2) may also interfere intermittently with the function of the midbrain reticular formation so that posture cannot be maintained and the patient thus suffers from 'drop attacks', in which he or she slumps heavily to the ground. Severe paroxysmal headaches of recent origin should always arouse suspicion of intermittent obstructive hydrocephalus.

Stenosis of the aqueduct leading from the third ventricle to the fourth may be a congenital malformation that does not produce any symptoms until some systemic infection causes proliferation of its ependymal lining, which then blocks the canal and produces an acute internal hydrocephalus. The aqueduct may also be obstructed by a tumour in the vicinity of the midbrain, such as a pinealoma or glioma (see Figure 18.1), or the aqueduct and fourth ventricle may be displaced or blocked by tumours in the posterior fossa.

Hydrocephalus may progress slowly from conditions in the region of the cisterna magna and foramen magnum. Tumours in this area, cysticercosis, a congenital cystic malformation known as the Dandy–Walker syndrome, platybasia (basilar impression) or Arnold–Chiari malformation (see Figure 18.2) may be responsible for obstruction of the flow of CSF. Platybasia is a flattening of the floor of the posterior fossa with rotation of the anterior parts of the atlas and axis upwards. It may be a congenital anomaly, often associated with spina bifida, or may develop through softening of the base of the skull in Paget's disease, osteoporosis or osteomalacia.

The condition is diagnosed by computerized tomography (CT scanning) (Figure 15.2) or magnetic resonance imaging (MRI). The offending lesion is removed when possible. If not, the pressure in the dilated ventricles can be relieved by a technique

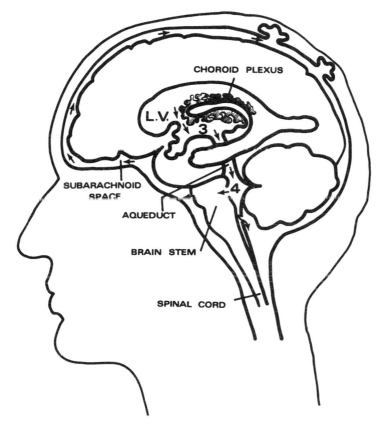

Figure 15.1 Cerebrospinal fluid circulation. (From Lance, 1986, by permission of the publishers, Charles Scribner's Sons, New York)

CSF flows from the choroid plexus in the lateral ventricles through the foramen of Monro into the third ventricle (3), aqueduct and fourth ventricle (4), emerging through the foramina of Magendie and Luschka into the subarachnoid space to be absorbed mainly by the arachnoid villi in the superior sagittal sinus.

using an operating microscope that punches a hole in the thinned floor of the third ventricle (third ventriculostomy), which permits the free flow of CSF into the subarachnoid space (see Figure 18.1). Alternatively, a catheter can be inserted into one lateral ventricle and run subcutaneously to the jugular vein and right atrium (ventriculoatrial shunt) or peritoneal cavity (ventriculoperitoneal shunt).

Communicating hydrocephalus

The conditions so far considered produce an internal hydrocephalus with dilatation of the ventricular system on the central side of the block. Less commonly, the fluid may emerge freely from the fourth ventricle by the foramina of Magendie and Luschka but be impeded from ascending through the basal cisterns and subarachnoid space because of adhesive arachnoiditis. It has long been recognized that this may be a cause of hydrocephalus in tuberculous or other meningitis, but the con-

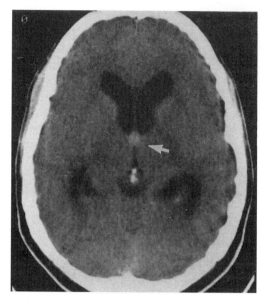

Figure 15.2 Internal hydrocephalus caused by obstruction of the foramen of Monro. A lesion in this site (arrowed) is commonly a colloid cyst of the third ventricle

dition may also develop quietly in older patients, causing dementia ('normal pressure' hydrocephalus). Progressive arachnoiditis may also follow head injury or subarachnoid haemorrhage.

Cerebral oedema

A sudden elevation of the blood pressure, as in malignant hypertension, may cause headache, presumably through the mechanism of cerebral oedema displacing pain-sensitive blood vessels, because the headache is relieved by the intravenous infusion of hypertonic solutions such as 50 per cent glucose but not when CSF pressure is reduced by lumbar puncture (Wolff, 1963). One hemisphere may swell following infarction, as a result of thrombosis of the internal carotid artery, or thrombosis or embolism of one of its main branches. Headache is commonly a symptom of cerebral infarction. Cerebral oedema may be sufficiently pronounced to cause papilloedema after internal carotid thrombosis, thus simulating an acute presentation of cerebral tumour.

Cerebral oedema used to be a major problem after craniotomy but is now controlled by the use of adrenal corticosteroids in high dosage, for example dexamethasone 32–64 mg daily. Potent diuretics, such as frusemide 40–120 mg daily, are also valuable in the control of cerebral oedema. The oral administration of urea and glycerol, and intravenous infusions of mannitol and glycerol, have enjoyed popularity at various times.

Hypocalcaemia may produce cerebral oedema, papilloedema and fits. Prolonged dosage with corticosteroids has been reported as causing headache, vomiting, papilloedema, diplopia and drowsiness. Addison's disease may also be responsible for cerebral oedema and papilloedema (Jefferson, 1956). Other causes of cerebral oedema are considered below under the heading 'Benign intracranial hypertension'.

Benign intracranial hypertension (idiopathic intracranial hypertension)

Elevation of CSF pressure without a demonstrable space-occupying lesion or obstruction of the CSF pathways is termed 'pseudotumor cerebri', 'benign intracranial hypertension' (BIH) or 'idiopathic intracranial hypertension'. A survey in the states of Iowa and Louisiana in the USA found an annual incidence of 0.9 per 100,000 persons (Durcan, Corbett and Wall, 1988). Among obese people, the incidence increased to 13 per 100,000 and in women aged 20–44 years who were more than 20 per cent over ideal weight, the incidence reached 19 per 100,000. The female to male ratio was 8 : 1 and the mean weight was 38 per cent above ideal weight for height. The disorder is clearly the prerogative of overweight women of childbearing age but no association was found with pregnancy or the use of oral contraceptives (Durcan, Corbett and Wall, 1988).

The condition usually presents with generalized headache (92 per cent), transient visual obscuration (72 per cent) and intracranial noises (60 per cent) (Wall and George. 1991). These noises were described as being like 'a rushing river', 'a waterfall', 'water inside a balloon', 'a rope twirling' or other buzzing, whistling or blowing sounds, and are presumably caused by turbulent venous flow. Wall and George (1991) prefer the term idiopathic intracranial hypertension because the course is not always benign. Of the 50 patients they studied, 26 per cent initially complained of visual impairment but over 90 per cent had some visual loss on perimetry. Over the follow-up period averaging 12 months, vision deteriorated in five patients and two became blind. In an earlier study of 57 patients followed up for 5–41 years (Corbett et al., 1982), 14 developed severe visual loss or became blind, with a much greater risk for patients with high blood pressure, of whom eight out of 13 lost their vision.

The insidious onset of headache is usually associated with papilloedema but monitoring of CSF pressure has disclosed some patients in whom pressure was elevated without producing papilloedema (Spence, Amacher and Willis, 1980; Marcelis and Silberstein, 1991). Paresis of one or both sixth cranial nerves develops in 10–40 per cent of cases, presumably because the nerves are displaced and compressed by cerebral oedema, and third nerve palsy has also been reported (Snyder and Frenkel, 1979; McCammon, Kaufman and Sears, 1981).

Foley (1955) described two groups of patients, one in which the condition followed non-specific infections and mild head injuries, and a larger group, mostly obese young women, in whom there was no obvious cause. Benign intracranial hypertension has also been reported as a reaction to certain drugs, such as tetracycline, nitrofurantoin and nalidixic acid, as the result of excessive intake of vitamin A and as a sequel to the withdrawal of corticosteroid therapy. The combination of low dosage tetracycline therapy and vitamin A, used in the treatment of acne, may increase the chances of the patient developing benign intracranial hypertension (Walters and Gubbay, 1981).

The condition must be clearly distinguished from otitic hydrocephalus, which it resembles closely. Benign intracranial hypertension appears to be caused by a reduction of CSF absorption because the production of CSF is normal while total CSF volume increases. Intracranial pressure builds up in waves followed by a sudden fall, suggesting that the increased pressure periodically forces fluid through the arachnoid villi. The various causative factors mentioned may all increase resistance to CSF flow across the villi (Johnston and Paterson, 1974). Cerebral blood volume is increased in benign intracranial hypertension (Mathew, Meyer and Ott, 1975) while the volume of the lateral and third ventricles is less than in normal controls, indicating that the brain is swollen by oedema or engorgement (Reid, Matheson and Teasdale, 1980). Chazal et al. (1979) confirmed a defect in the CSF resorption mechanism, the fault lying in the venous sinuses or in the arachnoid villi. The most plausible hypothesis is a vicious circle of defective CSF absorption, increased CSF pressure, venous engorgement and cerebral oedema, resulting in further reduction of CSF absorption.

The diagnosis is confirmed by the CT scan demonstration of normal or small ventricles and an elevated CSF pressure (above $250 \, mmH_2O$) with normal CSF constituents. Medical treatment consists of repeated lumbar puncture, acetazolamide 1000 mg daily to reduce CSF production and dietary advice to reduce weight. If visual loss progresses, a short course of corticosteroids is often prescribed and surgical procedures such as optic nerve sheath fenestration or a lumbar–subarachnoid shunt can be undertaken (Wall and George, 1991) if there is no improvement. Two-thirds of those patients with residual headache improve after the optic nerve sheath is slit (Corbett and Thompson, 1989). Corbett and Thompson emphasized the need for careful follow-up with perimetry, fundus photographs and measurements of intra-ocular pressure, and cautioned against relying on visual acuity and visual evoked potentials, which are relatively insensitive indices of deterioration.

Low cerebrospinal fluid pressure

Post-lumbar puncture headache

The headache that often follows lumbar puncture is probably caused by continued leakage of CSF from the subarachnoid space after the procedure, which lowers intracranial pressure, withdrawing support for the brain and thus causing traction upon intracranial vessels. Carbaat and van Crevel (1981) showed that the incidence of headache after lumbar puncture was not reduced by lying the patient flat for 24 hours and was almost 40 per cent whether the patient was kept in bed or allowed to walk about. Hilton-Jones et al. (1982) reported that 38 of their 76 patients developed post-lumbar puncture headache with no significant difference between those lying for 4 hours prone or supine, tilted head-up or head-down. In a series of 300 patients, headache with nausea was significantly more frequent in those kept at bed-rest for 6 hours, affecting 23 per cent compared with 13 per cent who were allowed to get up immediately (Vilming, Schrader and Monstad, 1988). The total headache incidence was 39 per cent in the recumbent and 35 per cent in the ambulant group. The incidence of post-lumbar puncture headache was reduced to 2.5 per cent by Engelhardt, Oheim and Neurdorfer (1991) in a series of 203 patients by the use of an 'atraumatic needle' with a conical tip and a side aperture.

Silberstein and Marcelis (1992), in their comprehensive review of CSF dynamics and headache associated with changes in CSF pressure, advocate bed-rest, an abdominal binder and the administration of caffeine as the initial management, followed by a short course of corticosteroids if headache persists. The headache resolves in less than 4 days in 53 per cent of cases and in less than 7 days in 72 per cent. Post-lumbar puncture headache may persist for months, with the characteristic postural headache being mistaken for a post-viral vascular headache (Lance and Branch, 1994). MRI of the brain shows uptake of gadolinium in the thickened meninges, probably caused by diapedesis of red cells inducing a fibrotic reaction (Figure 15.3) (Amor et al., 1996). If headache persists CSF isotope studies are indicated to determine the site of leakage (Figure 15.4) and consideration can be given to treatment by an epidural blood patch, a technique in which 10–20 ml of the patient's own blood is injected into the epidural space below the original lumbar puncture site. Seebacker et al. (1989) found that five out of six patients treated this way were relieved of headache within 2 hours whereas none of the six undergoing a sham procedure improved. All of the latter lost their headaches after a genuine blood patch.

An alternative is administration of caffeine (500 mg) intravenously which has been demonstrated to be effective (Sechzer and Abel, 1978).

Other low pressure syndromes

Intracranial hypotension may be caused by CSF rhinorrhoea as the result of trauma or bony erosion by a tumour, a spontaneous dural tear or spinal root avulsion. The trauma may be relatively trivial such as a sporting injury or following a roller-coaster ride (Schievink, Ebersold and Atkinson, 1996). Some cases have followed sexual intercourse (see Chapter 12). Silberstein and Marcelis (1992) also cite systemic medical illnesses, severe dehydration, hyperpnoea, meningoencephalitis, uraemia and infusion of hypertonic solutions as causes of low pressure syndromes.

Intracranial hypotension is classified as 'spontaneous' if no obvious source of CSF leakage is found for postural headache and CSF pressure remains below 60 mmH$_2$O. This condition, originally described as 'aliquorrhoea' by Schaltenbrand in 1938, may be diagnosed by the rapid transit of radionuclide from the CSF to the bladder without evidence of isotope leakage from the dural sac (Labadie, van Antwerp and Bamford, 1976). The headache may be accompanied by tinnitus and nausea. Small bilateral subdural haematomas may develop as a secondary phenomenon. Rando and Fishman (1992) reviewed this subject in presenting two patients with small CSF leaks from meningeal defects in spinal root sleeves. Treatment follows the same lines as for postlumbar puncture headache.

Intracranial infection

The headache of meningitis or encephalitis is often frontal or retro-orbital, associated with photophobia, nausea, drowsiness, neck stiffness, fever and general mal-

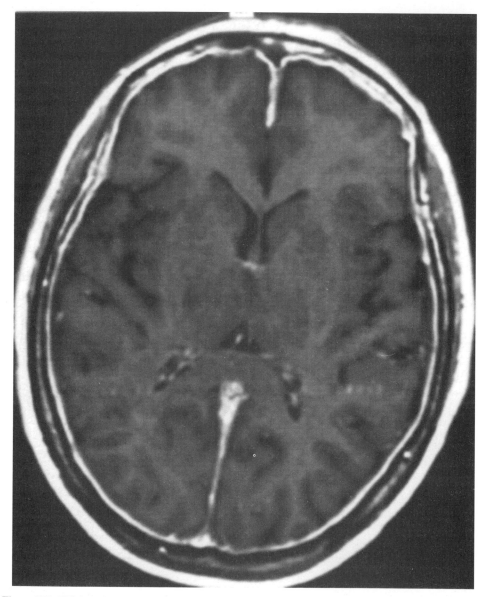

Figure 15.3 Thickened meninges enhanced by gadolinium in a low CSF pressure syndrome. (From Amor *et al.*, 1996, by permission)

aise. If the patient has signs of increased intracranial pressure it is advisable to have a CT scan of the brain to exclude subdural empyema, cerebral abscess or other space-occupying lesions before lumbar puncture, but this should not delay the administration of antibiotics when a pyogenic infection is suspected because delay can prove fatal.

The diagnosis is made by clinical assessment and lumbar puncture. The CSF

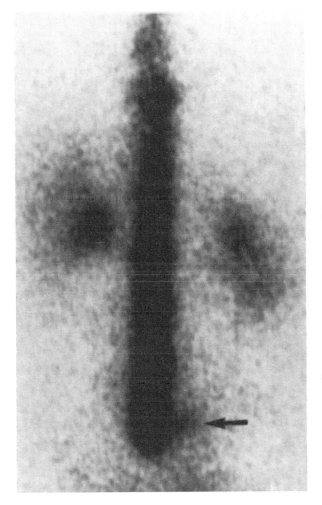

Figure 15.4 Isotope study showing leakage of the CSF from the lumbar sac

contains an excess of cells, mostly neutrophils, in pyogenic infections and in the acute phase of some cases of viral encephalitis. A purely lymphocytic pleocytosis usually indicates a viral infection but may be found in some cases of tuberculous or cryptococcal meningitis. A low CSF glucose value (in the absence of hypoglycaemia) means that the infecting organism is metabolizing glucose and indicates a pyogenic, tuberculous or cryptococcal infection. An exception to this rule is the unusual condition of meningitis carcinomatosis, in which the meninges are infiltrated and ensheathed with malignant cells that multiply so rapidly that the CSF glucose level drops.

Headache is a common complaint in patients with the acquired immunodeficiency syndrome (AIDS), commonly of infectious aetiology. Lipton *et al.* (1991) studied 49 patients infected with human immunodeficiency virus-1 (HIV-1) who presented with headache. The cause was found to be cryptococcal meningitis (19 patients), toxoplasmosis (eight patients), progressive multifocal leucoencephalopathy (one patient), syphilis (one patient) and lymphoma, brain abscess or undiagnosed mass lesions in nine cases. Factors contributing to headache in HIV-1 positive patients were discussed by Ramadan (1997).

Intracranial granuloma: sarcoidosis and Tolosa–Hunt syndrome

Sarcoidosis

The nervous system is involved in about 5 per cent of cases of sarcoidosis. Sarcoid granulomas may cause obstruction of the CSF pathways, resulting in hydrocephalus, or affect the region of the optic nerves, pituitary and hypothalamus (Thompson, 1991).

Tolosa–Hunt syndrome

Involvement of the superior orbital fissure by granuloma causes recurrent painful ophthalmoplegia (Tolosa–Hunt syndrome) that may be mistaken for ophthalmoplegic migraine and must be distinguished from other retro-orbital lesions such as intracranial aneurysms and sphenoid wing meningioma. The condition was described by Tolosa (1954) in a patient who died following surgical exploration for left retro-orbital pain associated with ophthalmoplegia and was found at autopsy to have granulomatous tissue surrounding the intracavernous portion of the internal carotid artery. Hunt el al. (1961) noted the responsiveness of the syndrome to steroid therapy. Although over 200 cases have been reported since then, there have been few with histological confirmation.

One of our own patients presented with severe left-sided headache, retro-orbital pain, nausea and diplopia (Goadsby and Lance, 1989) (Figure 5.3). After a 6-year history of recurrence of such episodes, sometimes with proptosis and paralysis of the left third and sixth cranial nerves, and repeated investigations, a positive CT scan was at last obtained. Biopsy disclosed a granuloma with some multinucleated giant cells.

Orbital phlebography in Tolosa–Hunt syndrome shows narrowing of the third segment of the superior ophthalmic vein, often combined with partial occlusion of the cavernous sinus (Hannerz, Ericson and Bergstrand, 1986). These authors examined 13 patients with Tolosa–Hunt syndrome and 83 other patients with the same sort of orbital pain characteristics. Of 50 patients who were found to have abnormal orbital phlebograms, 17 had orbital pain without neurological deficit, 20 had associated visual impairment and the remaining 13 had involvement of extra-ocular muscle innervation, one with additional optic nerve signs. The authors considered that retro-orbital vasculitis and granulomatous disease of presumably immunological origin is more common than reported cases of Tolosa–Hunt syndrome would suggest. Their view is supported by the fact that 39 of 41 patients treated with steroids lost their characteristic pain. A study by Hannerz (1992) emphasized that about one-third of patients with Tolosa–Hunt syndrome were subject to episodes of periorbital pain without ophthalmoplegia and that chronic fatigue and other systemic symptoms were not uncommon.

Headache associated with intrathecal injections

The chemical excitation of nerve endings in the meninges produces a reflex spasm of the neck extensors and sometimes of the lumbar muscles, which is analogous to the contraction of the abdominal wall resulting from peritoneal inflammation and is known as muscle 'guarding'. Muscle spasm consequent upon meningeal irritation gives rise to the physical signs of neck rigidity and Kernig's sign. This is encountered most often in subarachnoid haemorrhage, meningitis and encephalitis, but may also occur after the injection of air or chemical agents into the CSF.

The introduction of air into the subarachnoid space for diagnostic purposes (pneumoencephalography) has been out-moded by CT scanning and MRI. This procedure sometimes caused a sterile inflammatory reaction that rivalled meningoencephalitis in its severity and was associated with a CSF pleocytosis. The intrathecal injection of a contrast medium for myelography, or antibiotics, baclofen, long-acting steroids or other agents may sometimes cause a meningitic reaction with headache. The headache usually follows the injection within 5–72 hours, is present whether the subject is standing or lying and clears in a maximum of 14 days. There may be a CSF pleocytosis with negative culture.

Intracranial tumours

Unless a tumour or other space-occupying lesion affects a strategic position along the line of the drainage pathways of the cerebral ventricles, it is able to reach a considerable size before causing headache. Since intracranial vessels have to be pushed aside before pain is registered, infiltrating tumours, such as the gliomas, may extend throughout one hemisphere without causing headache, because the position of large vessels may remain undisturbed until the last stages of the disease. Tumours that compress the brain from outside, such as meningiomas, are likely to cause fits, focal cerebral symptoms, progressive impairment of intellectual function or other neurological deficit before they produce headache.

Of 163 patients with cerebral tumour reported by Iversen *et al.* (1987), 53 per cent suffered from headache, 16 per cent as the first symptom. Headache was twice as common in patients with gliomas and secondary tumours than in patients with meningiomas, and was related to the site rather than the size of the tumour, occurring more often with occipital, basal and posterior fossa tumours.

The headache of brain tumour or other space-occupying lesion progressively becomes more severe, aggravated by coughing, sneezing, straining or bending the head forward. Headache is the initial symptom of patients with posterior fossa tumours, except for those arising in the cerebellopontine angle, and is usually felt in the occipital region (Lavyne and Patterson, 1947). Supratentorial tumours cause frontal headache with extension to the occiput in about one-third of cases. A posterior fossa tumour may cause pain by direct compression of the fifth, seventh, ninth or tenth cranial nerves, which may refer pain to the face, ear or throat. Pain is experienced in the neck because of irritation of the dura, which is supplied by the upper three cervical nerve roots, and reflex spasm of neck muscles may cause the head to be held to one side (see Figure 5.2). Pain may also be referred to the eye and forehead by convergence of impulses from the upper cervical nerve roots upon neurones of the cervical cord, which also serve the trigeminal pathways. Finally, a generalized headache may be caused by blockage of the flow of CSF with a resulting increase in intracranial pressure.

The management of headache caused by intracranial tumour is obviously surgical removal of the cause whenever possible. Failing that, or as a preliminary to a definitive operation, a ventricular shunt may be inserted or corticosteroids prescribed to reduce intracranial pressure.

References

Amor, B. S., Maeder, P., Gudinchet, F. and Ingvar-Maeder, M. (1996). Syndrome d'hypotension intra-crânienne spontanée. *Rev. Neurol.* **152**, 611–614.

Bull. J. W. D., Nixon, W. L. B. and Pratt, R. T. C. (1955). The radiological criteria and familial occurrence of primary basilar impression. *Brain* **78**, 229–247

Carbaat, P. A. T. and van Crevel, H. (1981). Lumbar puncture headache: controlled study on the preventive effect of 24 hours bed rest. *Lancet* **ii**, 1133–1135

Chazal, J., Janny, P., Georget, A. M. and Colnet, G. (1979). Benign intracranial hypertension. A clinical evaluation of the CSF absorption mechanisms. *Acta Neurochir. Suppl.* **28**, 505–508

Corbett, J. J., Savino, S. J., Thompson, H. S. *et al.* (1982). Visual loss in pseudotumor cerebri: follow-up of 57 patients from 5 to 41 years and a profile of 14 patients with severe visual loss. *Arch. Neurol.* **39**, 461–474

Corbett, J. J. and Thompson, H. S. (1989). The rational management of benign intracranial hypertension. *Arch. Neurol.* **46**, 1049–1051

Durcan, F. J., Corbett, J. J. and Wall, M. (1988). The incidence of pseudotumor cerebri: Population studies in Iowa and Louisiana. *Arch. Neurol.* **45**, 875–877

Engelhardt, A., Oheim, S. and Neundorfer, B. (1991). Post-lumbar puncture headache: experiences with an 'atraumatic' needle. *Cephalalgia* **11** (Suppl. 11), 356–357

Foley, J. (1955). Benign forms of intracranial hypertension – 'toxic' and 'otitic' hydrocephalus. *Brain* **78**, 1–41

Goadsby, P. J. and Lance, J. W. (1989). Clinicopathological correlation in a case of painful ophthalmo-plegia. *J. Neurol. Neurosurg. Psychiat.* **52**, 1290–1293

Hannerz, J. (1992). Recurrent Tolosa–Hunt syndrome. *Cephalalgia* **12**, 45–51

Hannerz, J., Ericson, K. and Bergstrand, G. (1986). A new aetiology for visual impairment and chronic headache. The Tolosa–Hunt syndrome may be only one manifestation of venous vasculitis. *Cephalalgia* **6**, 59–63

Hilton-Jones, D., Harrad, R. A., Gill. M. W. and Warlow, C. P. (1982). Failure of postural manoeuvres to prevent lumbar puncture headache. *J. Neurol. Neurosurg. Psychiat.* **45**, 743–746

Hunt, W. E., Meagher, J. N., Le Fever, H. E. and Zeman, W. (1961). Painful ophthalmoplegia. Its relation to indolent inflammation of the cavernous sinus. *Neurology* **11**, 56–62

Iversen, H. K., Strange, P., Sommer, W. and Tjalve, E. (1987). Brain tumour headache related to tumour size, histology and location. *Cephalalgia* **7** (Suppl. 6), 394–395

Jefferson, A. (1956). A clinical correlation between encephalopathy and papilloedema in Addison's disease. *J. Neurol. Neurosurg. Psychiat.* **19**, 21–27

Johnston, I. and Paterson, A. (1974). Benign intracranial hypertension. 11. CSF pressure and circulation. *Brain* **97**, 301–312

Labadie, E. L., van Antwerp, J. and Bamford, C. R. (1976). Abnormal lumbar isotope cisternography in an unusual case of spontaneous hypoliquorrheic headache. *Neurology* **26**, 135–139

Lance, J. W. and Branch, G. B. (1994). Persistent headache after lumbar puncture. *Lancet* **343**, 414

Lavyne, M. H. and Patterson, R. H. Jr (1987). Headache associated with brain tumour. In *Wolff's Headache and Other Head Pain*, Ed. D. J. Dalessio. pp. 343–351. New York, Oxford University Press

Lipton, R. B., Feraru, E. R., Weiss, G. *et al.* (1991). Headache in HIV-1-related disorders. *Headache* **31**, 518–522

Marcelis, J. and Silberstein, S. D. (1991). Idiopathic intracranial hypertension without papilledema. *Arch. Neurol.* **48**, 392–399

Mathew, N. T., Meyer, J. S. and Ott, E. O. (1975). Increased cerebral blood volume in benign intracranial hypertension. *Neurology* **25**, 646–649

McCammon, A., Kaufman, H. H. and Sears, E. S. (1981). Transient oculomotor paralysis in pseudotumor cerebri. *Neurology (N.Y.)* **31**, 182–184

Ramadan, N. H. (1997). Unusual causes of headache. *Neurology* **48**, 1494–1499

Rando, T. A. and Fishman. R. A. (1992). Spontaneous intracranial hypotension: report of two cases and review of the literature. *Neurology* **42**, 481–487

Reid, A. C., Matheson, M. S. and Teasdale, G. (1980). Volume of the ventricles in benign intracranial hypertension. *Lancet* **ii**, 7–8

Schievink, W. I., Ebersold, M. J. and Atkinson, J. L. D. (1996). Roller-coaster headache due to spinal cerebrospinal fluid leak. *Lancet* **347**, 1409

Seebacher, J., Ribeiro. V., Le Guillou. J.-L. *et al.* (1989). Epidural blood patch as treatment for post-lumbar puncture headache – a double-blind controlled trial. *Cephalalgia* **9** (Suppl. 10), 185–186

Sechzer, P. H. and Abel, L. (1978). Post-spinal anesthesia headache treated with caffeine. Evaluation with demand method. *Curr. Therap. Res.* **24**, 307–312

Silberstein, S. D. and Marcelis, J. (1992). Headache associated with changes in intracranial pressure. *Headache* **32**, 84–91

Snyder, D. A. and Frenkel. M. (1979). An unusual presentation of pseudotumor cerebri. *Ann. Ophthalmol.* **11**, 1823–1827

Spence, J. D., Amacher, A. L. and Willis, N. R. (1980). Benign intracranial hypertension without papilledema: role of 24-hour cerebrospinal fluid pressure monitoring in diagnosis and management. *Neurosurgery* **7**, 326–336

Thompson, A. J. (1991). Sarcoidosis and the nervous system. In *Clinical Neurology*, Eds M. Swash and J. Oxbury. pp. 1725–1731. Edinburgh, Churchill-Livingstone

Tolosa, E. (1954). Periarteritic lesions of the carotid siphon with the clinical features of a carotid infra-clinoidal aneurysm. *J. Neurol. Neurosurg. Psychiat.* **17**, 300–302

Vilming, S. T., Schrader, H. and Monstad, I. (1988). Post-lumbar-puncture headache: the significance of body posture. A controlled study of 300 patients. *Cephalalgia* **8**, 75–78

Wall, M. and George. D. (1991). Idiopathic intracranial hypertension. A prospective study of 50 patients. *Brain* **114**, 155–180

Wolff, H. G. (1963). *Headache and Other Head Pain*, 3rd Edition. New York, Oxford University Press

Walters, B. N. J. and Gubbay, S. S. (1981). Tetracycline and benign intracranial hypertension: report of five cases. *Br. Med. J.* **282**, 19–20

Chapter 16

Disorders of the neck, cranial and extracranial structures

Cranium

It is remarkably uncommon to find a source of headache within the cranial bones, although some examples will be cited later of inflammatory or neoplastic lesions involving the sinuses or petrous temporal bones. Nevertheless it is always advisable to run one's hands over the scalp of anyone complaining of headache. Occasionally a scalp infection or osteomyelitis may give rise to pain that is described as headache. Any expanding lesion of bone, which stretches the periosteum, may cause local pain. Paget's disease of the skull may be associated with a vascular headache fluctuating in intensity, probably caused by increased cranial blood flow. The scalp may feel warm in Paget's disease because of arteriovenous shunting, which may reach such proportions that cardiac output is substantially increased. The softening of bone in Paget's disease may cause the base of the skull to be invaginated by the atlas and axis, giving rise to 'basilar impression' (platybasia). In this condition the posterior fossa is distorted and the flow of CSF may be impaired with an increase in intracranial pressure as described in Chapter 15.

Neck

John Hilton (1950) made the following remarks in the fourth of a series of 18 lectures given on 'Rest and Pain' between 1860 and 1862:

> Suppose a person to complain of pain upon the scalp, is it not very essential to know whether that pain is expressed by the fifth nerve or by the great or small occipital? Thus pain in the anterior and lateral part of the head, which are supplied by the fifth nerve, would suggest that the cause must be somewhere in the area of the distribution of the other portions of the fifth nerve. So if the pain be expressed behind, the cause must assuredly be connected with the great or small occipital nerve, and in all probability depends on disease of the spine between the first and second cervical vertebrae.
>
> John Hilton (1805–1878)

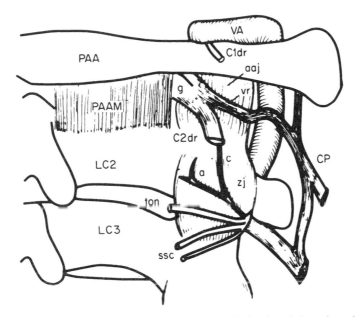

Figure 16.1 A line diagram of the right C2 ganglion and rami showing their major relations. (From Bogduk, 1981, by permission of the publishers, Adis Press, Sydney)

PAA = posterior arch of the atlas; LC2 = lamina of C2 vertebra; LC3 = lamina of C3 vertebra; PAAM = posterior atlantoaxial membrane; VA = vertebral artery; CP = cervical plexus; zj = C2–3 zygapophyseal joint; aaj = lateral atlantoaxial joint; C1dr = C1 dorsal ramus; C2dr = C2 dorsal ramus (cut proximal to its branching point); vr = C2 ventral ramus; g = C2 dorsal root ganglion; a = articular nerve; c = communicating branch C3 to C2; ssc = nerves to semispinalis capitus; ton = third occipital nerve.

Abnormalities of various structures in the neck have been implicated as a source of headache. These structures include the synovial joints, the intervertebral discs, ligaments, muscles, nerve roots and the vertebral artery (Edmeads, 1978). There is ample evidence that irritation of the upper three cervical roots causes pain in the occiput and may refer pain forwards to the orbit on the appropriate side. The most important contributor to the greater occipital nerve and hence to occipital sensation, including pain, is the second cervical root. The C2 dorsal root ganglion lies dorsal to the atlantoaxial joint (Figure 16.1). Lateral to this point, the C2 dorsal and ventral roots are fused to form a very short spinal nerve, which emerges around the lateral border of the posterior atlantoaxial membrane then divides into a dorsal and ventral ramus (Bogduk, 1981b). The ventral ramus gives branches to the lateral atlantoaxial joint on its way to enter the cervical plexus (Figure 16.1). The C2 dorsal ramus supplies various muscular branches, communicates with the C1 and C3 dorsal rami and becomes continuous with the greater occipital nerve, which emerges on to the scalp above an aponeurotic sling (Figure 16.2). For this reason the greater occipital nerve cannot be compressed by spasm of the trapezius, which would draw the aponeurotic sling away from the nerve. Bogduk (1981b) stresses that the C2 nerve is vulnerable to compression only in extreme rotation and extension of the atlas on its axis with dislocation of the lateral atlantoaxial joints. This is not the type of

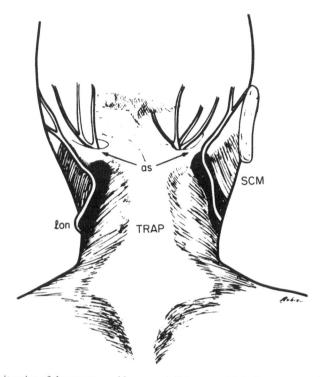

Figure 16.2 The exit point of the greater and lesser occipital nerves. Note the aponeurotic sling suspended from the superior nuchal line above which the nerves emerge. (From Bogduk, 1981b, by permission of the publishers, Adis Press, Sydney)

as = aponeurotic sling; lon = lesser occipital nerve; SCM = sternocleidomastoid; TRAP = trapezius.

movement in 'whiplash injury', which is more likely to cause damage to the lateral atlantoaxial joints and soft tissues than to the C2 root itself.

Several cervical syndromes have been described and these will now be described in turn.

Upper cervical syndrome

Pain can be referred from the upper neck and occiput forward to the orbital region by disorders of the upper cervical spine affecting the upper three cervical roots. Upper cervical instability following trauma, basilar impression (platybasia) and rheumatoid arthritis are clinical examples. Osteoarthrosis of the upper cervical zygapophyseal joints associated with reflex muscle contraction may also be a cause of occipital headache (Edmeads, 1978). Examination of the neck may show restriction of movement at a joint, a hypomobility lesion, probably caused by intra-articular adhesions, capsular contracture or local muscle spasm (Bogduk *et al.*, 1985). In contrast, some patients show hypermobility associated with laxity of the ligaments. Neck movement or palpation of the occipital nerves may induce occipital headache as well as local tenderness. Injection of a contrast medium into the cervical facet joints was found to replicate the patients' symptoms in about 50 per cent of cases (Dory, 1983) and triamcinolone 20–40 mg was then injected into the appropriate joint capsule after aspirating the contrast medium.

Treatment of most acute conditions is conservative with immobilization of the neck in a collar and the use of anti-inflammatory drugs and analgesics, but instability at the craniocervical junction or atlantoaxial joint may have to be treated surgically. In the absence of instability, pain arising from the zygapophyseal joints can often be managed by mobilization of the neck. Caution is advised for any manipulative procedures. Sudden or forceful neck manipulation can cause dissection of the cerebral arteries with brain stem infarction (see Chapter 14). The injection of local anaesthetic agents and steroids into tender areas is often helpful. Localization of facet joints responsible for pain is aided by the injection of local anaesthetic into the suspected joints or block of the second cervical ganglion (Bogduk, 1981c). Rarely, surgical treatment by coagulation or section of the nerve supply to facet joints, or section of the second and third dorsal roots, may be required for intractable occipital headaches of cervical origin.

Whiplash injury

Whiplash injury probably results from injury to structures like the transverse ligament of the atlas, the capsules of the upper cervical synovial joints and surrounding soft tissues. The occipital nerves may be damaged by a direct blow at the same time. The condition is considered in Chapter 13 on post-traumatic headache.

Third occipital nerve headache

A subvariety of the upper cervical syndrome is headache arising from the C2–3 facet joints mediated by the third occipital nerve. The C2–3 joints are a transition zone between the first and second cervical levels, which enable rotation of the head to take place, and the lower cervical spine, which is responsible for flexion and extension of the neck. Bogduk and Marsland (1986) describe the use of a radiologically controlled block of the nerves supplying the C2–3 facet joints in the diagnosis of occipital or suboccipital headache radiating to the forehead. All of the 10 patients studied had a history of neck injury, precipitation of pain by neck movement, or cervical tenderness. In seven out of 10 patients, the headache was relieved temporarily by the diagnostic nerve block. The injection of steroids provided relief extending from 2 weeks to 4 months, cryocoagulation for 3–6 weeks, radio-frequency coagulation for 3–12 months and open neurectomy for 18 months or more to the time of follow-up.

Cervicogenic headache

The term cervicogenic headache was coined by Sjaastad and his colleagues (Fredriksen, Hovdal and Sjaastad, 1987; Sjaastad, Fredriksen and Pfaffenrath, 1990) to describe episodic unilateral headaches, lasting from 3 hours to a week and recurring at intervals from 2 days to 2 months, that were considered to arise from the cervical spine. Although these headaches affected women more than men and were sometimes accompanied by migrainous features such as nausea, vomiting and photophobia, the authors distinguished them from migraine because they could be precipitated by neck movement, they usually started in the upper neck and the pain could be reproduced by pressure over the upper neck or occiput. The intimate relationship between trigeminal and upper cervical input to the central nervous system in the genesis of headache is well recognized. It is possible that 'cervicogenic headache' is a variety of migraine triggered from the upper cervical spine in a manner comparable with those triggered by other forms of afferent stimulation, such as glare and noise.

Cervical migraine

In the 1920s Barré and Lieou described a form of headache associated with cervical spondylosis, which they attributed to irritation of the vertebral nerve. Bärtschi-Rochaix (1968) wrote a monograph on the topic in 1949 entitled *Migraine Cervicale*. There is considerable doubt as to whether cervical migraine is an entity separate from vertebrobasilar migraine and whether it bears any relation to changes in the cervical spine. The headaches are described as bilateral, unilateral or alternating and are accompanied by giddiness, acoustic symptoms and blurring of vision or fortification spectra. Bärtschi-Rochaix (1968) considers that the symptoms are caused by impairment of flow in the vertebral arteries where they are displaced by osteophytes, in spite of the fact that only a minority of transient ischaemic attacks produced by this mechanism on head rotation are associated with headache.

Bogduk, Lambert and Duckworth (1981) studied the anatomy and physiology of the vertebral nerve to ascertain whether stimulation of this nerve could reduce blood flow in the vertebrobasilar arterial system. The 'vertebral nerve' in man and monkey consists of a series of neural arcades formed by communications between grey rami from the sympathetic trunk and ventral rami of the C3–7 segments. Above C3 the vertebral artery is accompanied by direct branches from the C1–3 ventral rami. From the C1 ventral ramus nerve, filaments (which have no detectable connection with those from lower levels) follow the vertebral artery across the atlas. Electrical stimulation of the vertebral nerve or cervical sympathetic trunk in the monkey reduced vertebral flow by only 18 per cent in contrast to the 70 per cent reduction in carotid blood flow produced by sympathetic stimulation. The lack of reactivity in the intact vertebrobasilar circulation is surprising in view of the reactivity of isolated segments *in vitro*. The fact that no single nerve accompanies the vertebral artery along its entire length and the unresponsiveness of the artery to sympathetic stimulation renders untenable any hypothesis linking irritation of the 'vertebral nerve' by osteophytes with migraine headache. A controlled trial of manipulation of the neck for the treatment of migraine did not demonstrate any significant decrease in frequency of headache (Parker, Tupling and Pryor, 1978).

Occipital neuralgia

Occipital neuralgia is characterized by an aching or paroxysmal jabbing pain in the area of distribution of the greater or lesser occipital nerves, usually accompanied by diminished sensation or dysaesthesiae of the affected area (Hammond and Danta, 1978). It may be accompanied by tenderness over the point where the nerve trunk crosses the superior nuchal line – the greater occipital nerve lies over this line midway between the mastoid process and the occipital protuberance while the lesser occipital nerve crosses it about 4 cm behind the ear (Figure 16.2).

If the occipital pain is continuous and there is no impairment of sensation, then it may be a referred pain from the atlantoaxial or C2–3 facet joints, from the posterior fossa or even from the first division of the trigeminal nerve, the descending spinal tract of which converges with the C2–3 afferent fibres on second-order neurones in the upper three segments of the spinal cord. The distinction can often be made by assessing the response to infiltration of the tender area by a local anaesthetic agent or blockade of the second cervical ganglion (Bogduk, 1981c). Caution must be exercised because the inadvertent injection of local anaesthetic into the cerebrospinal fluid via an underlying long nerve root sleeve may lead to respiratory arrest.

This condition obviously overlaps with the upper cervical and third occipital nerve syndromes described above. Ehni and Benner (1984) reported seven patients with occipital pain ('neuralgia') from degenerative disease at the atlantoaxial level relieved temporarily by local anaesthetic and steroid injection, and permanently by C2 dorsal rhizotomy.

The difficulty in differential diagnosis is illustrated by the 23 patients with occipital neuralgic pain reported by Hammond and Danta (1978), of whom nine had migrainous features, two suffered from rheumatoid arthritis and three from cervical spondylosis. Of the remainder, four had a history of direct trauma to the occipital region and eight of whiplash or other injury to the cervical spine.

Carbamazepine may relieve the pain if it is paroxysmal in nature. Transcutaneous nerve stimulation provides short-term relief and immobilization in a collar may ease the pain partially or completely (Hammond and Danta, 1978). Neurectomy of the appropriate nerve may stop the pain completely but pain may later recur with neuroma formation. Bogduk (1985) prefers nerve and facet joint blocks to determine the precise origin of occipital pain, with a view to the intra-articular injection of steroids or selective thermocoagulation of the appropriate nerve.

Neck–tongue syndrome

Lance and Anthony (1980) described an unusual syndrome affecting children or young adults on sudden rotation of the neck. The patient experiences a sharp pain in the upper neck or occiput, which may be accompanied by numbness or tingling in these areas. At the same time, the ipsilateral half of the tongue becomes numb. The explanation is that proprioceptive fibres from the tongue travel via communications from the lingual nerve to the hypoglossal nerve and thence to the second cervical root (Figure 16.3). Bogduk (1981a) has pointed out that, during rotation of the neck, the C2 central ramus is drawn over the atlantoaxial joint which it innervates. Transient subluxation of the atlantoaxial joint would produce local pain by stretching the joint capsule and numbness of the tongue by stretching the C2 ventral ramus, which contains proprioceptive fibres from the tongue.

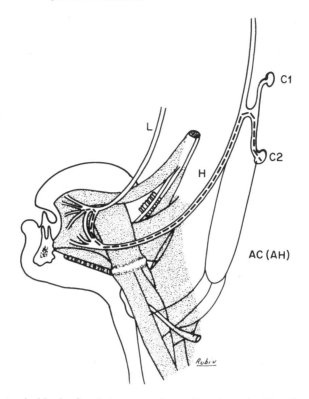

Figure 16.3 The anatomical basis of neck–tongue syndrome. Proprioceptive fibres from the tongue travel (dashed line) via the lingual nerve (L) and hypoglossal nerve (H) to the second cervical root (C2). AC (AH) = ansa cervicalis (ansa hypoglossi). (From Lance and Anthony,1980, by permission of the editor of *Journal of Neurology, Neurosurgery and Psychiatry*)

Other cases have been described in normal subjects (Lance 1984; Hankey, 1988) and in patients with degenerative spondylosis, ankylosing spondylitis and psoriatic arthritis (Webb, March and Tyndall, 1984; Bertoft and Westerberg, 1985). Bertoft and Westerberg reported that five of their seven non-rheumatic cases had a similarly affected parent or sibling, suggesting a genetically determined laxity of ligaments or joint capsules.

Some patients have been improved by cervical manipulation (Cassidy *et al.*, 1986; Terrett, 1988). The symptoms were abolished in one patient with upper cervical disease by fusion at the C2–3 level (Bertoft and Westerberg, 1985) and improved in another patient with more extensive symptoms by sectioning the second cervical spinal nerve (Elisevich *et al.*, 1984). Our own patients have not been sufficiently incapacitated by their symptoms to warrant any intervention.

Headache with cervical spinal cord lesions

Spierings, Foo and Young (1992) examined 20 patients with traumatic transection of the spinal cord between the C2–3 and C7–8 levels. Twelve of those patients were subject to generalized severe throbbing headaches caused by an acute increase in blood pressure associated with urinary obstruction or faecal impaction. These headaches were usually accompanied by other signs of sympathetic activity such as facial flushing, sweating and nasal congestion. Sixteen patients had experienced headaches other than bladder and bowel headaches but none had migrainous features. Only three of the 20 patients had never suffered from headache.

Eyes

Imbalance of the extra-ocular muscles (heterophoria), especially convergence weakness, or refractive errors, particularly uncorrected presbyopia, may set up 'eye-strain' headache, which is a form of tension headache following visual effort (Lyle, 1968). This condition is much overdiagnosed and it is uncommon for headache to be cured simply by the correction of a visual disturbance. Waters (1970) compared visual acuity and ocular muscle balance in groups of headache-prone and headache-free people. Hyperphoria with near vision was more common in migraine patients but no other difference was found. There are some odd ocular pains, which do not seem to be of any significance, known as ophthalmodynia (see Chapter 12). These are jabbing pains in one eye ball, which may be repetitive, without obvious cause. Angle-closure glaucoma may cause pain to be felt deeply in the eye and to radiate over the forehead in the area of distribution of the first division of the trigeminal nerve. There may not be mistiness of vision, coloured haloes seen around lights or circumcorneal injection to draw attention to the eye. Radiation of pain from eye to forehead should arouse suspicion of glaucoma in the middle-aged or elderly patient and lead to a full ophthalmological examination including measurement of the intra-ocular tension.

Pain in or behind the eye is a common feature of retrobulbar neuritis and may precede impairment of vision by a few hours or even days. The pain radiates to the frontal region of the same side. Sight becomes blurred and may be lost completely in the affected eye. The most common visual field defect is a central scotoma since the central part of the optic nerve containing fibres from the macula is more often affected by the demyelinating process. It is probable that retrobulbar neuritis is always caused by primary demyelination of the optic nerve, and more than half the patients who suffer an attack subsequently develop signs of demyelination elsewhere in the nervous system. The exact percentage of patients who progress to typical multiple sclerosis varies greatly from series to series depending upon the criteria of diagnosis and the length of follow-up.

During the acute attack, the eyeball is often tender to pressure and aches on eye movement. The optic fundi are usually normal on ophthalmoscopic examination unless the area of demyelination underlies the nerve head, when swelling of the optic disc is observed. This inflammatory oedema, termed papillitis, is said to give a reddish appearance to the disc as well as the characteristic appearance of papilloedema. Distinction between the two conditions does not present any difficulty because vision is seriously impaired or lost in papillitis, whereas there is usually no more than slight blurring of vision on head movement with papilloedema, even when the disc is grossly swollen. In a prospective study at 5 years follow-up 16% of patients with normal MRC head at baseline had developed clinically definite multiple sclerosis while 51% of patients with three or more lesions on MRI of the head had developed the disease (Optic Neuritis Study Group, 1997).

Both the pain and visual disturbance of retrobulbar neuritis usually respond rapidly to the use of adrenocorticotrophic hormone (ACTH) or corticosteroids.

Ears, nose, sinuses and throat

Vasomotor rhinitis is said to give rise to a midfrontal headache. This statement warrants scepticism because vasomotor rhinitis is a common disorder and affects many people without causing headache. It does, of course, predispose to sinusitis, which causes headache in the stage of active inflammation or when the ostium of a particular sinus is obstructed. Rhinological causes of headache and facial pain are discussed by Ryan and Kern (1978) who comment that chronic sinusitis rarely causes facial pain. Most patients who complain of recurrent 'sinus headache' are suffering from one of the varieties of migraine, which may be associated with nasal congestion (Blau, 1988).

The diagnosis of sinusitis rarely presents any difficulty when pain and tenderness are localized to the affected frontal or maxillary sinus or sinuses and percussion over the area increases the pain. Inflammation of the ethmoid or sphenoidal sinuses gives rise to a boring pain felt deeply in the midline behind the nose (Figure 16.4). The pain of sinusitis is made worse by bending the head forwards. If the ostium of the infected sinus is patent, blowing the nose or sneezing usually evokes a throb of pain. If the ostium is obstructed, the patient may awaken with a 'vacuum' headache caused by absorption of air from the blocked sinus.

One or both nostrils are usually blocked and the maintenance of a clear airway by decongestants will lead to discharge of mucopurulent material from the sinuses with subsequent relief of pain in most instances. The use of vasoconstrictor nose drops or nasal spray, such as neosynephrine 0.25 per cent every 2–3 hours, instilled first with the head postured backwards over the end of a bed, and then, after some minutes, with the head upright, will clear the airway in most patients. When the airway is clear, steam inhalation, followed by the application of radiant heat to the affected area, helps to clear the ostia. If symptoms of systemic disturbance appear, antibiotics may be required, but the first requirement is to ensure that the sinuses are draining freely. If this cannot be accomplished by the simple measures outlined, the advice of an ear, nose and throat surgeon should be obtained. Sinusitis is often taken lightly but may be treacherous if it persists, and lead to collections of pus in the extradural or subdural spaces, to cerebral abscess or to spread of infection through the bloodstream. A mucocele may develop in one frontal sinus if the ostium of the sinus is obstructed and can slowly expand, eroding bone until it projects into the orbit, causing proptosis.

The cranial nerves are invaded by nasopharyngeal carcinoma more often than by any other malignant growth in the head and neck because of the proximity of the nasopharynx to the foramina of the middle fossa. The condition is rare in communities of European origin but is common in China and South-East Asia. The trigem-

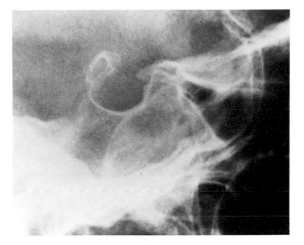

(a)

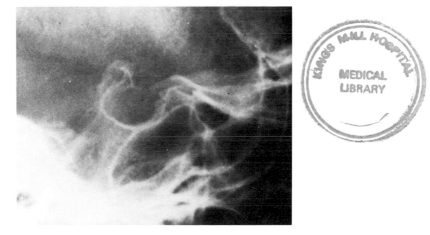

(b)

Figure 16.4 Sphenoidal sinusitis (a) before and (b) after treatment

inal nerve or its branches are involved in about half the cases, so that pain may be referred to the head. The sixth cranial nerve is also vulnerable and is destroyed in about 70 per cent of patients. In addition the ninth, tenth and eleventh cranial nerves may be invaded, causing hoarseness and dysphagia. Other symptoms include nasal obstruction, bloody nasal discharge and enlargement of cervical lymph nodes. About 40 per cent of patients present with headache.

Hippocrates warned that an association of headache with acute pain in the ear is to be dreaded 'for there is danger that the man may become delirious and die' (Adams, 1948). Otitis media may cause apical petrositis, thrombosis of the lateral sinus and otitic hydrocephalus (see Figure 14.3). Disease of the petrous temporal bone, whether infectious or neoplastic, can cause pain in the distribution of the first division of the trigeminal nerve and an ipsilateral sixth cranial nerve palsy (Gradenigo's syndrome). Intracranial abscesses from middle ear disease are uncommon nowadays, but may be found in the temporal lobe or cerebellum, and present with signs of raised intracranial pressure, focal neurological disturbance or meningeal irritation.

A rare clinical syndrome, retropharyngeal tendinitis, presents with severe pains in the back of the neck, aggravated by head movements and swallowing (Fahlgren, 1986). Patients may complain of swelling in the upper pharynx. Body temperature and erythrocyte sedimentation rate (ESR) are often elevated. Radiography demonstrates swollen prevertebral soft tissues and calcification at the level of the atlas and axis. Fahlgren reported 28 patients, but we have never encountered this syndrome.

Teeth

Dental caries or apical root infection can cause a neuralgic pain in the second or third divisions of the trigeminal nerve, with a constant aching component and superadded jabbing pains. The pain is made worse by hot or cold fluids in the mouth. Pains in the lower jaw are almost always of dental origin and warrant careful radiographs of the teeth as apical root infections may be missed in a routine examination. Pain resembling trigeminal neuralgia may be triggered by dental malocclusion (Blair and Gordon, 1973). Dental causes of pain are summarized by Heir (1987). Pains in the upper jaw are commonly of dental origin but can readily be produced by maxillary sinusitis. The pain of lower-half headache (facial migraine) and cluster headache often includes the upper teeth and gums. Atypical facial pain is often experienced in the nasolabial fold overlying the upper gum.

Temporomandibular joint disease

A common way for dental disturbance to refer pain to the upper part of the head is through dysfunction of one temporomandibular joint (Cawson, 1986). If the bite is unbalanced by premature contact of one or more teeth or by loss of molar teeth on one side, or if the bite is fixed so that the normal lateral or shearing movement of mastication is impossible, the patient adopts the most convenient chewing position, which commonly throws an abnormal strain on one temporomandibular joint. This may lead to pain which is felt in front of or behind the ear on the appropriate side with radiation to the temple, over the face, and down the neck on that side, and often associated with a blocked sensation in that ear (Costen's syndrome) (Costen, 1934). The condition is made worse by the patient becoming a chronic 'jaw clencher' if he or she was not one already, so that tension symptoms are set up in the temporal and other scalp muscles. Lateral pterygoid muscle dysfunction and tenomyositis of the masseter muscles may contribute to or be responsible for preauricular pain (Friedman, Agus and Weisberg, 1983). Ill-fitting dentures or any other source of discomfort in biting or chewing may evoke the same symptoms. In long-standing cases, crepitus may be heard or felt over the affected temporomandibular joint.

Palpation of the joint is readily done by a finger inserted into the external auditory canal with pressure being exerted anteriorly on to the joint. The diagnosis is confirmed if this procedure replicates the patient's pain. CT scanning of the temporomandibular joints did not find any correlation between pathological changes and pain (Tilds and Miller, 1987), but effusion into the painful joint has been demonstrated by a magnetic resonance study (Schellhas, Wilkes and Baker, 1989).

The management depends upon careful adjustment of the bite by a dental surgeon, but advice to the patient concerning relaxation of the temporal and masseter muscles and the administration of amitriptyline are also helpful. The problem is discussed further under the heading 'Tension-type headache' (Chapter 10).

The red ear syndrome

Some patients with temporomandibular joint dysfunction, glossopharyngeal neuralgia or irritation of the third cervical root may suffer from episodic burning pain in one ear lobe accompanied by obvious reddening of the affected ear (Lance, 1996). The condition may also occur without any apparent structural cause in response to touch or heat in susceptible subjects. The cause is uncertain but this could be an example of the ABC (Angry Back-firing C-nociceptor) syndrome described by Ochoa (1993) with the pain and increase in ear temperature being caused by the antidromic release of vasodilator peptides.

References

Adams, F. (1948). *The Genuine Works of Hippocrates*. p. 54. London, Sydenham Society

Bärtschi-Rochaix, W. (1968). Headaches of cervical origin. In *Handbook of Neurology*, Vol 5, Eds P. J. Vinken and G. W. Bruyn. pp. 192–203. Amsterdam, North Holland

Bertoft, E. S. and Westerberg, C. E. (1985). Further observations on the neck–tongue syndrome. *Cephalalgia* **5** (Suppl. 3), 312–313

Blair, G. A. S. and Gordon, D. S. (1973). Trigeminal neuralgia and dental malocclusions. *Br. Med. J.* **4**, 38–40

Blau, J. N. (1988). A note on migraine and the nose. *Headache* **28**, 495

Bogduk, N. (1981a). An anatomical basis for the neck–tongue syndrome. *J. Neurol. Neurosurg. Psychiat.* **44**, 202–208

Bogduk, N. (1981b). The anatomy of occipital neuralgia. *Clin. Exper. Neurol.* **17**, 167–184

Bogduk, N. (1981c). Local anaesthetic blocks of the second cervical ganglion: a technique with application in occipital headache. *Cephalalgia* **1**, 41–50

Bogduk, N. (1985). Greater occipital neuralgia. In *Current Therapy in Neurological Surgery*, Ed. D. M. Long. pp. 175–180. Toronto, B. C. Decker; Saint Louis, C. V. Mosby

Bogduk. N., Corrigan, B., Kelly, P., Schneider. G. and Farr, R. (1985). Cervical headache. *Med. J. Aust.* **143**, 202, 206–207

Bogduk, N., Lambert, G. A. and Duckworth, J. W. (1981). The anatomy and physiology of the vertebral nerve in relation to cervical migraine. *Cephalalgia* **1**, 11–24

Bogduk, N. and Marsland, A. (1986). On the concept of third occipital headache. *J. Neurol. Neurosurg. Psychiat.* **49**, 775–780

Cassidy, J. D., Diakow, P. R. P., De Korompay, V. L., Munkacsi, I. and Yong-Hing, K. (1986). Treatment of neck–tongue syndrome by spinal manipulation: a report of three cases. *Pain Clinic* **1**, 41–46

Cawson, R. A. (1986). Temporomandibular cephalalgia. In *Handbook of Clinical Neurology*, Vol. 4 (48), Ed. F. Clifford Rose. pp. 413–416. Amsterdam, Elsevier

Costen, J. B. (1934). A syndrome of ear and sinus symptoms dependent upon disturbed function of the temporomandibular joint. *Ann. Otol. Rhinol. Laryngol.* **43**, 1–15

Dory, M. A. (1983). Arthrography of the cervical facet joints. *Radiology* **148**, 379–382

Edmeads, J. (1978). Headaches and head pains associated with diseases of the cervical spine. *Med. Clin. N. Am.* **62**, 533–544

Ehni, G. and Benner, B. (1984). Occipital neuralgia and the C1–2 arthrosis syndrome. *J. Neurosurg.* **61**, 961–965

Elisevich, K., Stratford, J., Bray, G. and Finlayson, M. (1984). Neck–tongue syndrome: operative management. *J. Neurol. Neurosurg. Psychiat.* **47**, 407–409

Fahlgren, H. (1986). Retropharyngeal tendinitis. *Cephalalgia* **6**, 169–174

Fredrikson, T. A., Hovdal, H. and Sjaastad, O. (1987). 'Cervicogenic headache': clinical manifestations. *Cephalalgia* **7**, 147–160

Friedman, M. H., Agus, B. and Weisberg, J. (1983). Neglected conditions producing preauricular and referred pain. *J. Neurol. Neurosurg. Psychiat.* **46**, 1067–1072

Hammond, S. R. and Danta, G. (1978). Occipital neuralgia. *Clin. Exp. Neurol.* **15**, 258–270

Hankey, G. J. (1988). Neck–tongue syndrome on sudden neck rotation. *Aust. N.Z. J. Med.* **18**, 181

Heir, G. M. (1987). Facial pain of dental origin – a review for physicians. *Headache* **27**, 540–547

Hilton, J. (1950). *Rest and Pain*, Eds E. W. Walls and E. E. Philipp. p. 77. London, Bell

Lance, J. W. (1984). Unusual syndromes in neurological practice. *Med. J. Aust.* **140**, 409–416

Lance, J. W. and Anthony, M. (1980). Neck-tongue syndrome on sudden turning of the head. *J. Neurol. Neurosurg. Psychiat.* **43**, 97–101

Lance, J. W. (1996). The red ear syndrome. *Neurology* **47**, 617–620

Lyle, T. K. (1968). Ophthalmological headaches. In *Handbook of Clinical Neurology*, Vol. 5, Eds P. J. Vinken and G. W. Bruyn. pp. 204–207. Amsterdam, North Holland

Ochoa, J. L. (1993). The human sensory unit and pain: new concepts, syndromes and tests. *Muscle Nerve* **16**, 1009–1016

Optic Neuritis Study Group (1997). The five-year risk of MS after optic neuritis. *Neurology* **49**, 1404–1413

Parker, G. B., Tupling, H. and Pryor, D. S. (1978). A controlled trial of cervical manipulation for migraine. *Aust. N.Z. J. Med.* **89**, 589–593

Ryan, E. R. Jr and Kern, E. B. (1978). Rhinological causes of facial pain and headache. *Headache* **18**, 44–50

Schellhas, K. P., Wilkes, C. H. and Baker, C. C. (1989). Facial pain, headache, and temporomandibular joint inflammation. *Headache* **29**, 228–231

Sjaastad, O., Fredriksen, T. A. and Pfaffenrath, V. (1990). Cervicogenic headache: diagnostic criteria. *Headache* **30**, 725–726

Spierings, E. L. H., Foo, D. K. and Young, R. R. (1992). Headaches in patients with traumatic lesions of the cervical spinal cord. *Headache* **32**, 45–49

Terrett, A. G. I. (1988). Neck–tongue syndrome and spinal manipulative therapy. In *Upper Cervical Syndrome: Chiropractic Diagnosis and Treatment*, Ed. H. Vernon. pp. 223–239. Baltimore, Williams and Wilkins

Tilds, B. N. and Miller, P. R. (1987). Radiographic pathology of the temporomandibular joints, and head pain. *Headache* **27**, 427–430

Waters, W. E. (1970). Headache and the eye. A community study. *Lancet* **ii**, 1–4

Webb, J., March, L. and Tyndall, A. (1984). The neck–tongue syndrome: occurrence with cervical arthritis as well as normals. *Rheumatology* **11**, 530–533

Chapter 17

Cranial neuralgias and pain of central origin

Persistent pain of cranial nerve origin

The first division of the trigeminal nerve may be compressed in the orbit, the superior orbital fissure, cavernous sinus or near the apex of the petrous temporal bone. Tumours, such as a meningioma growing from the sphenoid wing or a pituitary tumour, may refer pain to the forehead associated with diminished sensibility over the area supplied by the first division of the trigeminal nerve. The sudden onset of severe pain behind and above one eye may indicate the enlargement of an aneurysm of the internal carotid or posterior communicating artery. The Gasserian ganglion may also be compressed by meningioma. A neuroma may arise from the fifth nerve. Trigeminal nerve compression is often painless. When pain is present it may be constant or stabbing in quality, often associated with sensory impairment in the appropriate area of distribution.

Involvement of the nervus intermedius refers pain to the external auditory canal, the glossopharyngeal nerve to the base of the tongue and tonsillar fossa, and the vagus nerve to a region in or behind the ear.

Raeder's paratrigeminal neuralgia

The term Raeder's syndrome is applied to pain of trigeminal distribution, usually the ophthalmic division, in association with an ocular (post-ganglionic) sympathetic deficit comprising ptosis, miosis and impairment of sweating over the medial aspect of the forehead but not elsewhere on the face. Since this combination may have many different causes, the syndrome simply serves to draw attention to the region of the carotid siphon as the site of disturbance, but the nature of the disturbance must be determined by the history and special investigations.

Two of the five patients described by Raeder in 1924 did not have pain as a presenting symptom. One had a parasellar tumour, two cases resulted from trauma and the cause in two cases was unknown (Mokri, 1982). The many descriptions in the literature since then have been summarized by Mokri (1982) and Sjaastad *et al.* (1994). They fall into two groups; those with episodic pain that we now recognize as cluster headache and those with aneurysms, neoplasms, inflammation or trauma involving the internal carotid artery and impinging on the first division of the trigeminal nerve. Sjaastad *et al.* (1994) distinguish the features of Raeder's syndrome from the supra-orbital fissure syndrome of Tolosa–Hunt and the posterior cavernous sinus syndrome of Gradenigo. The concept of Raeder's syndrome has some localizing value but no more than that.

Gradenigo's syndrome

Lesions of the apex of the petrous temporal bone cause pain referred to the fronto-temporal region and ear in conjunction with a paralysis of the sixth cranial nerve, which runs across the bone at that point. Gradenigo's syndrome was originally described as a complication of middle ear infection but may also be found with tumours arising from or invading this area.

Neuralgias

Post-herpetic neuralgia

Herpes zoster is caused by reactivation of the varicella zoster virus, which is thought to lie dormant in the trigeminal, geniculate and dorsal root ganglia after chicken-pox infection in early life. The incidence of post-herpetic neuralgia is about 10 per cent when all age groups are considered, but increases with age, reaching 50 per cent by the age of 60 years. The distribution of the rash and subsequent pain follows trigeminal distribution in about 23 per cent of cases (Watson, 1990), mostly affecting the ophthalmic division. The rash may also involve the external auditory meatus, the soft palate or the area supplied by the upper cervical roots. Paralysis of the third, fourth or sixth cranial nerves, or a facial palsy may accompany the herpetic eruption (Ragozzino *et al.*. 1982). The combination of an herpetic rash in the external auditory canal and a facial palsy results from invasion of the geniculate ganglion and is known as Ramsay–Hunt syndrome. An unpleasant burning pain often precedes the skin eruption by 2–4 days. Pain in the area of distribution of the first division of the trigeminal nerve may cause diagnostic difficulties when it appears several days before the rash or, on rare occasions, without any rash at all.

Post-herpetic neuralgia has been defined as pain persisting beyond the crusting of lesions or beyond a certain limit, usually longer than 1 month after onset of the rash. The pain is characteristically burning with occasional stabbing components and the lightest touch over the affected area may be felt as painful (allodynia). Nurmikko and Bowsher (1990) found that the sensory threshold for warmth, cold, touch, pinprick and vibration was diminished over the affected areas in those patients whose rash was followed by neuralgic pain but not in those who escaped post-herpetic neuralgia. Allodynia was present in 87 per cent of the patients with post-herpetic neuralgia and extended to the maxillary division in half of the patients after ophthalmic herpes. The fact that all modalities of sensation were affected is against the view that neuralgic pain depends upon the selective destruction of large afferent fibres.

In a review of the gate-control theory of pain, Nathan (1976) summarized the conflicting views expressed in various reports of the pathological changes wrought by herpes zoster, concluding that the condition cannot be explained by the selective fall-out of a certain range of nerve fibres. Skin and nerve are involved by fibrous tissue with degeneration of large fibres followed by smaller fibres. The genesis of the pain is presumably related to a disturbance in the pattern of afferent impulses and the removal of some central inhibitory influence because pain usually persists after section of the trigeminal nerve or medullary tractotomy. The descending (spinal) tract of the trigeminal nerve is the direct rostral continuation of the tract of Lissauer in the spinal cord. Like the tract of Lissauer, the ventrolateral portion of the descending trigeminal tract exerts a suppressor effect on sensory transmission in its neighbouring segments, and the dorsomedial portion has a facilitatory effect (Denny-Brown and Yanagisawa, 1973). Fibres from the ophthalmic division of the trigeminal nerve lie in the ventrolateral segment so it is conceivable that the virus of herpes zoster could selectively damage this inhibitory area, thus permitting unrestrained outflow of afferent impulses responsible for post-herpetic neuralgia.

Whether post-herpetic neuralgia can be prevented by the administration of corticosteroids or acyclovir at the onset of herpes zoster remains controversial (Portenoy, Duma and Foley, 1986, Watson, 1990, editorial, 1990). Eaglstein, Katz and Brown (1970) reported that triamcinolone 48 mg daily, reducing dosage over 3 weeks, was more effective than placebo in a small controlled trial. The usual practice is to prescribe a course of steroids at the onset in any patient who is not immunosuppressed. Watson (1990) recommends prednisone 60 mg daily with gradual reduction in dosage over 2 weeks.

When the rash is extensive or ophthalmic herpes threatens sight, acyclovir should be prescribed. There are reports that 800 mg five times daily for 7–10 days will reduce the incidence of post-herpetic neuralgia (Editorial, 1990). Whereas there are publications claiming that steroids alone or acyclovir alone will help to prevent post-herpetic neuralgia, it is clear that the administration of both agents together does not confer any additional advantage (Esmann et al., 1987). Time and further trials may tell us the best method of preventing this unpleasant condition.

Once post-herpetic neuralgia is established, what then? Blockade of peripheral nerves, roots or the sympathetic nervous system and various surgical procedures are of no proven benefit (Portenoy et al., 1986). Amitriptyline has proved useful in the management of persistent pain since its effectiveness was established for chronic tension headache (Lance and Curran, 1964). Watson et al. (1982) demonstrated its benefit in post-herpetic neuralgia in a double-blind crossover study in which 16 out of 24 patients were relieved by a (median) dose of 75 mg daily. The tablets are best given at night to minimize daytime drowsiness and the dosage should be increased gradually as described in Chapter 10. For those patients who are unable to tolerate amitriptyline, imipramine can be useful. Carbamazepine helps to control the stabbing component of post-herpetic pains but not the constant burning pain. We have recently found gabapentin to be useful in some patients.

The topical application of a cream containing capsaicin (usually starting with 0.025 per cent) has been reported as being successful in open trials but not in one double-blind trial (Editorial, 1990). The theoretical basis for its use is that it discharges substance P from nerve terminals, thereby desensitizing them.

Shanbrom (1961) reported that an intravenous drip of 500 ml of 0.1–0.2 per cent procaine repeated up to 10 times if necessary relieved 13 out of 16 patients. We have used a lignocaine (lidocaine) drip, 1 g of lignocaine being added to 500 ml of 5 per cent glucose in N/5 saline and administered at the rate of 2 mg/minute (1 ml/minute) as in the treatment of patients with cardiac dysrhythmias after myocardial infarction. This drip may be repeated daily for 3 days or more. Diminution of post-herpetic pain often outlasts the duration of the infusion and is sometimes permanent.

Bates and Nathan (1980) used transcutaneous electrical nerve stimulation in 74 patients with post-herpetic neuralgia resistant to other forms of therapy, with the electrodes being placed above and below the scarred area. Continuing benefit was derived by one-third of the patients for 1 year and one-quarter for 2 years or more.

Trigeminal neuralgia

The prevalence of trigeminal neuralgia has been estimated as 155 per million of the population (Selby, 1975). It affects women more than men in the ratio of 1.6 : 1. Its alternative name 'tic douloureux' (a painful spasm) came into use in the mid-eighteenth century. The term 'tic douloureux' should be pronounced in the French manner as Anglicization to 'tic doloroo' gives pain to the Francophile scarcely less severe than the condition itself. The onset of the disorder usually occurs after the age of 40 years, with a mean varying from 50 to 58 years in different reported series. Familial occurrence is rare.

The pain is strictly limited to some part of the distribution of the trigeminal nerve, involving the right side more than the left in the ratio 3 : 2. It usually starts in the second or third divisions, affecting the cheek or chin. Less than 5 per cent start in the first division. All three divisions have been involved in 10–15 per cent of reported cases and the pain has become bilateral in 3–5 per cent.

The pain is sudden, intense and stabbing in quality, lasting only momentarily but often recurring in repeated paroxysms. The patient can always identify trigger factors such as talking, chewing, swallowing, or touching the face or gums as in shaving or cleaning the teeth. There may also be trigger points, areas around the nose or lips, which are particularly liable to evoke a paroxysm if touched, the pain commonly being in the same division as the trigger point. The pain may recur daily for weeks or months and then remit for a period of time, even for years, before returning. This periodicity sometimes leads to confusion between trigeminal neuralgia and cluster headache. There have indeed been reported instances of the two conditions being associated but this is rare and the characteristic lancinating pain of trigeminal neuralgia bears little resemblance to the boring pain of cluster headache, which lasts for 10 minutes or more each time. The overlap with the SUNCT syndrome (Chapter 11) is yet to be fully defined (Benoliel and Sharav, 1998). Trigeminal neuralgia may occasionally occur with glossopharyngeal neuralgia so that pain is referred to the ear and throat as well as the area of trigeminal distribution. There is a tendency for trigeminal neuralgia to become progressively worse in frequency and severity of episodes. There is usually no sensory loss in 'idiopathic' trigeminal neuralgia so that other conditions, such as neuroma or multiple sclerosis, must be considered if sensation is found to be impaired.

Facial flushing may sometimes be observed after repeated jabs of neuralgia, probably caused by the release of vasodilator peptides. Drummond, Gonski and

Lance (1983) found flushing of the face in the area of cutaneous distribution of the appropriate division after thermocoagulation of the Gasserian ganglion for the relief of trigeminal neuralgia, while the levels of calcitonin gene-related peptide (CGRP) and substance P rose in external jugular venous blood (Goadsby, Edvinsson and Ekman, 1988).

Fromm *et al.* (1990) have described prodromal symptoms of pain resembling sinusitis or toothache that may precede the onset of typical trigeminal neuralgia by some days. Such pains may last for several hours and be triggered by jaw movements, or by hot or cold fluids, which may lead to unnecessary dental procedures.

What is the aetiology of trigeminal neuralgia? Fromm, Terrence and Maroon (1984) summarized the situation neatly by ascribing the aetiology to a peripheral cause and a central pathogenesis. The peripheral cause is most commonly an aberrant vessel compressing the trigeminal root where it enters the pons. Compression of the divisions, mainly second and third, by the internal carotid artery and the possibility of degenerative changes or herpes simplex infection of the Gasserian ganglion have been considered as possible causes but these theories have little to support them. In 1932, Dandy reported the results of dividing the sensory root of the trigeminal nerve by a posterior fossa approach in 250 patients with trigeminal neuralgia. Dandy (1934) later recorded his personal observations in 215 of the operated cases. He found a gross lesion distorting the trigeminal nerve in 60 per cent of patients, the most common being the impingement on the nerve of a hardened superior cerebellar artery (66 cases) or a branch of the petrosal vein (30 cases). other causes included acoustic neuromas, cholesteatomas, an osteoma, basilar artery aneurysms, angiomas and adhesion of the sensory root to the brain stem.

Jannetta (1976) refined the posterior fossa approach to the trigeminal nerve, using microsurgical techniques, and concluded that *all* tic douloureux is 'symptomatic tic douloureux'. The trigeminal root entry zone was compressed or distorted by a branch of the anterior inferior cerebellar artery in the 4 per cent of patients in whom the first division was primarily affected, while the superior cerebellar artery was responsible when the second and third divisions were affected. In 100 consecutive patients with trigeminal neuralgia, Jannetta found tumours in 6 per cent, plaques of multiple sclerosis in 4 per cent, atrophic areas of nerve in 2 per cent and vascular compression of the trigeminal nerve in the remaining 88 per cent. Richards, Shawdon and Illingworth (1983) explored the posterior fossa in 52 patients. Compression of the trigeminal root was caused by arterial loops in 37 (71 per cent) and by clinically unsuspected tumours in three cases. Progressive elongation and tortuosity of arterial loops is thought to account for the condition becoming more common with advancing age. Haines, Jannetta and Zorub (1980) examined the trigeminal nerves in 20 cadavers of patients known to have been free of trigeminal neuralgia. Of the 40 nerves, 11 were in contact with an artery but only four of these were distorted by it. An additional four nerves were compressed by veins. In contrast, of 40 trigeminal nerves surgically exposed for the treatment of trigeminal neuralgia, 31 were compressed by adjacent arteries and eight by veins.

Somatosensory evoked potentials were obtained by stimulating the lips in 17 patients with unoperated trigeminal neuralgia (Stöhr, Petruch and Scheglmann, 1981). The latency of the response was delayed on the affected side in seven patients by about 2 msec, confirming compression of the trigeminal nerve or ganglion on that side. A comparison of responses evoked from the lower lip in 10 patients treated by retro-Gasserian glycerol injection with 20 normal controls demonstrated diminished amplitude and prolonged latency of responses on the operated side (Dalessio *et al.*, 1990). Trigeminal evoked potentials can therefore be used either as an indication for posterior fossa operation or as a check on the success of any destructive procedure.

Experimental demyelination of the trigeminal root in cats and monkeys has been shown to follow about 3 weeks after the insertion of sutures through the root and at this time the nerve was found to be hyperexcitable (Burchiel, 1980). Multiple discharges were evoked by a single stimulus and an after-discharge by afferent volleys. Action potentials were generated at the site of the lesion, and were enhanced by hyperventilation and suppressed by diphenylhydantoin. Such lesions could be caused in the peripheral or central trigeminal pathways of man by vascular or other compression or by primary demyelination, as in multiple sclerosis, so that the use of anticonvulsants to damp down neural hyperexcitability has logical application in the control of trigeminal neuralgia in man.

Diphenylhydantoin (Dilantin) was used in the medical management of trigeminal neuralgia but has been supplanted by carbamazepine (Tegretol) 200 mg, the dose being increased slowly from half a tablet to up to two tablets three times daily to reach a blood level that will control the pain without inducing giddiness and ataxia. Carbamazepine nearly always causes some degree of leucopenia. For this reason patients should be warned to report for a blood count should they develop any infection. The blood may be checked every 3 months as a routine but it is doubtful whether regular blood counts really fulfil any useful function since leucopenia of clinical significance is rare and may appear quite suddenly. Tomson *et al.* (1980) found the optimum blood level for control of pain to lie between 24 and 43 µmol/litre (5.7–10.1 µg/ml). Carbamazepine is best administered in divided doses three times daily, as trigeminal neuralgia tends to recur 6–9 hours after each dose (Tomson and Ekbom, 1981).

The second choice of medication for those patients not responding to carbamazepine is baclofen (Lioresal). Baclofen proved superior to placebo in a crossover trial (Fromm, Terrence and Chattha, 1984) and relieved 74 per cent of patients in an open trial with a dosage of 40–80 mg daily. Of 50 patients, 37 were free of pain after 2 weeks. Six patients were unable to tolerate baclofen because of drowsiness and nausea. Eighteen patients remained controlled on baclofen for a mean duration of 3 years, although 12 of these required the addition of carbamazepine or phenytoin. L-Baclofen is more effective and has less side-effects than racemic baclofen (Lioresal) (Fromm and Terrence, 1987) but is not currently available for clinical use.

Clonazepam (Rivotril, Clonopin) 0.5–2.0 mg three times daily is also effective in suppressing trigeminal neuralgia but drowsiness and mood changes limit its use. The painful paroxysms of trigeminal neuralgia can be controlled temporarily by the intravenous infusion of lignocaine (lidocaine) but mexiletine, a lidocaine derivative administered orally in doses of 10 mg/kg body weight daily, has not proved of benefit (Pascual and Berciano, 1989).

If the condition persists in spite of medical treatment, a surgical approach becomes necessary. Operations were devised to decompress the Gasserian ganglion or sensory root, giving temporary relief, or to compress these structures, giving more lasting relief, but alcohol injection or section of the sensory root became the preferred surgical procedures. In more recent times, controlled thermocoagulation of the Gasserian ganglion by a probe inserted in the same manner as for alcohol injection has provided relief of pain with less impairment. The technique offers hope of sparing the corneal reflex and thus preventing ocular complications and is effective in 90 per cent of cases, but 17 per cent are left with troublesome dysaesthesiae and 3 per cent with 'anaesthesia dolorosa' (Illingworth, 1986). Jannetta (1976) advocated posterior fossa exploration, using a binocular microscope to examine the nerve at the point of entry into the pons. Dissection of any compressing artery or vein away from the trigeminal root and placement of a small piece of polyvinyl chloride sponge between the nerve and the offending vessel was followed by a sudden or gradual abatement of pain in all but four of Jannetta's patients followed for periods of up to 94 months. This procedure is usually the treatment of choice in younger patients since facial sensation is spared, but thermocoagulation of the Gasserian ganglion (radio-frequency trigeminal ganglionolysis) or glycerol injection around the ganglion are less invasive procedures (Illingworth, 1986) for the older patient not responding to medication.

More recently still, fine-beam radiotherapy ('gamma knife radiosurgery') has been advocated for the relief of trigeminal neuralgia (Young *et al.*, 1997). Of 51 patients treated, 38 became free of pain and seven were substantially improved. Eight of another nine patients in whom the pain was caused by a tumour were relieved.

Glossopharyngeal neuralgia

Glossopharyngeal neuralgia is about 100 times less common than trigeminal neuralgia, and causes a similar type of lancinating pain in the ear, base of the tongue, tonsillar fossa or beneath the angle of the jaw (Chawla and Falconer, 1967). The distribution is not only in the sensory area of the glossopharyngeal nerve but also those of the auricular and pharyngeal branches of the vagus nerve. It is provoked by swallowing, talking or coughing. Of 217 cases reported by Rushton, Stevens and Miller (1981), 25 also had trigeminal neuralgia. Pain may predominate in the pharynx or in the ear, presenting as pharyngeal or otalgic forms of neuralgia (Bruyn, 1986a). Glossopharyngeal neuralgia may be secondary to compression of the nerve by neoplasms, infections or blood vessels. Cardiovascular disturbances such as bradycardia, hypotension and even transient asystole have been reported to accompany glossopharyngeal neuralgia on occasions (Bruyn, 1986a). The ear on the affected side occasionally becomes red and painful (Lance, 1996) and, as mentioned at the end of Chapter 16, glossopharyngeal neuralgia can be a cause of the red ear syndrome.

If the pain does not respond to carbamazepine, phenytoin or baclofen, microvascular decompression or intracranial section of the glossopharyngeal nerve and the upper two rootlets of the vagus nerve is usually undertaken.

Nervus intermedius neuralgia

Sensation from the external auditory canal and part of the external ear is mediated by the nervus intermedius, part of the facial nerve. Pain in the associated area of distribution may be experienced in geniculate herpes (Ramsay–Hunt syndrome). It remains doubtful as to whether stabbing pains in the ear can ever be ascribed to the nervus intermedius or whether they represent the otalgic variation of glossopharyngeal neuralgia (Bruyn, 1986b).

Superior laryngeal neuralgia

This is a rare disorder characterized by severe pain in the lateral aspect of the throat, submandibular region and under the ear, brought on by swallowing, shouting or turning the head. The pain may be constant or lancinating, triggered by pressure on the side of the throat. It may occasionally follow respiratory infections, tonsillectomy or carotid endarterectomy (Bruyn, 1986c). The diagnosis is confirmed by local anaesthetic block of the superior laryngeal nerve and the condition relieved by neurectomy.

Sluder's sphenopalatine neuralgia

Sluder (1910) reported 60 patients in whom symptoms and signs indicated a disturbance of the sphenopalatine ganglion. He described pain at the root of the nose, involving also the eye, jaws, teeth and ear. On the affected side he noticed diminished sensibility of the soft palate, a higher arch of the palate and diminished taste sensation. Pain was relieved by application of cocaine 20 per cent to the mucosa overlying the sphenopalatine ganglion.

Sluder cited examples of a woman aged 27 with episodes of such pain recurring from three times weekly to once every 3 months (which may have been 'facial migraine'), patients with pain accompanying respiratory infections and one whose pain extended down the arm and leg. The International Headache Society Classification Committee considered this condition to be a synonym for cluster headache, but it appears more likely to be a collection of facial pains of differing aetiology. The literature on the syndrome is reviewed by Bruyn (1986d).

Vail's vidian neuralgia

Vail (1932) considered that many of the cases described by Sluder had pain arising from the vidian nerve rather than the sphenopalatine ganglion and ascribed the cause to inflammation of the sphenoid sinus. He described 31 cases, 28 of whom were female, between the ages of 24 and 59 years of age. The attacks often came on between 2 and 3 a.m., suggesting that many of these patients may have had migraine or cluster headache. The diagnosis, like that of Sluder's neuralgia, is of historical interest only.

Charlin's nasociliary neuralgia

Charlin described paroxysms of severe pain in the inner angle of the eye and nostril associated with corneal lesions or iridocyclitis, conjunctival injection, nasal congestion and sweating on the nose or forehead (Bruyn, 1986e). Trigger areas are situated over the infratrochlear and external nasal nerves and pain is said to be relieved by the intranasal application of cocaine.

Central causes of head and facial pain

Multiple sclerosis

Trigeminal neuralgia has been a symptom of multiple sclerosis in 1–8 per cent of cases in reported series (Selby, 1975). From the other point of view, 2–3 per cent of patients with trigeminal neuralgia have multiple sclerosis. In 80–90 per cent of the documented cases, other symptoms of multiple sclerosis preceded the onset of tri geminal neuralgia by 1–29 years. In the remainder, the facial pain was the presenting symptom and other signs of multiple sclerosis followed 1 month to 6 years later. Of patients with multiple sclerosis and trigeminal neuralgia, the pain becomes bilateral in 11–14 per cent compared with 3–4 per cent of patients with the idiopathic form. The pain is caused by a plaque of multiple sclerosis in the pons at the entry zone of the trigeminal nerve. Jannetta (1976) observed such plaques in 4 per cent of patients subjected to posterior fossa exploration for trigeminal neuralgia. Watkins and Espir (1969) reported that migrainous headache was more common in patients with multiple sclerosis, affecting 27 per cent of patients compared with 12 per cent of a control group. This supports the concept of a central origin for migraine. See also page 70 and Figure 7.3.

Anaesthesia dolorosa

This unpleasant and intractable condition consists of pain or other disagreeable sensations being experienced in a body area that is numb as the result of some deafferenting disease or procedure, comparable with a phantom limb. It is as though central pain pathways, being deprived of their normal afferent input, discharge spontaneously to convey a false message of perceived pain to higher centres. After radio-frequency lesions of the Gasserian ganglion, anaesthesia dolorosa has been reported in up to 3 per cent of patients and other disturbing sensations in another 17 per cent (Illingworth, 1986).

Thalamic pain

Pain and burning sensations in the face and scalp may be caused by central lesions involving the second-order trigeminal neurones, the quintothalamic tract, or the ventrobasal nuclei of the thalamus. These pathways or nuclei may be damaged by vascular disease or multiple sclerosis and, less commonly, by syringomyelia or glioma. The pain often extends to the limbs and trunk on the affected side and diminished sensibility to pinprick and temperature can usually be detected over the painful half of the body. Touching the hypaesthetic area may evoke pain (allodynia).

The condition is notoriously difficult to control. Tricyclic antidepressants like amitriptyline and anticonvulsants, such as carbamazepine, clonazepam and sodium valproate, may be helpful in management (Miles and Bowsher, 1991). Baclofen is also worth a trial.

Atypical facial pain

By definition, this term embraces all of those patients whose symptoms do not fit in with a recognized pattern of headache or neuralgic symptoms. In practice, there is a distinctive group of patients with what might be called typical atypical facial pain. This commonly affects patients in their thirties or forties, women more often than men (Clough, 1991). The most common sites are in the nasolabial fold or on the chin overlying the lower gum. The pain is usually constant, fluctuating in intensity, and aching or boring in quality. It could be said that it bears the same relationship to 'lower-half headache' as tension headache does to migraine. It often starts after some apparently innocuous dental procedure or minor facial trauma.

The condition has been considered in the past as an hysterical conversion phenomenon or symptom of depression. Lascelles (1966) could find no justification for the former view in his study of 93 patients but considered that the majority had depressive symptoms with fatigue, agitation and sleep disorders. It is important to note that most of the patients had good premorbid personalities so that their psychological symptoms may well be a reaction to their depressing illness. Kerr (1979) considered that atypical facial pain could be initiated by a small neuroma at the site of trauma, which then became a self-perpetuating pain phenomenon.

We regard the condition as an organic syndrome of central origin for the following reasons:

1. The pain is remarkably similar in site and quality from patient to patient and would be consistent with hyperexcitability of the trigeminal nerve, commonly the second division, or its central connections.
2. The most common sites of pain coincide with trigger points for trigeminal neuralgia.
3. The pain often starts after dental procedures, bringing up the possibility that some infection could be introduced at that time or that herpes simplex virus, a permanent resident in the second and third trigeminal divisions of many people, might be activated to involve central pain pathways and to set up a reaction akin to the neuralgia following herpes zoster.
4. Thermographic assessment of the facial circulation in nine of our patients with unilateral atypical facial pain demonstrated increased heat loss from the cheek of the affected side in six patients and from the orbit in 4 (Drummond, 1988). This suggests a reflex vasodilator response to activity in the trigeminal system and supports the concept of an organic basis for this disorder.

Jaegher, Singer and Kroening (1988) reported two patients, one with intense unilateral facial pain following extraction of an upper molar tooth and the other with pain following sinus operations, who improved after stellate ganglion block. They described this syndrome as 'reflex sympathetic dystrophy of the face'.

Surgical measures do not usually help atypical facial pain and may make it worse. The regular administration of imipramine, amitriptyline and dothiepin often eases the pain, with the monoamine oxidase inhibitor, phenelzine, being reserved for resistant cases. We have also found baclofen useful in some instances. Electroconvulsive therapy has improved some patients who were severely depressed (Lascelles, 1966).

References

Bates, J. A. V. and Nathan, P. W. (1980). Transcutaneous nerve stimulation for chronic pain. *Anaesthesia* **35**, 817–823

Benoliel, R. and Sharav, Y. (1998). Trigeminal neuralgia with lacrimation or SUNCT syndrome? *Cephalalgia* **18**, 85–90

Bruyn, G. W. (1986a). Glossopharyngeal neuralgia. In *Handbook of Clinical Neurology*, Eds P. J. Vinken, G. W. Bruyn and H. L. Klawans, Vol. 4 (48): *Headache*, Ed. F. Clifford Rose. pp. 459–473. Amsterdam, Elsevier

Bruyn, G. W. (1986b). Nervus Intermedius neuralgia (Hunt). In *Handbook of Clinical Neurology*, Eds P. J. Vinken, G. W. Bruyn and H. L. Klawans, Vol. 4 (48): *Headache*, Ed. F. Clifford Rose. pp 487–494. Amsterdam, Elsevier

Bruyn, G. W. (1986c). Superior laryngeal neuralgia. In *Handbook of Clinical Neurology*, Eds. P. J. Vinken, G. W. Bruyn and H. L. Klawans, Vol. 4 (48): *Headache*, Ed. F. Clifford Rose. pp. 495–500. Amsterdam, Elsevier

Bruyn, G. W. (1986d). Sphenopalatine neuralgia (Sluder). In *Handbook of Clinical Neurology*, Eds P. J. Vinken, G. W. Bruyn and H. L. Klawans, Vol. 4 (48): *Headache*, Ed. F. Clifford Rose. pp 475–487. Amsterdam, Elsevier

Bruyn, G. W. (1986e). Charlin's neuralgia. In *Handbook of Clinical Neurology*, Eds P. J. Vinken, G. W. Bruyn and H. L. Klawans, Vol. 4 (48): *Headache*, Ed. F. Clifford Rose. pp. 483–486. Amsterdam, Elsevier

Burchiel, K. J. (1980). Abnormal impulse generation in focally demyelinated trigeminal roots. *J. Neurosurg.* **53**, 674–683

Chawla, J. C. and Falconer, M. A. (1967). Glossopharyngeal and vagal neuralgia. *Br. Med. J.* **3**, 529–531

Clough, C. G. (1991). Atypical facial pain. In *Clinical Neurology*, Eds M. Swash and J. Oxbury. pp. 370–372. Edinburgh, Churchill Livingstone

Dalessio, D. J., Mclsaac, H., Aung, M. and Polich, J. (1990). Non-invasive trigeminal evoked potentials : normative data and application to neuralgia patients. *Headache* **30**, 696–700

Dandy, W. E. (1934). Concerning the cause of trigeminal neuralgia. *Am. J. Surg.* **24**, 447–455

Denny-Brown, D. and Yanagisawa, N. (1973). The function of the descending root of the fifth nerve. *Brain* **96**, 783–814

Drummond, P. D. (1988). Vascular changes in atypical facial pain. *Headache* **28**, 121–123

Drummond, P. D., Gonski, A. G. and Lance, J. W. (1983). Facial flushing after thermocoagulation of the Gasserian ganglion. *J. Neurol. Neurosurg. Psychiat.* **46**, 611–616

Eaglstein, W. H., Katz, R. and Brown, J. A. (1970). The effects of early corticosteroid therapy on the skin eruption and pain of herpes zoster. *J. Am. Med. Assoc.* **211**, 1681–1683

Editorial (1990). Postherpetic neuralgia. *Lancet* **336**, 537–538

Esmann, V., Geil, J. P., Kroon, S. *et al.* (1987). Prednisolone does not prevent post-herpetic neuralgia. *Lancet* **ii**, 126–129

Fromm, G. H., Graff-Radford, S. B., Terrence, C. F. and Sweet, W. H. (1990). Pre-trigeminal neuralgia. *Neurology* **40**, 1493–1495

Fromm, G. H. and Terrence, C. F. (1987). Comparison of L-baclofen and racemic baclofen in trigeminal neuralgia. *Neurology* **37**, 1725–1728

Fromm, G. H., Terrence, C. F. and Chattha, A. S. (1984). Baclofen in the treatment of trigeminal neuralgia: double-blind study and long-term follow-up. *Ann. Neurol.* **15**, 240–244

Fromm, G. H.. Terrence, C. F. and Maroon, J. C. (1984). Trigeminal neuralgia. Current concepts regarding etiology and pathogenesis. *Arch. Neurol.* **41**, 1204–1207

Goadsby, P.J., Edvinsson, L. and Ekman, R. (1988). Release of vasoactive peptides in the extracerebral circulation of man and the cat during activation of the trigeminovascular system. *Ann. Neurol.* **23**, 193–196

Haines, S. J., Jannetta, P. J. and Zorub, D. S. (1980). Microvascular relations of the trigeminal nerve. An anatomical study with clinical correlation. *J. Neurosurg.* **52**, 381–386

Illingworth, R. (1986). Trigeminal neuralgia: surgical aspects. In *Handbook of Clinical Neurology*, Eds P. J. Vinken. G. W. Bruyn and H. L. Klawans, Vol. 4 (48): *Headache*, Ed. F. Clifford Rose. pp. 449–458. Amsterdam, Elsevier

Jaeger, B., Singer, E. and Kroening, R. (1986). Reflex sympathetic dystrophy of the face. Report of two cases and a review of the literature. *Arch. Neurol.* **43**, 693–695

Jannetta, P. J. (1976). Microsurgical approach to the trigeminal nerve for tic douloureux. *Progr. Neurol. Surg.* **7**, 180–200.

Kerr, F. W. L. (1979). Craniofacial neuralgia. In *Advances in Pain Research and Therapy*, Eds J. J. Bonica, J. C. Liebeskind and D. G. Albe-Fessard. pp. 283–295. New York, Raven Press

Lance, J. W. (1996). The red ear syndrome. *Neurology* **47**, 617–620

Lance, J. W. and Curran, D. A. (1964). Treatment of chronic tension headache. *Lancet* **i**, 1236–1239

Lascelles, R. G. (1966). Atypical facial pain and depression. *Br. J. Psychiat.* **112**, 651–659

Miles, J. B. and Bowsher, D. (1991). Chronic pain syndromes. In *Clinical Neurology*, Eds M. Swash and J. Oxbury. pp. 649–657. Edinburgh, Churchill Livingstone

Mokri, B. (1982). Raeder's paratrigeminal syndrome. Original concept and subsequent deviations. *Arch. Neurol.* **39**, 395–399

Nathan, P. W. (1976). The gate-control theory of pain. A critical review. *Brain* **99**, 123–158

Nurmikko, T. and Bowsher, D. (1990). Somatosensory findings in postherpetic neuralgia. *J. Neurol. Neurosurg. Psychiat.* **53**, 135–141

Pascual, J. and Berciano, J. (1989). Failure of mexiletine to control trigeminal neuralgia. *Headache* **29**, 517–518

Portenoy, R. K., Duma, C. and Foley, K. M. (1986). Acute herpetic and postherpetic neuralgia: clinical review and current management. *Ann Neurol.* **20**, 651–661

Ragozzino, M. W., Melton III, L. J., Kurland, L. T., Chu. C. P. and Perry, H. O. (1982). Population based study of herpes zoster and its sequelae. *Medicine* **61**, 310–316

Richards, P., Shawdon, H. and Illingworth, R. (1983). Operative findings on microsurgical exploration of the cerebello-pontine angle in trigeminal neuralgia. *J. Neurol. Neurosurg. Psychiat.* **46**, 1098–1101

Rushton, J. G., Stevens, J. C. and Miller, R. H. (1981). Glossopharyngeal (vagoglossopharyngeal) neuralgia. A study of 217 cases. *Arch. Neurol.* **38**, 201–205

Selby. G. (1975). Diseases of the fifth cranial nerve. In *Peripheral Neuropathy*, Eds P. J. Dyck, P. K. Thomas and E. H. Lambert. pp. 533–569. Philadelphia, Saunders & Co

Shanbrom, E. (1961). Treatment of herpetic pain and postherpetic neuralgia with intravenous procaine. *J. Am. Med. Assoc.* **176**, 1041–1043

Sjaastad, O., Elsås, T., Shen, J.-M., Joubert, J. and Fredriksen, T.A. (1994). Raeder's syndrome : 'anhidrosis', headache, and a proposal for a new classification. *Funct. Neurol.* **9**, 215–234

Sluder, G. (1910). The syndrome of sphenopalatine-ganglion neurosis. *Am. J. Med. Sci.* **140**, 868–878

Stöhr, M., Petruch, F. and Scheglmann, K. (1981). Somatosensory evoked potentials following trigeminal nerve stimulation in trigeminal neuralgia. *Ann. Neurol.* **9**, 63–66

Tomson, T. and Ekbom, K. (1981). Trigeminal neuralgia: time-course of pain in relation to carbamazepine dosing. *Cephalalgia* **1**, 91–97

Tomson, T., Tybring. G., Bertilsson, L., Ekbom, K. and Rane, E. (1980). Carbamazepine therapy in trigeminal neuralgia. Clinical effects in relation to plasma concentration. *Arch. Neurol.* **37**, 699–730

Vail, H. H. (1932). Vidian neuralgia. *Ann. Otol. Rhinol. Laryngol.* **41**, 837–856

Watkins, S. M. and Espir, M. (1969). Migraine and multiple sclerosis. *J. Neurol. Neurosurg. Psychiat.* **32**, 35–37

Watson, C. P. N. (1990). Postherpetic neuralgia: clinical features and treatment. In *Pain Syndromes in Neurology*, Ed. H. L. Fields. pp. 223–238. London, Butterworths

Watson, C. P., Evans, R. J., Reed, K., Merskey, H., Goldsmith, L. and Warsh J. (1982). Amitriptyline versus placebo in postherpetic neuralgia. *Neurology* **32**, 671–673

Young, R. F., Vermeulen, S. S., Grimm, P., Blasko, J. and Posewitz, A. (1997). Gamma knife radiosurgery for treatment of trigeminal neuralgia – idiopathic and tumour related. *Neurology* **48**, 608–614

Chapter 18

The investigation and general management of headache

A systematic case history (Chapter 2) and the interpretation of the history (Chapter 4) is usually sufficient for the diagnosis of migraine, cluster and tension-type headache. When headaches are of recent onset, of uncertain pattern, or if they are associated with progressive neurological signs or systemic disturbance, investigation becomes obligatory. The clinical approach depends on the length of the headache history and the mode of presentation.

Differential diagnosis

The acute severe headache

The abrupt onset of a severe headache ('thunderclap headache') usually requires immediate investigation (Day and Raskin, 1986; Wijdicks, Kerkhoff and van Gijn, 1988). The following possibilities have to be considered:

With neck rigidity
Subarachnoid haemorrhage
Meningitis, encephalitis
Systemic infections ('meningism')

Without neck rigidity
Pressor responses (e.g. phaeochromocytoma, reaction while on MAO inhibitors, 'benign sex headache' at orgasm)
Acute obstructive hydrocephalus (e.g. colloid cyst of the third ventricle)
Expanding intracranial aneurysm
Carotid or vertebral artery dissection
Migraine
Occipital neuralgia

Wijdicks, Kerkhoff and van Gijn (1988) followed up 71 patients with such headaches and concluded that angiography was not indicated if CT scan and CSF study were normal.

The subacute onset of headache

The recent development of headache may be of sinister import. The following are possible causes:

An expanding intracranial lesion (e.g. haematoma, tumour, abscess)
Progressive hydrocephalus
Temporal arteritis in patients over 55 years of age
Benign intracranial hypertension

Recurrent discrete episodes of headache or facial pain

Migraine, including 'lower-half' headache (facial migraine)
Cluster headache
Trigeminal neuralgia
Transient ischaemic attacks
Intermittent obstructive hydrocephalus
Paroxysmal hypertension (e.g. phaeochromocytoma)
Tolosa–Hunt syndrome
Benign cough, exertional and sex headaches
Ice-cream headache
Ice-pick pains
Sinusitis (rarely a cause of episodic headache)

Chronic headache or facial pain (more than 1 year duration)

Tension-type headache
Migraine
Post-traumatic headache
Atypical facial pain
Post-herpetic neuralgia

It is unlikely that headache caused by intracranial lesions or temporal arteritis should persist for as long as this without diagnosis.

Investigation

Only a small proportion of headache patients require investigation, other than a careful history and physical examination. Clinical judgement will determine which of these tests are necessary.

Blood count and erythrocyte sedimentation rate (ESR)

These are routine tests for patients admitted to hospital and should be done in general practice when there have been symptoms of systemic disorder, or signs of infection or meningeal reaction, or when dealing with a patient above the age of 55 years in whom the possibility of temporal arteritis must be ruled out. Polycythaemia may be associated with haemangioblastoma of the cerebellum. Leukaemia may present with intracranial deposits. Anaemia may indicate neoplasia or other systemic disease, and may accentuate any tendency to headache. A high ESR also directs attention to some locus of infection, hidden malignancy, multiple myeloma, one of the collagen diseases or subacute bacterial endocarditis, all of which may produce intracranial manifestations.

Plain X-rays

Simple radiography of the skull is rarely needed in the investigations of headache unless one is seeking evidence of sinusitis, mastoiditis, a skull fracture or platybasia.

Opinions differ about the significance of certain findings. Hyperostosis frontalis interna is regarded by some European authors as an inflammatory condition producing headache. It is a common variation of the normal from middle-age onwards, particularly in female patients. 'Thumbing', a beaten-copper appearance of the cranial vault, may be a normal variation, although it alerts the observer to the possibility of long-standing raised intracranial pressure. The sutures should be observed carefully in the young child as they separate when intracranial pressure is increased.

In most patients with headache, the appearance of the skull radiograph will be normal. If an intracranial lesion is suspected, a chest X-ray should also be obtained to exclude primary or secondary carcinoma, tuberculosis, sarcoid, bronchiectasis or other conditions of relevance.

Computerized axial tomography (CT scan)

In developed countries, it is difficult to dissuade anybody with any sort of headache from having a CT scan of the brain. The injection of a contrast agent carries the risk of an allergic reaction although, with non-ionic contrast media, the risk is small. One should always enquire about a patient's response to the injection of contrast media on any previous occasion and about a history of allergic reactions of any kind in the past history.

A CT scan has become the initial investigation for patients with suspected subarachnoid haemorrhage, intracranial space-occupying lesions or hydrocephalus. The interpretation of particular CT appearances may vary from country to country. For example, an enhancing lesion that would be diagnosed as a glioma in Western countries would more likely prove to be a tuberculoma in India. Cysticercosis is a possible cause of obstructive hydrocephalus in some South American, Mediterranean or Asian countries.

CT scanning can give a greater resolution of temporomandibular joint degeneration, sinus pathology and fractures of the temporal and facial bones than conventional radiology, which might be of particular value in the management of post-traumatic headache and facial pain.

Selby (1987) gives the following as indications for CT scanning in migraine patients:

1. Persistence of focal neurological deficits.
2. Definite EEG evidence of a focal cerebral lesion.
3. Hemicrania always on the same side and associated with contralateral neurological symptoms.
4. An orbital bruit suggestive of an arteriovenous malformation.
5. History of partial (focal) seizures.
6. A recent change in the frequency, severity or clinical features of the migraine attacks, or the finding of abnormal signs on neurological examination.
7. An anxious patient doubting the diagnosis of migraine and its therapeutic limitations.

Abnormalities shown by CT scanning of migraine patients are referred to in Chapter 7. The CT appearances of a third ventricular tumour is illustrated in Chapter 15 (Figure 15.2).

Magnetic resonance imaging (MRI)

MRI complements CT scanning in defining the outline and determining the nature of intracranial lesions. It is particularly helpful in localizing the site of obstruction of CSF pathways (Figure 18.1) and in detecting Arnold–Chiari syndrome (Figure 18.2). It is useful in assessing whether an arteriovenous malformation has bled previously by the presence or absence of haemosiderin surrounding it, and in depicting posterior fossa tumours and white matter lesions.

MRI can demonstrate thrombosis of the superior sagittal or other venous sinuses (Donohoe, Waldman and Resor, 1987; Salvati, 1990). Dissection of the internal carotid artery is clearly displayed because a dark flow void can be seen surrounded by the bright signal caused by a subintimal clot (Cox, Bertorini and Laster, 1991).

MRI of patients with basilar artery migraine (Jacome and Leborgne, 1990) and cluster headache (Sjaastad and Rinck, 1990) has not shown any specific abnormality. Small lesions have been found in the white matter of migraine patients more often than in control subjects (Igasashi et al, 1991). Magnetic resonance angiography has substantially reduced the need for conventional arteriograms.

Carotid and vertebral angiography

Angiography demonstrates arterial dissection (see Figure 14.1) and stenosis or occlusion (Figure 18.3) of the major arteries in the investigation of transient ischaemic attacks. Cerebral angiography determines the site of origin of aneurysms, the feeding vessels of arteriovenous malformations and the vascular supply of brain tumours. It can sometimes show bilateral subdural haematomas that may have been missed by CT scanning when in their isodense phase. Clots in the superior sagittal sinus can often be shown better by MRI than angiography.

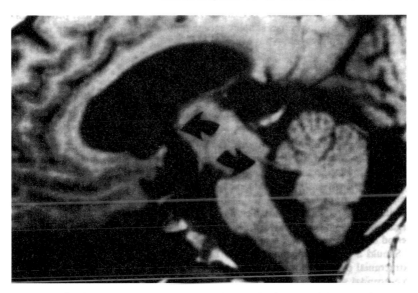

Figure 18.1 Obstructive hydrocephalus relieved by third ventriculostomy. (Photograph courtesy of the Departments of Neurosurgery and Radiology, Prince of Wales Hospital, Sydney)

MRI showing obliteration of the aqueduct (caudal end indicated with lower arrow) by a glioma of the midbrain tectum. Pressure in the dilated lateral and third ventricles has been reduced by making a communication between the posterior part of the distended floor of the third ventricle and the subarachnoid space. A flow void indicates passage of CSF through the foramen of Monro and the ventriculostomy (upper arrow)

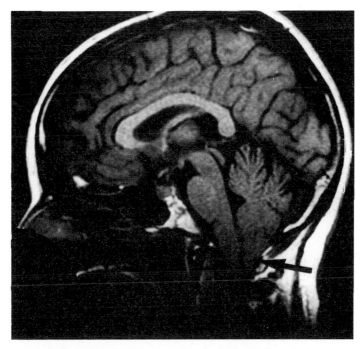

Figure 18.2 Arnold–Chiari malformation. A tongue of cerebellum extends down to the C2 level

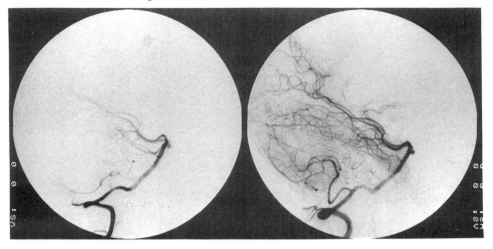

Figure 18.3 PICA thrombosis. The sparse filling of the vertebrobasilar circulation and the absence of the posterior inferior cerebellar artery (PICA) on the left contrasts with the normal circulation on the right

Electroencephalography

Electroencephalography (EEG) is rarely required for the diagnosis of headache, unless there are accompanying epileptic features. The association of migraine with epilepsy is discussed in Chapters 6 and 7, and the rare occurrence of headache as an ictal phenomenon is mentioned in Chapter 12. Occasionally, EEG may prove helpful in a suspected case of herpes simplex encephalitis in which the CT scan is normal by showing a temporal slow-wave focus.

Lumbar puncture

Lumbar puncture is undertaken when the clinical suspicion of subarachnoid hae-morrhage is high but a CT scan of the brain is normal. It is also indicated for the diagnosis of meningitis or encephalitis, and for the measurement of CSF pressure (for example, in benign intracranial hypertension).

It is always advisable to have a CT scan of the brain done before performing lumbar puncture if there is any indication of raised intracranial pressure or possi-bility of an intracranial space-occupying lesion. When a CT scanner is readily avail-able, patients with suspected meningitis can be started on antibiotic therapy immediately, transferred to the CT scan unit and the CSF sample obtained once the result of the CT scan is available. The identification and culture of the infecting organism will not be affected by the administration of antibiotics for such a short period but delay in starting antibiotics can prove fatal in fulminating meningitis. Should a lumbar puncture have to be done urgently in a patient with raised intra-cranial pressure, for example one with papilloedema and possible meningitis in a hospital without ready access to CT scanning, it is a worthwhile precaution to have at hand a 20-ml syringe filled with normal saline. If signs of coning develop after lumbar puncture, saline can be injected intrathecally and the foot of the bed elevated.

A small point concerning the technique of lumbar puncture which one of the authors has found useful is to infiltrate the skin with local anaesthetic 1–2 cm laterally to the midline at the selected intervertebral disc space and to angulate the lumbar puncture needle towards the midline as it is inserted from this point. The suggested track passes through soft tissues until the needle touches the spine. A gentle tapping movement of the needle will indicate to the examiner whether the needle is in contact with bone or with the elastic interlaminar ligament. If the latter, the needle can be inserted through the ligament with confidence that CSF will emerge when the stilette is removed. The advantages of this oblique approach are that it is usually painless and permits tactile sensibility of the position of the needle point. These advantages are lost with the firm pressure required to penetrate the interspinous ligament in the midline approach, making it difficult to know when the lumbar sac is entered.

CSF isotope studies

The insertion of a radionuclide tracer into the CSF to locate the site of leakage in low pressure syndromes is mentioned in Chapter 15 (Figure 15.4).

General principles of management

What do patients with headache expect from their doctors? Will they leave the consulting room content or with their expectations unfulfilled?

Fitzpatrick and Hopkins (1981) found that dissatisfaction was more common in migraine patients than those with tension headache, in those with headache duration of longer than 1 year, and those with significant psychiatric symptoms. Common criticisms were that patients were not told what their diagnosis meant, and that there was no discussion of the causes of their disorder or of means of avoiding or alleviating episodes.

When the history has been taken and the examination completed, the doctor has to take sufficient time to show that he or she understands the problem and to explain why investigations are or are not necessary for that particular patient. If the history is typical of migraine, cluster or tension headache, this should be explained to the patient so that fears of cerebral tumour can be dispelled at the outset. Sometimes one has to succumb to pressure and order a CT scan of the brain to complete the process of reassurance.

Some patients hope to find a simple cause for their headaches and a simple cure. For those patients with no discernible structural basis for their headaches, it may be helpful to explain that they have been born with a sensitive nervous system that responds to various stimuli by producing a painful reaction in the blood vessels of the brain and scalp. They should also be told that they can reduce the frequency and severity of attacks by physical and mental relaxation, and avoiding trigger factors, but that most patients benefit from pharmacological agents other than analgesics.

Because some people are reluctant to use medication of any sort it is worthwhile taking the trouble to explain that preventive treatment is designed to build up the body's own pain control pathway to prevent attacks recurring and that acute therapy is aimed at constricting blood vessels and turning off nerves to stop the painful process.

Once treatment has been prescribed and the rationale for it clarified, the patient should be warned of any common side-effect, advised to start with small doses and requested to attend again to report progress. It should be understood that no medication benefits everyone who takes it and that the earnest endeavour to control headaches depends on the continuing collaboration between patient and doctor. As the efficacy of our management improves so will the compliance and satisfaction of our patients.

References

Cox, L. K., Bertorini, T. and Laster, R. E. (1991). Headache due to spontaneous internal carotid artery dissection. Magnetic resonance imaging evaluation and follow up. *Headache* **31**, 12–16

Day, J. W. and Raskin, N. H. (1986). Thunderclap headache: symptom of unruptured cerebral aneurysm. *Lancet* **ii**, 1247–1248

Donohoe, C. D., Waldman, S. D. and Resor, L. D. (1987). Magnetic resonance imaging in cerebral venous thrombosis. *Headache* **27**, 155–157

Fitzpatrick, R. and Hopkins, A. (1981). Referrals to neurologists for headaches not due to structural disease. *J. Neurol. Neurosurg. Psychiat.* **44**, 1061–1067

Igarashi, H., Sakai, F., Kan, S., Okada, J. and Tazaki, Y. (1991). Magnetic Resonance Imaging of the brain in patients with migraine. *Cephalalgia* **11**, 69–74

Jacome, D. D. and Leborgne, J. (1990). MRI studies in basilar artery migraine. *Headache* **30**, 88–90

Salvati, C. A. (1990). Cerebral venous thrombosis shown by MRI. *Headache* **30**, 650–651

Selby, G. (1987). Investigating migraine: when, why and how. In *Migraine. Clinical and Research Aspects*, Ed. J. N. Blau. pp. 77–90. Baltimore, Johns Hopkins University Press

Sjaastad. O. and Rinck, P. (1990). Cluster headache: MRI studies of the cavernous sinus and the base of the brain. *Headache* **30**, 350–351

Wijdicks, E. F. M., Kerkhoff, H. and van Gijn, J. (1988). Long-term follow-up of 71 patients with thunderclap headache mimicking subarachnoid haemorrhage. *Lancet* **ii**, 68–70

An explanation of hyperventilation

Anxiety attacks with hyperventilation (overbreathing) are commonly associated with headache. They can be overcome by:

- recognizing the cause and
- obeying a few simple rules.

What are the symptoms?

- light-headedness, dizziness, faintness, 'giddiness'
- tightness or pain in the chest
- dry mouth
- heart beating faster
- blurring of vision
- sweating
- trembling of hands and legs
- weakness ('jelly legs')
- pins and needles in hands, feet and around mouth
- headache
- anxiety, fear or panic
- sensation of being unable to breathe
- a feeling of having a heart attack, passing out, losing control or of being about to die.
- spasms of hands and feet (in prolonged episodes).

When you overbreathe you may swallow air, causing:

- distension of the stomach
- burping
- passing wind.

What do you mean by overbreathing?

- deep sighing breaths

- yawning often
- rapid shallow breathing
- deep breathing.

When is this most likely to happen?

- when you are tense, bored or depressed
- in crowds, at a party or in a supermarket.

How does this cause symptoms?
Normally nature takes care of the rate and depth of breathing. The carbon dioxide (CO_2) in your blood makes you breathe enough to eliminate it and get sufficient oxygen.

If you override nature and breathe too much you wash out too much CO_2. This reduces the blood flow to your brain and makes you feel dizzy. It also reduces the available calcium in the blood, which can cause 'pins and needles' and make the hands and feet spasm.

Adrenaline increases in the bloodstream causing a feeling of anxiety, sweating and trembling, and makes the heart beat faster.

Contraction of muscles causes pain and tightness in the chest and headache.

How can you stop it?
Look for the first signs of sighing or yawning.

Do not:

- open the windows
- run outside
- take deep breaths.

Instead:

- sit down
- hold your breath and count to 10
- breathe out slowly and say 'relax' to yourself
- then breathe in and out slowly every 6 seconds (10 breaths per minute)
- as soon as possible forget about your breathing and let nature do it for you.

General principles

- Take it easy. It is not a disaster if you forget someone's name, burn the dinner or don't have time to mow the lawn. Talk more slowly. Walk more slowly. You have plenty of time.
- Think positively. You can handle a problem as well as the next person. All the people you meet in the street or around a conference table have their problems too. Spread out your workload through the day. Give yourself enough time for each task.
- Remain calm.

- Don't bottle up your feelings – discuss any worries or things that make you angry or upset.
- Eat regular meals and don't hurry them.
- Limit yourself to five cups of tea or coffee each day.
- Cut out smoking or reduce it to less than 10 cigarettes per day.
- Learn to recognize any tendency to overbreathe.
- Learn to relax your muscles – no frowning or jaw-clenching.
- Take regular exercise.
- Take time out for social activities and holidays.

You can control your attacks completely by following these rules.

Relaxation exercises: instructions issued to patients with migraine or tension-type headaches

What has muscle contraction to do with headache?

The blood vessels and nerve fibres of the scalp lie in muscle. Place your fingers on each temple and clench your jaw. You will feel the muscle belly of the temporal muscle swell as it contracts. Let the jaw go loose and the muscle becomes flat again. Many people contract these muscles all day without realizing it so they are working continuously, which may set up a constant dull ache in the temples. The vessels which run through the muscles often constrict while the muscle is contracting. During sleep the muscles may relax and the vessels dilate so that a person may wake in the middle of the night or the early morning with a throbbing headache in the temples. Some others may grind their teeth at night during sleep and may therefore wake up with aching jaws and a raw tender spot on their upper gum caused by sideways movement of the jaw during sleep. Over-contraction of the jaw muscles is very common in tense or anxious people, who often do not realize that their muscles are not relaxed.

Do you feel the jaw muscles aching at the end of the day, or after an unpleasant or difficult conversation, or after an argument? Do you feel an ache in one or both temples at these times or wake up with a headache in this area? If the headache is in one temple only, check your bite to see if you chew equally and evenly on both sides and can move the jaw freely from side to side. If you have back teeth missing on one side or the other, the strain of chewing is thrown on to the other side, which causes an ache in the hinge-joint of the jaw and in the temple. If this is the case you should see your dentist about balancing the bite, as this can be a very important factor in excessive jaw-clenching.

Just as chronic jaw-clenching is a common cause of aching in the temples, chronic frowning is a common cause of pain in the forehead. Do others say to you that you frown a lot or look worried most of the time? This can be an indication that you are using your scalp muscles without being aware of it.

Pain in the neck can also result from muscle contraction. Some people walk about holding their neck stiffly as though it were a solid block of wood. This may be an attempt to protect the neck because of the sensation of grating in the neck on movement or the discovery on X-ray that some of the discs in the neck have degenerated. Disc degeneration is quite common even in young people and is almost universal in older age groups. If there has been a whiplash injury to the neck or attention is drawn to the neck in any way, the muscles may contract to splint the neck and a vicious cycle is set up of pain leading to muscle spasm which leads to more pain.

Muscle-contraction or tension headache is usually a constant tight pressing feeling in the forehead, temples or back of the head and may spread all around the head 'like a tight band'. Because the scalp muscles are linked together by a sheet of strong tissue which passes over the skull, muscle contraction may also cause the feeling of pressure on top of the head. Sharp jabbing pains may also be felt because scalp nerves are compressed by muscle contraction.

Over-contraction of muscle is a faulty habit which develops over the years and often starts in childhood. About one in seven patients with tension headache can remember having similar headaches under the age of 10 years. It may be associated with mental tension and anxiety but may have become an automatic reaction which continues even when there are no obvious problems of any sort.

Are you able to relax?

The most natural form of treatment is to train the muscles of the body to relax and the first step is to realize that you are not as relaxed as you think you are. Try these simple tests.

1. Sit in a chair and lean back. Ask someone to lift your arm in the air in a comfortable position as though it were resting on the side of an armchair. Take your time and relax completely. Then ask your friend to take away his hands, which have been supporting your arm. When the supporting hands are taken away, what does your arm do? If it flops lifelessly downwards, you are indeed relaxed. If it stays in the air, or you move it slowly downwards, you are not relaxed. Your muscles are contracting continuously *without you realizing it.*
2. Lie on a bed or couch with your head on a pillow and try to relax completely. When you consider that you have achieved this, ask your accomplice to pull the pillow away from under your head. Does your head drop limply on to the bed? Or does it stay poised in midair as though the pillow was still there? If you are still holding your head in the air above an invisible pillow, your muscles must be contracting *without you realizing it.*

Once you have acknowledged that excessive muscle contraction is playing a part in the aching of your head or neck, and that you do not really know whether the muscles are contracting or not, you are ready to start relaxation exercises.

Paradoxically, you cannot relax about relaxing. It is not a passive process. It is no use saying to someone 'relax' and imagining that they can do it without further thought. You cannot say to yourself 'relax' and then do it unless you have carefully practised the art of 'switching off' the nerve supply to the muscles. This is a voluntary action as deliberate as turning off a light switch and must be practised until it can be done at will and done rapidly.

At first it is necessary to set aside at least 10 minutes night and morning for the exercises. It is a great help to have someone with you in the early stages to ensure that you are completely relaxed when you think you are. This person will be referred to below as the 'assistant'. It is obviously a great advantage if the assistant can be a trained physiotherapist or occupational therapist but this is not always practicable and a well-motivated husband or wife, relative or friend can be of enormous value in ensuring that the exercises are performed conscientiously and that relaxation is practised until it becomes complete.

The sequence of relaxation exercises

Lie down on a firm surface such as a carpeted floor. A bed with an inner spring mattress will do, but not one with a soft, sagging mattress. A pillow can be used to support the head at first but may be discarded later as relaxation becomes easier. For the first few sessions only a short-sleeved shirt and shorts should be worn so that muscle contraction can be seen as well as felt. Lie on the back with the legs slightly separated and the arms comfortably flexed at the elbow so that the elbows are by the sides with the hands resting on the body. Various muscles will be contracted and relaxed in turn.

Legs. Contract the leg muscles so that the legs become rigid pillars. The muscle bellies will be seen to stand out as the muscles contract. Concentrate on the sensation set up by the muscles contracting, and the feeling of tension in them. Then, suddenly and deliberately, 'switch off the power supply' so that the muscles become limp. Concentrate on whether any sensation is coming from the muscles now. Are they completely relaxed? At this point it is helpful for an assistant to put his hand behind the subject's knees and lift them up sharply to see if the leg is completely floppy and that the muscles do not contract again as soon as the limb is moved passively. If they are not completely relaxed, or if they contract again when the limb is touched or moved, the sequence should be repeated.

Many people only half relax on the first few attempts. This can be detected by watching the muscles closely. After the first relaxation, the muscle bellies are not as prominent as they were but there may be some contraction remaining. Try again to 'switch off' and this second attempt may be rewarded by seeing the muscle become completely flaccid. The legs may then be bent at the knee by the assistant, moved about, or rolled backwards and forwards with the feet flailing 'like a rag doll'. This sequence may be completed by lifting one leg, letting it drop downwards like an inanimate object, then doing the same with the other.

Arms. Brace the arms so that the elbows are forced downwards on the couch (or on the assistant's hand if he is checking the degree of relaxation). The arms are held rigidly and the muscle contraction is suddenly stopped so that the arms become limp and lifeless. The assistant should then be able to bounce the elbow up and down without any resistance being offered. This sequence should be repeated until the subject is aware of the sensation of muscle contraction and the contrast with the feeling of relaxation, and the assistant is satisfied that the arm becomes truly flaccid.

Neck. Lift the head from the pillow and then allow it to drop backwards. The assistant may provide resistance by pressing on the forehead until the subject feels the contraction of the muscles in the front of the neck. When the head is dropped backwards, the assistant can rock it gently to and fro to make certain that there is no residual activity in the muscles. Now push the head backwards into the pillow and register the sensation of contraction of the muscles in the back of the neck. Stop the contraction suddenly so that the head may be rotated freely on the neck by the assistant. Repeat this until relaxation is satisfactory.

Forehead. Frown upwards so that the brow is furrowed. If there is difficulty in doing this, look upwards as far as the eyes will move and the forehead will become creased. Again, feel the sensation of tension in the muscles, then close the eyes and let the forehead muscles relax. The assistant can detect the presence or absence of contraction by seeing whether the skin of the forehead moves freely with his hand.

Eyes. Screw the eyes up tightly and become aware of the sensation of tension, then relax the muscles and lie with the eyes lightly closed. Make sure that there is no trembling or flickering of the closed eyelids and that the eye muscles feel entirely relaxed .

Jaws. Clench the jaw firmly and concentrate on feeling the sense of tightness in the temples as well as in the jaw itself. Then switch off and let the jaw fall open. Push the jaw open, perhaps against the pressure of the assistant's hand, then relax completely. Move the jaw sideways to the right as far as it will go and experience the sensation which this gives to the jaw and temple before relaxing. Then do the same to the left. Complete the sequence by clenching the jaw firmly again, and let the jaw drop open loosely. The assistant should then be able to hold the tip of the jaw with his fingers and waggle the jaw up and down rapidly without any opposition from the jaw muscles.

This is the hardest of all relaxation procedures to achieve and you must not be disappointed if you are unsuccessful on the first occasion. It may require repeated practise to enable the jaw muscles to cease all activity so that the jaw may be moved easily by the assistant. It is most important that you persevere until you accomplish this because over-contraction of jaw muscles is the most common factor in tension headache and the 'switching-off' process must be thoroughly learned.

Whole body relaxation. Once you are able to relax the legs, arms, neck, forehead, eye and jaw muscles in order, lie for 5 minutes with all muscles relaxed. Once you have achieved total relaxation, the process becomes negative rather than positive. In other words. you permit natural relaxation to continue rather than willing yourself to relax actively. At this stage, it is helpful to think of some beautiful and tranquil scene, to imagine yourself lying on a grassy bank on a warm summer's day with the drowsy sounds of summer in the background. Everyone has some particular sound he or she associates with peace and tranquillity. It may be the rippling of a trout stream, the humming of bees, the song of birds, the soughing of wind in the trees or distant music. Choose your own theme and your own mental picture and live in that scene for a few minutes. As you do so, feel the sensation of heaviness creep over your legs, trunk and arms, then spread to your neck and head, eyes and face. Lie completely inert, with all muscles relaxed, a feeling of heaviness throughout the body and a pleasant scene pictured in the mind. Feel the sensation of freedom in the mind and in the head. This can become a permanent freedom if your muscles obey you all the time as well as they do at that moment.

After relaxation exercises are finished

The final and most important step is to carry the art of relaxation into your everyday life. Watch the way you stand, the way you sit, the way in which you speak on the telephone, talk to people, write, type or perform any other activity of a typical day. Check that all the muscles which are not essential to the task of the moment are in a state of relaxation. You can handle any situation, irrespective of the degree of mental stress, without physical tension once you become accustomed to the idea. You actually perform more efficiently if you tackle any problem in an orderly fashion without excessive and useless muscle contraction. If you notice any warning sensations of tension in the scalp, jaw or neck muscles, you must pause a moment to ensure that these muscles are 'switched off' in the manner you have practised. In this way you will finish the day feeling much fresher and with much less chance of headache making your day a misery.

Keep practising

There is no point in performing the exercise routine religiously for a week and then forgetting the whole thing. If you do, unless you are a very exceptional person, the old habits of muscle contraction will assert themselves again. Keep practising, stay relaxed and free yourself from headache.

Index